T0259592

Cholestatic Liver Diseases

Editor

CYNTHIA LEVY

CLINICS IN LIVER DISEASE

www.liver.theclinics.com

Consulting Editor
NORMAN GITLIN

May 2013 • Volume 17 • Number 2

ELSEVIER

1600 John F. Kennedy Boulevard • Suite 1800 • Philadelphia, Pennsylvania, 19100-2000

http://www.theclinics.com

CLINICS IN LIVER DISEASE Volume 17, Number 2
May 2013 ISSN 1089-3261, ISBN-13: 978-1-4557-7113-4

Editor: Kerry Holland

Developmental Editor: Donald Mumford

Clinics in Liver Disease (ISSN 1089-3261) is published quarterly by Elsevier Inc., 360 Park Avenue South, New York, NY 10010-1710. Months of issue are February, May, August, and November. Business and Editorial Offices: 1600 John F. Kennedy Blvd., Ste. 1800, Philadelphia, PA 19103-2899. Customer Service Office: 3251 Riverport Lane, Maryland Heights, MO 63043. Periodicals postage paid at New York, NY and additional mailing offices. Subscription prices are $282.00 per year (U.S. individuals), $139.00 per year (U.S. student/resident), $387.00 per year (U.S. institutions), $374.00 per year (foreign individuals), $192.00 per year (foreign student/ resident), $465.00 per year (foreign instituitions), $326.00 per year (Canadian individuals), $192.00 per year (Canadian student/resident), and $465.00 per year (Canadian institutions). Foreign air speed delivery is included in all *Clinics* subscription prices. All prices are subject to change without notice. **POSTMASTER:** Send address changes to *Clinics in Liver Disease*, Elsevier Health Sciences Division, Subscription Customer Service, 3251 Riverport Lane, Maryland Heights, MO 63043. **Customer Service: Telephone: 1-800-654-2452 (U.S. and Canada); 314-447-8871 (outside U.S. and Canada). Fax: 314-447-8029. E-mail: journalscustomer service-usa@elsevier.com (for print support); journalsonlinesupport-usa@elsevier.com (for online support).**

Reprints. For copies of 100 or more of articles in this publication, please contact the Commercial Reprints Department, Elsevier Inc., 360 Park Avenue South, New York, NY 10010-1710. Tel.: 212-633-3812; Fax: 212-462-1935; E-mail: reprints@elsevier.com.

Clinics in Liver Disease is covered in *MEDLINE/PubMed (Index Medicus)*, Science Citation Index Expanded, Journal Citation Reports/Science Edition, and Current Contents/Clinical Medicine.

Printed and bound by CPI Group (UK) Ltd, Croydon, CR0 4YY

Transferred to digital print 2013

Contributors

CONSULTING EDITOR

NORMAN GITLIN, MD, FRCP (LONDON), FRCPE (EDINBURGH), FACG, FACP
Formerly, Professor of Medicine, Chief of Hepatology, Emory University; Currently, Consultant, Atlanta Gastroenterology Associates, Atlanta, Georgia

EDITOR

CYNTHIA LEVY, MD
Associate Professor of Clinical Medicine, Division of Hepatology, University of Miami Miller School of Medicine, Miami, Florida

AUTHORS

ANNA BAGHDASARYAN, MD, PhD
Fellow, Division of Gastroenterology and Hepatology, Department of Internal Medicine III, Medical University of Vienna, Vienna, Austria; Laboratory of Experimental and Molecular Hepatology, Division of Gastroenterology and Hepatology, Department of Internal Medicine, Medical University of Graz, Graz, Austria

ULRICH BEUERS, PhD, MD
Tytgat Institute for Liver and Intestinal Research, Department of Gastroenterology and Hepatology, Academic Medical Center, University of Amsterdam, Amsterdam, The Netherlands

KALYAN RAM BHAMIDIMARRI, MD, MPH
Division of Hepatology, Department of Medicine, University of Miami Miller School of Medicine, Miami, Florida

EINAR S. BJORNSSON, MD, PhD
Professor of Gastroenterology and Hepatology, Division of Gastroenterology and Hepatology, The National University Hospital of Iceland, Reykjavik, Iceland

RUTH BOLIER, MD
Tytgat Institute for Liver and Intestinal Research, Department of Gastroenterology and Hepatology, Academic Medical Center, University of Amsterdam, Amsterdam, The Netherlands

ANDRES F. CARRION, MD
Division of Gastroenterology, Department of Medicine, University of Miami Miller School of Medicine, Miami, Florida

FRANK CZUL, MD
Department of Medicine, University of Miami Miller School of Medicine, Miami, Florida

ANDREW S. DELEMOS, MD
Clinical and Research Fellow in Medicine, Gastrointestinal Unit, Massachusetts General Hospital; Research Fellow in Medicine, Harvard Medical School, Boston, Massachusetts

LAWRENCE S. FRIEDMAN, MD
Professor of Medicine, Harvard Medical School, Tufts University School of Medicine; Assistant Chief of Medicine, Massachusetts General Hospital, Boston, Massachusetts; Chair, Department of Medicine, Newton-Wellesley Hospital, Newton, Massachusetts

PAUL GISSEN, MD, PhD
MRC Laboratory for Molecular Cell Biology, UCL Institute of Child Health, London, United Kingdom

ANDREA A. GOSSARD, MS, CNP
Assistant Professor of Medicine, Associate in Gastroenterology and Hepatology, Cholestatic Liver Disease Study Group, Division of Gastroenterology and Hepatology, Mayo Clinic, Rochester, Minnesota

EMINA HALILBASIC, MD
Fellow, Division of Gastroenterology and Hepatology, Department of Internal Medicine III, Medical University of Vienna, Vienna, Austria

JANE L. HARTLEY, MBChB, MRCPCH, MMedSci, PhD
Liver Unit, Birmingham Children's Hospital, Birmingham, United Kingdom

GIDEON M. HIRSCHFIELD, MB BChir, PhD, FRCP
Senior Lecturer, NIHR Biomedical Research Unit, Centre for Liver Research, Institute of Biomedical Research, The Medical School, University of Birmingham, Birmingham, United Kingdom

MOHAMAD H. IMAM, MBBS
Cholestatic Liver Diseases Study Group, Division of Gastroenterology and Hepatology, Mayo Clinic, Rochester, Minnesota

JON GUNNLAUGUR JONASSON, MD
Professor of Pathology, Department of Pathology, The National University Hospital of Iceland, Reykjavik, Iceland

DEIRDRE A. KELLY, MD, FRCPI, FRRCP, FRCPCH
Liver Unit, Birmingham Children's Hospital, Birmingham, United Kingdom

CYNTHIA LEVY, MD
Associate Professor of Clinical Medicine, Division of Hepatology, University of Miami Miller School of Medicine, Miami, Florida

KEITH D. LINDOR, MD
Executive Vice Provost, College of Health Solutions, Arizona State University, Phoenix, Arizona

MARLYN J. MAYO, MD
Associate Professor of Internal Medicine, Division of Digestive and Liver Diseases, UT Southwestern, Dallas, Texas

RONALD P.J. OUDE ELFERINK, PhD
Tytgat Institute for Liver and Intestinal Research, Department of Gastroenterology and Hepatology, Academic Medical Center, University of Amsterdam, Amsterdam, The Netherlands

ADAM PEYTON, DO
Division of Hepatology, University of Miami Miller School of Medicine, Miami, Florida

MARINA G. SILVEIRA, MD
Assistant Professor of Medicine, Division of Gastroenterology and Hepatology, Louis Stokes Cleveland VAMC, Case Medical Center, Cleveland, Ohio

JAYANT A. TALWALKAR, MD, MPH
Cholestatic Liver Diseases Study Group, Division of Gastroenterology and Hepatology, Mayo Clinic, Rochester, Minnesota

MICHAEL TRAUNER, MD
Professor and Chair of Gastroenterology and Hepatology, Division of Gastroenterology and Hepatology, Department of Internal Medicine III, Medical University of Vienna, Vienna, Austria

CLAUDIA O. ZEIN, MD, MSc
Department of Gastroenterology and Hepatology, Digestive Disease Institute, Cleveland Clinic, Cleveland, Ohio

Contents

Preface: Cholestatic Liver Diseases   xiii

Cynthia Levy

Genetic Determinants of Cholestasis   147

Gideon M. Hirschfield

> Cholestasis is an overarching term applied for conditions whereby biliary constituents are found in the circulation because of impairment to bile flow. A variety of processes can lead to cholestasis, be they acute or chronic injuries to hepatocytes, cholangiocytes, or the broader biliary tree itself. Such injuries may be driven by rare but highly informative primary genetic abnormalities, or may be seen in individuals with a prior genetic predisposition when confronted by specific environmental challenges such as drug exposure. This review provides a broad outline of some fundamental primary genetic cholestatic syndromes and an update on varying genetic predisposition underlying several acquired cholestatic processes.

Nuclear Receptors as Drug Targets in Cholestatic Liver Diseases   161

Emina Halilbasic, Anna Baghdasaryan, and Michael Trauner

> Cholestatic liver diseases encompass a wide spectrum of disorders with different causes, resulting in impaired bile flow and accumulation of bile acids and other potentially hepatotoxic cholephils. The understanding of the molecular mechanisms of bile formation and cholestasis has recently improved significantly through new insights into nuclear receptor (patho) biology. Nuclear receptors are ligand-activated transcription factors, which act as central players in the regulation of genes responsible for elimination and detoxification of biliary constituents accumulating in cholestasis. They also control other pathophysiologic processes such as inflammation, fibrogenesis, and carcinogenesis involved in the pathogenesis and disease progression of cholestasis liver diseases.

Drug-Induced Cholestasis   191

Einar S. Bjornsson and Jon Gunnlaugur Jonasson

> Cholestasis caused by drugs is an important differential diagnosis in patients presenting with a biochemical cholestatic pattern. The extent of serologic tests and radiological imaging depends on the clinical context. The underlying condition of the patient and detailed information on drug use, results of rechallenge, and the documented hepatotoxicity of the drug are important to establish a diagnosis of drug-induced liver injury (DILI). Most cases of cholestatic DILI are mild, but in rare cases, ductopenia and cholestatic cirrhosis can develop. Approximately 10% of patients with cholestatic jaundice caused by drugs develop liver failure.

Primary Sclerosing Cholangitis   211

Claudia O. Zein

> Primary sclerosing cholangitis (PSC) is a chronic, progressive, cholestatic liver disease characterized by multifocal strictures of intra and extrahepatic bile ducts. PSC occurs more commonly in men and is often associated with inflammatory bowel disease. At present, there is no effective medical therapy for PSC. Current management of patients with PSC is centered on endoscopic therapy of biliary strictures, management of complications of chronic cholestasis and of progressive liver disease, and close clinical monitoring for development of cholangiocarcinoma, as well as for timely referral for liver transplantation.

Primary Biliary Cirrhosis: Therapeutic Advances   229

Frank Czul, Adam Peyton, and Cynthia Levy

> Primary biliary cirrhosis (PBC) is a chronic and slowly progressive cholestatic liver disease characterized by destruction of the interlobular bile ducts, which, if untreated, leads to fibrosis, biliary cirrhosis, and liver failure. Because liver transplantation remains the only curative option for PBC, the goals of treatment are to slow the rate of progression, to alleviate related symptoms, and to prevent complications. Ursodeoxycholic acid is the only US Food and Drug Administration–approved medical treatment of PBC. Several agents are undergoing evaluation as monotherapy or as an adjuvant to ursodeoxycholic acid. This review summarizes current therapeutic advances in the care of patients with PBC.

Cholestatic Liver Disease Overlap Syndromes   243

Marlyn J. Mayo

> Primary biliary cirrhosis and primary sclerosing cholangitis share some clinical features with autoimmune hepatitis, but when features of autoimmune hepatitis are present, prognosis can be affected and immunosuppressive treatment warranted. The presence of severe interface hepatitis in primary biliary cirrhosis portends a worse prognosis and should prompt evaluation for possible autoimmune hepatitis overlap and treatment with immunosuppression. Specific models to identify which subjects benefit most from the addition of immunosuppression need to be developed. Drug-induced liver injury and IgG4 disease may masquerade as autoimmune hepatitis or primary sclerosing cholangitis and are important to consider in the differential diagnosis of the overlap or variant syndromes.

IgG4-Associated Cholangitis   255

Marina G. Silveira

> IgG4-associated cholangitis is the hepatobiliary manifestation of a recently characterized inflammatory systemic disease, associated with increased IgG4 serum levels and IgG4-positive lymphoplasmacytic infiltration. Often, patients present with obstructive jaundice, and imaging reveals stenoses of the extrahepatic or intrahepatic bile ducts, often in association with parenchymal pancreatic findings and irregularities of the pancreatic duct. The histologic findings include lymphoplasmacytic infiltrates, on

occasion resulting in tumefactive lesions (which can mimic malignancy), obliterative phlebitis, and fibrotic changes. Steroid treatment is the mainstay of management, but relapse is common after discontinuation of therapy or during tapering of steroids and may require further treatment.

Secondary Sclerosing Cholangitis: Pathogenesis, Diagnosis, and Management   269

Mohamad H. Imam, Jayant A. Talwalkar, and Keith D. Lindor

Secondary sclerosing cholangitis (SSC) is an aggressive and rare disease with intricate pathogenesis and multiple causes. Understanding the specific cause underlying each case of SSC is crucial in the clinical management of the disease. Radiologic imaging can help diagnose SSC and hence institute management in a timely manner. Management may encompass simple interventions, such as supportive therapy, antibiotics, and monitoring, or more serious measures, such as surgery, endoscopic intervention, or liver transplantation. Patients with AIDS cholangiopathy have limited therapeutic options and worsened survival. The disease should always be highly suspected in patients with primary sclerosing cholangitis with questionable diagnosis.

Alagille Syndrome and Other Hereditary Causes of Cholestasis   279

Jane L. Hartley, Paul Gissen, and Deirdre A. Kelly

Neonatal conjugated jaundice is a common presentation of hereditary liver diseases, which, although rare, are important to recognize early. Developments in molecular genetic techniques have enabled the identification of causative genes, which has improved diagnostic accuracy for patients and has led to a greater understanding of the molecular pathways involved in liver biology and pathogenesis of liver diseases. This review provides an update of the current understanding of clinical and molecular features of the inherited liver diseases that cause neonatal conjugated jaundice.

Systemic Causes of Cholestasis   301

Andrew S. deLemos and Lawrence S. Friedman

Systemic causes of cholestasis constitute a diverse group of diseases across organ systems. The pathophysiology of cholestasis in systemic disease can be a consequence of direct involvement of a disease process within the liver or extrahepatic biliary system or secondary to immune-mediated changes in bile flow. Evaluating a patient with cholestasis for a systemic cause requires an understanding of the patient's risk factors, clinical setting (eg, hospitalized or immunosuppressed patient), clinical features, and pattern of laboratory abnormalities.

Advances in Pathogenesis and Treatment of Pruritus   319

Ruth Bolier, Ronald P.J. Oude Elferink, and Ulrich Beuers

The pathogenesis of itch during cholestasis is largely unknown and treatment options are limited. Lysophosphatidate, female steroid hormones, and endogenous opioids are among the agents discussed as potential pruritogens in cholestasis. The itch-alleviating action of guideline-based therapeutic interventions with anion exchanger resins, rifampicin, opioid antagonists, and serotonin reuptake inhibitors are studied to unravel the molecular pathogenesis of itch. Still, a considerable part of the patients is in need of alternative experimental therapeutic approaches (eg, UV-B phototherapy, extracorporeal albumin dialysis, nasobiliary drainage), providing additional information about the enigmatic pathophysiology of cholestatic pruritus.

Care of the Cholestatic Patient

331

Andrea A. Gossard

Cholestasis is defined as impairment of bile formation or bile flow. Care of the patient with cholestatic features is dependent on identifying the cause of the cholestasis, initiating appropriate treatment of reversible conditions, and the recognition and management of cholestasis-specific complications. Cholestasis may include extrahepatic ducts and intrahepatic bile ducts, or may be limited to one or the other. Jaundice and pruritus are the hallmarks of cholestasis clinically but biochemical evidence may, and often does, precede the clinical manifestations.

Liver Transplant for Cholestatic Liver Diseases

345

Andres F. Carrion and Kalyan Ram Bhamidimarri

Cholestatic liver diseases include a group of diverse disorders with different epidemiology, pathophysiology, clinical course, and prognosis. Despite significant advances in the clinical care of patients with cholestatic liver diseases, liver transplant (LT) remains the only definitive therapy for end-stage liver disease, regardless of the underlying cause. As per the United Network for Organ Sharing database, the rate of cadaveric LT for cholestatic liver disease was 18% in 1991, 10% in 2000, and 7.8% in 2008. This review summarizes the available evidence on various common and rare cholestatic liver diseases, disease-specific issues, and pertinent aspects of LT.

Index

361

CLINICS IN LIVER DISEASE

FORTHCOMING ISSUES

August 2013
Hepatitis B Virus
Tarik Asselah, MD, and
Patrick Marcellin, MD, *Editors*

November 2013
Drug Hepatotoxicity
Nikolaos T. Pyrsopoulos, MD, PhD, MBA,
Editor

February 2014
The Impact of Nutrition and Obesity on Chronic Liver Diseases
Zobair M. Younossi, *Editor*

RECENT ISSUES

February 2013
Novel and Combination Therapies for Hepatitis C Virus
Paul J. Pockros, MD,
Editor

November 2012
A Practical Approach to the Spectrum of Alcoholic Liver Disease
David Bernstein, MD, AGAF, FACP, FACG,
Editor

August 2012
Nonalcoholic Fatty Liver Disease
Arun J. Sanyal, MBBS, MD, *Editor*

RELATED INTEREST

Infectious Disease Clinics of North America, December 2012, (Vol. 26, No. 4)
Care of the Patient with Hepatitis C Virus Infection
Barbara H. McGovern, MD, *Editor*

NOW AVAILABLE FOR YOUR iPhone and iPad

Preface

Cholestatic Liver Diseases

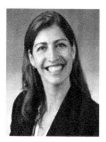

Cynthia Levy, MD
Editor

Over the past 2 decades, our understanding of cholestatic liver diseases has deepened. Genetic predisposition, for instance, is increasingly recognized as a major contributor to susceptibility or severity of various cholestatic diseases. In this issue of *Clinics in Liver Diseases,* Dr Gideon Hirschfield reviews the role of genetic determinants in both rare genetic syndromes and the more common autoimmune and drug-induced presentations. Drs Hallibasic, Baghdasaryan, and Trauner then methodically discuss the role of nuclear receptors in the pathogenesis and disease progression in cholestasis, as well as their use as important therapeutic targets. These 2 articles set the stage for a detailed survey of cholestatic liver diseases, beginning with a state-of-the-art summary on drug-induced liver injury with an emphasis on cholestatic presentations by Drs Jonasson and Bjornsson. Dr Claudia Zein examines the complex and controversial management of patients with primary sclerosing cholangitis, while Drs Czul, Peyton, and I explore the most recent advances and novel therapies for primary biliary cirrhosis. The nuances and challenges regarding the specific diagnosis and treatment of patients with overlap syndromes are lucidly discussed by Dr Marlyn Mayo. One of the most active areas of clinical investigation has been the differential diagnosis of sclerosing cholangitis. IgG4-associated cholangitis is reviewed by Dr Marina Silveira, and other secondary causes, including the newly recognized entity of sclerosing cholangitis in critically ill patients, are presented by Drs Iman, Talwalkar, and Lindor. Drs Hartley, Gissen, and Kelly highlight developments in the Pediatric arena, especially with respect to identification of causative genes and the multiple clinical phenotypes potentially associated with the same gene. Drs deLemos and Friedman describe the multiple systemic causes of cholestasis and present a very useful diagnostic algorithm for clinical practice. Drs Bolier, Oude Elferink, and Beuers discuss the current understanding of the pathogenosis of pruritus, exploring the role of the recently described autotoxin and its product, lysophosphatidic acid. We then turn to the management of extrahepatic complications from longstanding cholestasis, addressed by Andrea Gossard, as most cholestatic liver diseases do not have a definitive therapy. Lastly, for those whose condition progresses to end-stage liver disease, liver transplantation remains the only

Clin Liver Dis 17 (2013) xiii–xiv
http://dx.doi.org/10.1016/j.cld.2013.01.001
1089-3261/13/$ – see front matter © 2013 Published by Elsevier Inc.

curative option. The closing article by Drs Carrion and Bhamidimarri describes the available data on liver transplantation for both common and rare cholestatic diseases.

I would like to thank all the contributors for their willingness to share their expertise, Kerry Holland for her invaluable editorial assistance, and Dr Norman Gitlin for giving me the opportunity to edit this issue of *Clinics in Liver Diseases.*

Cynthia Levy, MD
Center for Liver Diseases
Division of Hepatology
University of Miami Miller School of Medicine
1500 NW 12th Avenue, Suite 1101E
Jackson Medical Towers
Miami, FL 33136, USA

E-mail address:
clevy@med.miami.edu

Genetic Determinants of Cholestasis

Gideon M. Hirschfield, MB BChir, PhD, FRCP

KEYWORDS

- Cholestasis • Genetics • Biliary transporters

KEY POINTS

- Cholestasis is the consequence of any impairment in bile flow that leads to abnormal retention of constituents of bile in the liver and serum.
- Bile acids are inherently cytotoxic, and cholestatic liver disease is therefore frequently a cause of progressive liver fibrosis if untreated.
- Rare genetic syndromes with functional mutations in critical bile transporters have proved highly insightful into the broad pathogenesis of cholestasis.
- More common autoimmune, as well as drug-induced, cholestatic syndromes also have made a broad genetic contribution.
- Therapies based on better molecular appreciation of cholestasis may ultimately prove useful for patients.

INTRODUCTION

The major functions of bile are solubilization of lipid in the bowel along with the faecal removal of waste metabolites. Bile is able to function in this way through a mixed composition that includes bile acids, cholesterol, phospholipids, proteins, and other organic molecules, as well as ions. Cholestasis occurs when there is a pathologic failure at any point along the hepatobiliary tree that leads to impaired secretion of bile, such that biliary constituents spill into blood. Such instances occur as a result of injuries (congenital and acquired) spanning a range of sites along the hepatobiliary tree from the hepatocyte to the draining bile ducts (**Fig. 1**).[1,2]

Complete output of hepatic bile acid includes primary bile acids derived from de novo synthesis and active ileal reabsorption, alongside secondary bile acids that are formed and passively reabsorbed in the colon after bacterial dehydroxylation (eg, ursodeoxycholic acid). The rate-determining step during bile formation is canalicular (apical) excretion of osmotically active bile acids by adenosine triphosphate

Disclosures: None relevant.
NIHR Biomedical Research Unit and Centre for Liver Research, Institute of Biomedical Research, The Medical School, University of Birmingham, Wolfson Drive, Birmingham B15 2TT, UK
E-mail address: g.hirschfield@bham.ac.uk

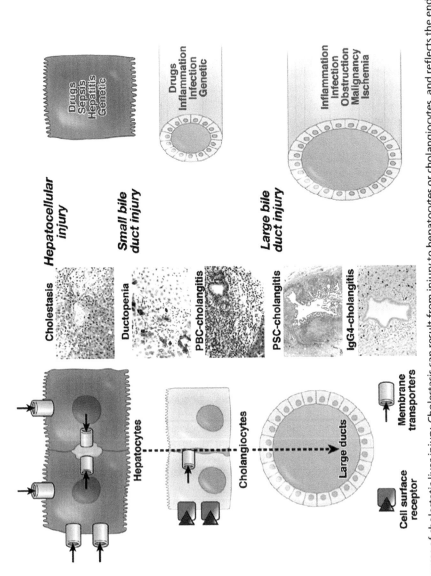

Fig. 1. Sites and sources of cholestatic liver injury. Cholestasis can result from injury to hepatocytes or cholangiocytes, and reflects the end result of many potential injuries. IgG4, immunoglobulin G4; PBC, primary biliary cirrhosis; PSC, primary sclerosing cholangitis. (*Reproduced from* Hirschfield GM, Heathcote EJ, Gershwin ME. Pathogenesis of cholestatic liver disease and therapeutic approaches. Gastroenterology 2010;139(5):1481–96; with permission.)

(ATP)-binding cassette transporters, which is followed by water moving across aquaporin channels and tight junctions. The main biliary lipids are secreted across the canalicular membrane of hepatocytes by specific transmembrane transporters: ABCB11 (also known as bile salt export pump [BSEP]), ABCG5/ABCG8 (obligate heterodimer that facilitates cholesterol efflux), and ABCB4 (multidrug-resistance gene MDR3/MDR2 in man/mice, which pumps phospholipids, mostly phosphatidyl-choline). The transporter ATP8B1 (FIC1) maintains the asymmetry of phospholipid species to promote the required lipid architecture of the canalicular membrane.[3] Bile acids additionally help canalicular secretion of phospholipids and cholesterol in the formation of mixed biliary micelles. Secretory and absorptive processes, mainly bicarbonate secretion by cholangiocytes, modify canalicular bile during its passage along the biliary tree.[4,5] Genetic determinants of cholestasis can be clini-cally relevant directly because of their role in biliary transport, or indirectly as genetic variation predisposing to biliary injury (eg, autoimmune disease or drug-induced liver injury). This short review outlines some of the pertinent genetic insights to date that are of importance to clinicians looking after patients with cholestatic liver disease.

INHERITED CHOLESTATIC SYNDROMES

Rare genetic syndromes have proved insightful as regards the molecular mechanisms of cholestasis. New knowledge has led advances in understanding the molecular mechanisms underpinning diseases whereby fundamental biliary transporters fail to function normally and detergent bile is retained within the liver, with resultant inherent cytotoxicity and progressive liver fibrosis.

Progressive Familial Intrahepatic Cholestatic Syndromes

A rare progressive familial intrahepatic cholestatic (PFIC) disease was described by Clayton and colleagues[6] in 1969 and eponymously named Byler disease, after the original Amish kindred, in whom intrahepatic cholestasis was lethal. In-depth family studies ultimately led to appreciation of the 3 major primary active transport proteins required for normal canalicular bile flow.[7,8] A group of mutations in the transporters have over time been causally related to different types of autosomal recessive PFIC, with inactivating mutations in the transporters ATP8B1, ABCB11, or ABCB4 resulting in PFIC syndrome types 1, 2, or 3, respectively (**Table 1**). With molecular appreciation better understood, increasingly these diseases are better described through their molecular terminology, even if the term PFIC remains in common usage. It is also increasingly clear that a spectrum of cholestatic disease caused by variants in *ABCB11*, *ABCB4*, and *ATP8B1* is seen, and this spans the severe phenotype of PFIC to milder, often later-onset or intermittent forms of cholestasis, such as drug-induced cholestasis, benign recurrent intrahepatic cholestasis, or intrahepatic chole-stasis of pregnancy (ICP).

The 3 classic syndromes present as cholestasis usually in the first year of life; affected children are commonly growth restricted given their failure to absorb dietary fat normally, and run the risk of direct complications from malabsorption of vitamins A, D, E, and K. This process parallels an often progressive and notably symptomatic (itch) liver disease related to bile acid retention, often leading to a need for complex biliary diversion for symptom control as well as liver transplantation for more definitive management. However, if molecular insights can be improved it remains possible that medical treatments that improve bile transporter function may be of use, with inevitable potential for use beyond the narrow constraints of rare genetic cholestatic syndromes.[9]

Table 1
Progressive familial intrahepatic cholestatic (PFIC) syndromes

	PFIC1	PFIC2	PFIC3
Onset	Childhood	Childhood	Childhood and adults
Serum findings	Low/normal GGT; high bile acids	Low/normal GGT; high bile acids	Elevated GGT; normal bile acids
Bile acids	Very low, phosphatidylserine present	Absent	Normal but devoid of phosphatidylcholine
Hepatic changes	Granular bile with canalicular cholestasis	Giant cell hepatitis	Bile duct proliferation
Clinical observations	Intense itch; significant extrahepatic manifestations (pancreatitis, diarrhea, deafness)	Intense itch; Pseudorecurrence post liver transplant (antibody mediated); hepatocellular carcinoma risk	Moderate itch; biliary cirrhosis
Gene	*ATP8B1*	*ABCB11* (BSEP)	*ABCB4* (MDR3)
Gene function	Aminophospholipid translocase	Bile salt export	Phosphatidylcholine exchange
Broader clinical spectrum	Benign recurrent intrahepatic cholestasis; intrahepatic cholestasis of pregnancy	Benign recurrent intrahepatic cholestasis; drug-induced liver injury	Intrahepatic cholestasis of pregnancy; drug-induced liver injury; low phospholipid–associated cholelithiasis

Abbreviations: BSEP, bile salt export pump; GGT, γ-glutamyltransferase.

Of note, clinically PFIC3 patients may be distinguished by a raised serum γ-glutamyltransferase (GGT) (PFIC1 and PFIC2 being classically described as so-called low or normal-GGT syndromes), and although immunohistochemistry can be invaluable to establish whether specific transporters are implicated in disease etiology, definitive clinical diagnosis generally now assumes that genetic testing be performed. For example, in PFIC2 patients BSEP immunoreactivity is absent from the canalicular membrane; however, in PFIC3 canalicular MDR3 immunoreactivity can remain detectable, meaning that whereas PFIC2 may be reliably diagnosed by immunofluorescence, the diagnosis of PFIC3 requires gene sequencing.[10–12]

PFIC1/FIC1 deficiency
PFIC1/FIC1 deficiency is an autosomal recessive childhood-onset disease caused by mutations in *ATP8B1*, which encodes an aminophospholipid flippase that is widely expressed, not just in the liver. As a consequence, in addition to severe pruritus, diarrhea, pancreatic disease, rickets, pneumonia, abnormal sweat tests, hearing impairment, and poor growth are more common in FIC1 patients than in BSEP patients (which has a hepatic pattern of expression).[13] Liver transplantation therefore only partially reverses the clinical phenotype.

PFIC2/BSEP deficiency
This condition presents similarly to FIC1 deficiency but is the result of mutations in *ABCB11*, which encodes a distinct canalicular transporter.[14] In contrast to *ATP8B1*, BSEP has hepatic expression only, with no extrahepatic manifestations being

described. It is characterized by cholestasis, gallstones, and a higher incidence of hepatocellular carcinoma, normally extremely rare in pediatric practice.[15] At presentation, serum aminotransferase and bile salt levels are higher in BSEP than in FIC1 deficiency, whereas serum alkaline phosphatase values are higher and serum albumin values lower in FIC1 patients.[13] In one clinical series of 62 children with normal-GGT PFIC based on genetic testing, 13 patients were PFIC1 and 39 PFIC2; PFIC type remained undefined in 10 individuals. PFIC2 patients were more likely to develop neonatal cholestasis. High-serum alanine aminotransferase and α-fetoprotein, severe lobular lesions with giant hepatocytes, early liver failure, cholelithiasis, hepatocellular carcinoma, very low biliary bile acid concentration, and negative BSEP canalicular staining suggested PFIC2, whereas an absence of these signs and/or presence of extrahepatic manifestations suggested PFIC1. Not unusually for even apparently monogenetic disease, PFIC1 and PFIC2 phenotypes were not clearly correlated with mutation patterns. Clinically the combination of ursodeoxycholic acid, biliary diversion, and liver transplantation meant that nearly 90% of patients were alive at a median age of 10.5 years, half of these without liver transplantation.[16] Intriguingly BSEP patients, when transplanted, can develop a recurrent cholestatic syndrome that is a consequence of humoral immunity to de novo allograft expressed BSEP.[17]

PFIC3/MDR3 deficiency
This inherited cholestatic syndrome is also an autosomal recessive trait, which results in defective biliary phospholipid secretion and generation of more toxic bile. Although it may present in early life with cholestasis (elevated GGT), it has a broader range of presentations including recurrent choledocholithiasis in older children and adults, some cases of ICP (see later discussion), and reports of familial idiopathic biliary cirrhosis.[18–21]

Intrahepatic Cholestasis of Pregnancy

This syndrome is collectively the result of a variety of abnormalities in biliary transport, and has a multifactorial basis that includes hormonal, environmental, and genetic risks.[22] Clinically pruritus is characteristic, alongside a transaminitis secondary to bile acid retention, and less commonly jaundice; elevated serum bile acids are found, typically starting in the third trimester of pregnancy, and ICP resolves after delivery but has a significant recurrence rate in following pregnancies. Cholestasis that fails to resolve requires investigation to establish a cause (eg, underlying autoimmune cholestatic liver disease exacerbated by pregnancy). Epidemiologically there is an association with an increased incidence of fetal distress, premature delivery, and stillbirth, hence the proactive management of such individuals by obstetricians. Ursodeoxycholic acid is frequently prescribed, and a recent meta-analysis concluded that therapy was effective in reducing pruritus and improving liver biochemistry as well as possibly benefiting fetal outcomes.[23]

As many as 15% of those with ICP may have associated mutations in the MDR3 (ABCB4) gene,[24,25] a gene for which the consequences of mutations cover a spectrum of clinical disorders from ICP and low-phospholipid–associated cholelithiasis (LPAC), to PFIC3 as already described.[26] LPAC is a condition characterized by gallstones, high serum GGT, intrahepatic microlithiasis, and recurrent biliary symptoms despite cholecystectomy (usually notably at a young age), and affected women frequently report prior cholestasis of pregnancy. ICP-associated variants were first highlighted in a case report,[27] in which the mother of a child with PFIC3 was found to carry a heterozygous single-nucleotide deletion and, along with female relatives, gave a positive history of ICP. However, across populations MDR3 mutations may not be as relevant with other genes implicated: mutations in *ATP8B1* occur rarely[28] as does genetic variation in *BSEP*.[29] There are also reports of involvement of another biliary transporter, *ABCC2*, which encodes the multidrug-resistance related protein 2 (MRP2).[30] MRP2 exports organic anions including bilirubin into the bile, and is more classically associated with the benign Dubin-Johnson syndrome, an autosomal recessive disorder characterized by direct hyperbilirubinemia and abnormal urinary coproporphyrin excretion, but not elevated bile acids. In a South American report a polymorphism in exon 28 of *ABCC2* was associated with ICP. The farnesoid X receptor (FXR) encoded by *NR1H4* is the principal bile acid receptor and regulates hepatic bile acid synthesis and transport. One study has described 4 heterozygous variants within FXR that are associated with ICP, 3 of which are functional.[31]

Alagille Syndrome

In neonates, Alagille syndrome (ALGS) is the most common inherited cause of conjugated hyperbilirubinemia.[32,33] ALGS is a multisystem autosomal dominant disorder characterized by cholestatic liver disease and bile duct paucity on liver biopsy, congenital cardiac defects, typically peripheral pulmonary stenosis, renal anomalies, vascular abnormalities, characteristic facies (broad forehead, deep-set eyes, and a pointed chin), posterior embryotoxon of the eye on slip-lamp examination and skeletal anomalies, commonly butterfly vertebrae. In most patients (>93%) a mutation in *JAGGED1* (NOTCH pathway ligand) can be identified, whereas a smaller number of ALGS individuals have mutations in *NOTCH2* (receptor). Mutations are inherited in 40% and de novo in the remainder. The offspring of an individual with ALGS develops disease in 50% of cases yet, intriguingly, the genotype-phenotype correlation within families is not strong, with disease-modifier genes remaining to be better defined. The Notch pathway is crucial for a wide variety of developmental processes, including the formation of tissue boundaries. At least 5 ligands and 4 Notch receptors are expressed in humans. Cholestasis is a major manifestation of mutations, and histologically bile duct paucity is seen although ductal proliferation is occasionally evident neonatally, usually with portal inflammation, which may lead to a misdiagnosis of biliary atresia. Bile duct paucity is progressive in some patients, and may be more common in late infancy and early childhood compared with early infancy. Progressive liver disease, however, eventually causing cirrhosis and failure and requiring liver transplantation, is uncommon, occurring in only 15% of patients. Although there is no reliable way of predicting which infants are at high risk, those who subsequently manifest progressive liver disease have been shown to have chronically elevated total bilirubin, conjugated bilirubin, and cholesterol. A small proportion of patients have no manifestations of liver disease.

Cystic Fibrosis

As many as 10% of patients with cystic fibrosis (CF) develop multilobular biliary cirrhosis during their first decade of life.[34] Complications include portal hypertension, nutritional failure and, occasionally, liver failure. The CF transmembrane regulator protein is expressed in the cholangiocyte, and subsequent altered biliary transport causes a focal obstruction to bile flow, retention of bile acids, and peribiliary fibrogenesis driven by inflammation. Recent studies have suggested that the Z allele of *SERPINA1* (α1-antitrypsin) is a risk factor for liver disease in CF, although the role of this and other genetic modifiers remains to be clarified.[35]

Given that a sclerosing cholangiopathy is encountered in CF liver disease, a role for *CFTR* variants in primary sclerosing cholangitis (PSC) has been proposed, but never clearly proved.[36] In a subset of PSC patients with inflammatory bowel disease, an increased prevalence of CFTR abnormalities was described, and experimental induction of colitis in *CFTR* knockout mice results in the development of bile duct injury. In a recent PSC genome scan, the G-protein–coupled bile acid receptor 1 (also known as *TGR5*) was identified as a potential candidate gene. This molecule is involved in bile acid–induced fluid secretion in biliary epithelial cells and can be found colocalized with CFTR and the apical sodium-dependent bile salt uptake transporter, suggesting a functional coupling of TGR5 to bile acid uptake and chloride secretion. Intriguingly it has also been identified in cholangiocyte cilia, where it might couple biliary bile acid concentration and composition to ductular bile formation.[37]

Miscellaneous

Arthrogryposis, renal dysfunction, and cholestasis (ARC) syndrome is caused by mutations in the *VPS33* gene, which has a role in vacuolar protein sorting and lysosomal function.[38] Mutations in the gene encoding VIPAR, which interacts with VPS33, have also been shown to cause ARC syndrome in a minority of patients. The VPS33B-VIPAR complex appears to have diverse functions in the pathways regulating apical-basolateral polarity in the liver and kidney. Other rarer causes of sclerosing cholangitis also reinforce cellular themes for cholestatic liver injury, particularly the importance of cell-junction integrity. In the liver, tight junctions separate bile flow from plasma and are composed of strands of claudins and occludin. The observation, therefore, that *claudin-1* gene mutations are found in neonatal sclerosing cholangitis, in association with ichthyoids, implicates independently how hepatocyte and bile duct injuries secondary to increased paracellular bile regurgitation function may be relevant.[39] Aagenaes syndrome is a very rare autosomal recessive condition that presents with chronic and severe lymphedema and severe neonatal cholestasis. The neonatal cholestasis usually reduces during early childhood and subsequently becomes intermittent. The genetic cause of lymphedema cholestasis syndrome (LCS) remains unknown but is localized in one pedigree to a locus, LCS1, on chromosome 15q.[40]

ACQUIRED CHOLESTATIC SYNDROMES

Acquired cholestatic syndromes are prevalent and are usually the consequence of environmental exposure in individuals at broad genetic risk. The environmental exposure may be readily apparent as a drug or toxin, or more speculative, as in autoimmune liver disease. Appreciation of some of the accompanying genetic risk factors has shed light on important pathways involved in biliary injury, different for example to those understood from detailed analysis of rare PFIC pedigrees.

Primary Biliary Cirrhosis

Before the advent of genome-wide association studies, only human leukocyte antigen (HLA) was robustly associated with primary biliary cirrhosis (PBC), a classically autoimmune liver disease, with striking biliary specificity, despite attempts at candidate gene studies. Studies from northern and southern Europe, as well as North America, show that HLA-DR8 (DRB1*0801) is significantly overrepresented in patients with PBC relative to controls. The application of genetic array technology brought the new insight that PBC has shared genetic risks with other autoimmune diseases. The data from the author and those of colleagues suggest that several immune pathways contribute to the development of PBC.[41–47] Of note, a strong implied role for the interleukin (IL)-12 signaling axis arose from associations including *IL12A* (IL-12p40), *IL12RB2*, *STAT4*, *IRF5*, *SOCS1*, and *NFκB*, which implicate IL-12/interferon (IFN)-γ–dominated type 1 immune responses, and the IL-23 pathway in the development of antigen specific autoreactivity in PBC (**Fig. 2**). The association with *CXCR5* is also notable given that high expression of CXCR5 is a defining hallmark of T follicular helper cells, a CD4 T-helper (Th) cell subset that promotes germinal center reactions and the selection and affinity maturation of B cells. The binding of IL-12 to its receptor modulates autoimmune responses by evoking IFN-γ production, which is characteristic of Th1-driven immune

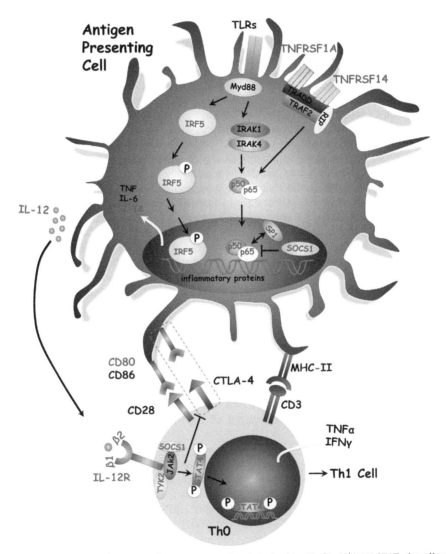

Fig. 2. Immunoregulatory pathways across the interleukin-12 (IL-12)/JAK-STAT signaling pathway are implicated in the risk of developing primary biliary cirrhosis. Genetic studies of primary biliary cirrhosis (PBC) now suggest varied immunoregulatory pathways particularly related to IL-12 signaling as relevant to risk of developing PBC in Caucasian populations. Abbreviations as per http://www.ncbi.nlm.nih.gov.

responses, but this can in turn modulate IL-23–driven induction of IL-17–producing helper T lymphocytes. The specific cellular effects of IL-12 are mediated via its ability to induce activation of the transcription factor STAT4, which promotes IFN-γ production, and in addition to triggering Th1 responses contributes to loss of tolerance in several models of autoimmunity. STAT4 activation stabilizes the transcription factor t-bet, which is required for Th1 differentiation. Through activation of IRF5, INF-γ promotes polarization of M1 macrophages that produce proinflammatory cytokines and contribute to tissue destruction. M1 macrophages are characterized by IRF5 expression, with forced IRF5 expression in M2 macrophages driving global expression of M1-specific cytokines, chemokines, and costimulatory molecules as well as potent T_H1–T_H17 responses. The importance of this pathway in PBC is emphasized by the finding of a strong genetic association with *IRF5*, as well as the association of this locus across autoimmune disease.

At present, however, the genetic risk for PBC has focused on the pathogenesis of loss of tolerance rather than on clinical cholestatic phenotype or response to treatment by the bile acid ursodeoxycholic acid. A different pattern of genetic risk is therefore likely to explain symptoms such as pruritus, or biochemical stratification such as is seen in response to ursodeoxycholic acid. To date robust associations are lacking, but previous data has alluded, for example, to AE2 variants as risk factors for disease severity.[48]

Primary Sclerosing Cholangitis

Recent genetic approaches through studies of large cohorts has allowed common genetic variation in disease predisposition to also be probed robustly for this autoimmune large bile duct cholangiopathy, and the observations made suggest predisposing subtle changes to pathways that mediate inflammation (eg, *HLA, IL2/IL2RA, IL21, REL, CARD9, BCL2L11, MST1*), cholangiocyte biology (eg, *TGR5, CFTR, GPC5/6*), liver fibrosis (eg, *SXR, MMP3*) and malignancy risk (eg, *NKG2D, GPC5, GPX1*).[49–52] Similar to many autoimmune disorders, the predominant attributable risk factors are found within the major histocompatibility complex on chromosome 6p21, particularly at HLA-B variants, but with a complex association signal including the class II region. This very significant HLA association, however, is not understood more than superficially and represents an important research bottleneck that must be broken before the antigen specificity and triggers of this autoimmune disease are understood.

Weaker, but nevertheless insightful, non-HLA associations are detected for multiple inflammatory bowel disease (IBD)-related and autoimmunity loci. The overlap with IBD is not complete, and the majority of risk loci of both ulcerative colitis and Crohn disease do not confirm associations with PSC. Although this may change as power to detect association strengthens with increased cohort size, it nevertheless mirrors clinical practice whereby the IBD of PSC demonstrates distinguishing features in comparison with classic colitis (eg, rectal sparing, backwash ileitis, right-sided predominance). Individual loci raise specific interest such as, for example, in the locus on chromosome 2q35, which harbors the bile acid receptor TGR5, raising a tantalizing angle on an association between PSC and CFTR variations that remains clearer in mice than in man (see earlier discussion). The IL-2 axis is highlighted as potentially of relevance to disease etiology, with obvious implications raised for regulatory T-cell function in pathogenesis, and thereby potentially therapy, as well as animal models highlighting biliary phenotypes. Furthermore, these gene associations across IL-2 signaling are mirrored by increasing awareness of the role of T-regulatory and Th17 cells in autoimmune liver disease generally, both cell populations having been specifically implicated in autoimmune cholestatic syndromes.

Drug-Induced Liver Injury

Drugs associated with a cholestatic pattern of liver injury seem able to inhibit bile secretion and bile acid transport at many levels. This action includes effects on uptake and efflux across the sinusoidal membrane, as well as canalicular efflux. Although the toxin exposure is key, genetic risk appears to be relevant, with important advances made in defining, for example, patterns of HLA risk for certain drug injuries. For example, susceptibility to liver injury with amoxicillin/clavulanic acid is highly HLA restricted, with high-resolution HLA genotyping confirming associations with HLA-A*0201 and HLA-DQB1*0602.[53] In addition, in an analysis of autoimmune-related genes, rs2476601 in the gene *PTPN22* was also associated. Similarly the HLA-B*5701 genotype is a major determinant of drug-induced liver injury caused by flucloxacillin.[54]

More broadly, it is clear that drug injury interferes with bile acid transporters. Although not a drug transporter, MDR3 plays a key role in the biliary secretion of phosphatidylcholine (see earlier discussion), and genetic variants in MDR3 and BSEP may predispose individuals to drug-induced cholestasis.[55–57] Drugs such as rifampicin, cyclosporine A, bosentan, and erythromycin can all experimentally inhibit Bsep, while sulindac competitively inhibits canalicular bile acid transport and ethinylestradiol-17β-glucuronide is secreted into bile by Mrp2 and then inhibits Bsep from the luminal side of the canalicular membrane. Two nonsynonymous single-nucleotide polymorphisms in *BSEP* have been described, c.1331T>C (p.V444A) in exon 13 and c.2029A>G (p.M677V) in exon 17, with frequencies that are higher than 0.5%. Individuals with the p.V444A variant have lower BSEP expression, and this variant is considered a risk factor for drug-induced cholestasis. For example, one study of contraceptive-induced cholestasis revealed an association with BSEP 1331T>C polymorphism as a susceptibility factor. Other examples of genetically determined drug-induced cholestasis have been reported. A study from the United Kingdom found that allelic variants of *UGT2B7*, *CYP2C8*, and *ABCC2* (thought to predispose to the formation and accumulation of reactive diclofenac metabolites) were associated with diclofenac hepatotoxicity.[58] Other similar work identified a *PXR* polymorphism as a risk factor for flucloxacillin-induced liver injury.[59]

SUMMARY

Although cholestatic liver disease remains a multifactorial process in which environmental risk is very important, rare syndromes and some more common clinical diseases have been able to shed light on the underpinning genetic risks. This research may ultimately help in the development of better diagnostic and therapeutic approaches for treating patients with a variety of cholestatic diseases.

REFERENCES

1. Hirschfield GM, Heathcote EJ, Gershwin ME. Pathogenesis of cholestatic liver disease and therapeutic approaches. Gastroenterology 2010;139(5):1481–96.
2. Paumgartner G. Biliary physiology and disease: reflections of a physician-scientist. Hepatology 2010;51(4):1095–106.
3. Groen A, Romero MR, Kunne C, et al. Complementary functions of the flippase ATP8B1 and the floppase ABCB4 in maintaining canalicular membrane integrity. Gastroenterology 2011;141(5):1927–1937.e1–e4.
4. Wagner M, Zollner G, Trauner M. New molecular insights into the mechanisms of cholestasis. J Hepatol 2009;51(3):565–80.

5. Halilbasic E, Claudel T, Trauner M. Bile acid transporters and regulatory nuclear receptors in the liver and beyond. J Hepatol 2013;58:155–68.
6. Clayton RJ, Iber FL, Ruebner BH, et al. Byler disease. Fatal familial intrahepatic cholestasis in an Amish kindred. Am J Dis Child 1969;117(1):112–24.
7. Nicolaou M, Andress EJ, Zolnerciks JK, et al. Canalicular ABC transporters and liver disease. J Pathol 2012;226(2):300–15.
8. Kubitz R, Droge C, Stindt J, et al. The bile salt export pump (BSEP) in health and disease. Clin Res Hepatol Gastroenterol 2012;36:536–53.
9. Gonzales E, Grosse B, Cassio D, et al. Successful mutation-specific chaperone therapy with 4-phenylbutyrate in a child with progressive familial intrahepatic cholestasis type 2. J Hepatol 2012;57(3):695–8.
10. Jansen PL, Strautnieks SS, Jacquemin E, et al. Hepatocanalicular bile salt export pump deficiency in patients with progressive familial intrahepatic cholestasis. Gastroenterology 1999;117(6):1370–9.
11. Keitel V, Burdelski M, Warskulat U, et al. Expression and localization of hepatobiliary transport proteins in progressive familial intrahepatic cholestasis. Hepatology 2005;41(5):1160–72.
12. Evason K, Bove KE, Finegold MJ, et al. Morphologic findings in progressive familial intrahepatic cholestasis 2 (PFIC2): correlation with genetic and immunohistochemical studies. Am J Surg Pathol 2011;35(5):687–96.
13. Pawlikowska L, Strautnieks S, Jankowska I, et al. Differences in presentation and progression between severe FIC1 and BSEP deficiencies. J Hepatol 2010;53(1):170–8.
14. Strautnieks SS, Byrne JA, Pawlikowska L, et al. Severe bile salt export pump deficiency: 82 different ABCB11 mutations in 109 families. Gastroenterology 2008;134(4):1203–14.
15. Knisely AS, Strautnieks SS, Meier Y, et al. Hepatocellular carcinoma in ten children under five years of age with bile salt export pump deficiency. Hepatology 2006;44(2):478–86.
16. Davit-Spraul A, Fabre M, Branchereau S, et al. ATP8B1 and ABCB11 analysis in 62 children with normal gamma-glutamyl transferase progressive familial intrahepatic cholestasis (PFIC): phenotypic differences between PFIC1 and PFIC2 and natural history. Hepatology 2010;51(5):1645–55.
17. Jara P, Hierro L, Martinez-Fernandez P, et al. Recurrence of bile salt export pump deficiency after liver transplantation. N Engl J Med 2009;361(14):1359–67.
18. Davit-Spraul A, Gonzales E, Baussan C, et al. Progressive familial intrahepatic cholestasis. Orphanet J Rare Dis 2009;4:1.
19. Ziol M, Barbu V, Rosmorduc O, et al. ABCB4 heterozygous gene mutations associated with fibrosing cholestatic liver disease in adults. Gastroenterology 2008;135(1):131–41.
20. Gotthardt D, Runz H, Keitel V, et al. A mutation in the canalicular phospholipid transporter gene, ABCB4, is associated with cholestasis, ductopenia, and cirrhosis in adults. Hepatology 2008;48(4):1157–66.
21. Pasmant E, Goussard P, Baranes L, et al. First description of ABCB4 gene deletions in familial low phospholipid-associated cholelithiasis and oral contraceptives-induced cholestasis. Eur J Hum Genet 2012;20(3):277–82.
22. Geenes V, Williamson C. Intrahepatic cholestasis of pregnancy. World J Gastroenterol 2009;15(17):2049–66.
23. Bacq Y, Sentilhes L, Reyes HB, et al. Efficacy of ursodeoxycholic acid in treating intrahepatic cholestasis of pregnancy: a meta-analysis. Gastroenterology 2012;143:1492–501.

24. Wasmuth HE, Glantz A, Keppeler H, et al. Intrahepatic cholestasis of pregnancy: the severe form is associated with common variants of the hepatobiliary phospholipid transporter ABCB4 gene. Gut 2007;56(2):265–70.
25. Bacq Y, Gendrot C, Perrotin F, et al. ABCB4 gene mutations and single-nucleotide polymorphisms in women with intrahepatic cholestasis of pregnancy. J Med Genet 2009;46(10):711–5.
26. Rosmorduc O, Poupon R. Low phospholipid associated cholelithiasis: association with mutation in the MDR3/ABCB4 gene. Orphanet J Rare Dis 2007; 2:29.
27. Jacquemin E, Cresteil D, Manouvrier S, et al. Heterozygous non-sense mutation of the MDR3 gene in familial intrahepatic cholestasis of pregnancy. Lancet 1999; 353(9148):210–1.
28. Mullenbach R, Bennett A, Tetlow N, et al. ATP8B1 mutations in British cases with intrahepatic cholestasis of pregnancy. Gut 2005;54(6):829–34.
29. Dixon PH, van Mil SW, Chambers J, et al. Contribution of variant alleles of ABCB11 to susceptibility to intrahepatic cholestasis of pregnancy. Gut 2009; 58(4):537–44.
30. Sookoian S, Castano G, Burgueno A, et al. Association of the multidrug-resistance-associated protein gene (ABCC2) variants with intrahepatic cholestasis of pregnancy. J Hepatol 2008;48(1):125–32.
31. Van Mil SW, Milona A, Dixon PH, et al. Functional variants of the central bile acid sensor FXR identified in intrahepatic cholestasis of pregnancy. Gastroenterology 2007;133(2):507–16.
32. Kamath BM, Loomes KM, Piccoli DA. Medical management of Alagille syndrome. J Pediatr Gastroenterol Nutr 2010;50(6):580–6.
33. Penton AL, Leonard LD, Spinner NB. Notch signaling in human development and disease. Semin Cell Dev Biol 2012;23(4):450–7.
34. Herrmann U, Dockter G, Lammert F. Cystic fibrosis-associated liver disease. Best Pract Res Clin Gastroenterol 2010;24(5):585–92.
35. Bartlett JR, Friedman KJ, Ling SC, et al. Genetic modifiers of liver disease in cystic fibrosis. JAMA 2009;302(10):1076–83.
36. Pall H, Zielenski J, Jonas MM, et al. Primary sclerosing cholangitis in childhood is associated with abnormalities in cystic fibrosis-mediated chloride channel function. J Pediatr 2007;151(3):255–9.
37. Keitel V, Cupisti K, Ullmer C, et al. The membrane-bound bile acid receptor TGR5 is localized in the epithelium of human gallbladders. Hepatology 2009;50(3): 861–70.
38. Smith H, Galmes R, Gogolina E, et al. Associations among genotype, clinical phenotype, and intracellular localization of trafficking proteins in ARC syndrome. Hum Mutat 2012;33:1656–64.
39. Grosse B, Cassio D, Yousef N, et al. Claudin-1 involved in neonatal ichthyosis sclerosing cholangitis syndrome regulates hepatic paracellular permeability. Hepatology 2012;55(4):1249–59.
40. Bull LN, Roche E, Song EJ, et al. Mapping of the locus for cholestasis-lymphedema syndrome (Aagenaes syndrome) to a 6.6-cM interval on chromosome 15q. Am J Hum Genet 2000;67(4):994–9.
41. Hirschfield GM, Liu X, Xu C, et al. Primary biliary cirrhosis associated with HLA, IL12A, and IL12RB2 variants. N Engl J Med 2009;360(24):2544–55.
42. Walker EJ, Hirschfield GM, Xu C, et al. CTLA4/ICOS gene variants and haplotypes are associated with rheumatoid arthritis and primary biliary cirrhosis in the Canadian population. Arthritis Rheum 2009;60(4):931–7.

43. Hirschfield GM, Liu X, Han Y, et al. Variants at IRF5-TNPO3, 17q12-21 and MMEL1 are associated with primary biliary cirrhosis. Nat Genet 2010;42(8): 655–7.
44. Liu X, Invernizzi P, Lu Y, et al. Genome-wide meta-analyses identify three loci associated with primary biliary cirrhosis. Nat Genet 2010;42(8):658–60.
45. Mells GF, Floyd JA, Morley KI, et al. Genome-wide association study identifies 12 new susceptibility loci for primary biliary cirrhosis. Nat Genet 2011;43(4):329–32.
46. Hirschfield GM, Xie G, Lu E, et al. Association of primary biliary cirrhosis with variants in the CLEC16A, SOCS1, SPIB and SIAE immunomodulatory genes. Genes Immun 2012;13(4):328–35.
47. Juran BD, Hirschfield GM, Invernizzi P, et al. Immunochip analyses identify a novel risk locus for primary biliary cirrhosis at 13q14, multiple independent associations at four established risk loci and epistasis between 1p31 and 7q32 risk variants. Hum Mol Genet 2012;21:5209–21.
48. Poupon R, Ping C, Chretien Y, et al. Genetic factors of susceptibility and of severity in primary biliary cirrhosis. J Hepatol 2008;49(6):1038–45.
49. Melum E, Franke A, Schramm C, et al. Genome-wide association analysis in primary sclerosing cholangitis identifies two non-HLA susceptibility loci. Nat Genet 2011;43(1):17–9.
50. Janse M, Lamberts LE, Franke L, et al. Three ulcerative colitis susceptibility loci are associated with primary sclerosing cholangitis and indicate a role for IL2, REL, and CARD9. Hepatology 2011;53(6):1977–85.
51. Folseraas T, Melum E, Rausch P, et al. Extended analysis of a genome-wide association study in primary sclerosing cholangitis detects multiple novel risk loci. J Hepatol 2012;57(2):366–75.
52. Naess S, Shiryaev A, Hov JR, et al. Genetics in primary sclerosing cholangitis. Clin Res Hepatol Gastroenterol 2012;36:325–33.
53. Lucena MI, Molokhia M, Shen Y, et al. Susceptibility to amoxicillin-clavulanate-induced liver injury is influenced by multiple HLA class I and II alleles. Gastroenterology 2011;141(1):338–47.
54. Daly AK, Donaldson PT, Bhatnagar P, et al. HLA-B*5701 genotype is a major determinant of drug-induced liver injury due to flucloxacillin. Nat Genet 2009; 41(7):816–9.
55. Lang C, Meier Y, Stieger B, et al. Mutations and polymorphisms in the bile salt export pump and the multidrug resistance protein 3 associated with drug-induced liver injury. Pharmacogenet Genomics 2007;17(1):47–60.
56. Dawson S, Stahl S, Paul N, et al. In vitro inhibition of the bile salt export pump correlates with risk of cholestatic drug-induced liver injury in humans. Drug Metab Dispos 2012;40(1):130–8.
57. Padda MS, Sanchez M, Akhtar AJ, et al. Drug-induced cholestasis. Hepatology 2011;53(4):1377–87.
58. Daly AK, Aithal GP, Leathart JB, et al. Genetic susceptibility to diclofenac-induced hepatotoxicity: contribution of UGT2B7, CYP2C8, and ABCC2 genotypes. Gastroenterology 2007;132(1):272–81.
59. Andrews E, Armstrong M, Tugwood J, et al. A role for the pregnane X receptor in flucloxacillin-induced liver injury. Hepatology 2010;51(5):1656–64.

Nuclear Receptors as Drug Targets in Cholestatic Liver Diseases

Emina Halilbasic, MD[a], Anna Baghdasaryan, MD, PhD[a,b],
Michael Trauner, MD[a,*]

KEYWORDS

- Cholestatic liver disease • Nuclear receptors • Cholestasis • Bile acids

KEY POINTS

- Nuclear receptors (NRs) regulate ligand-activated transcription factor networks of genes for the elimination and detoxification of potentially toxic biliary constituents accumulating in cholestasis.
- Activation of several NRs also modulates fibrogenesis, inflammation, and carcinogenesis as sequels of cholestasis.
- Impaired NR signaling may be involved in the pathogenesis of cholestasis and genetic variants of NR-encoding genes are associated with susceptibility and progression of cholestatic disorders.
- NRs represent attractive targets for pharmacotherapy of cholestatic disorders, because their activation may orchestrate several key processes involved in the pathogenesis of cholestatic liver diseases.
- Several already available drugs may exert their beneficial effects in cholestasis via NR activation (eg, ursodeoxycholic acid via glucocorticoid receptor and pregnane X receptor; rifampicin via pregnane X receptor; fibrates via PPARα; budesonide via glucocorticoid receptor) and novel therapeutic developments target NRs (obeticholic acid - farnesoid X receptor).

INTRODUCTION

Cholestasis may be best defined as an impairment of bile flow whereby bile reaches the duodenum in insufficient amounts.[1] The cause of different cholestatic diseases

This work was supported by grants F3008-B05 and F3517-B20 from the Austrian Science Foundation (to MT).

a Division of Gastroenterology and Hepatology, Department of Internal Medicine III, Medical University of Vienna, Vienna, Austria; b Laboratory of Experimental and Molecular Hepatology, Division of Gastroenterology and Hepatology, Department of Internal Medicine, Medical University of Graz, Graz, Austria

* Corresponding author. Division of Gastroenterology and Hepatology, Department of Internal Medicine III, Medical University of Vienna, Waehringer Guertel 18-20, A-1090 Vienna, Vienna, Austria.

E-mail address: michael.trauner@meduniwien.ac.at

is quite diverse, comprising hereditary and acquired diseases caused by genetic and environmental factors (discussed in previous articles in this volume). Independent of their cause, the main features of cholestatic liver disorders include an accumulation of cholephils such as bile acids (BAs) in the liver and systemic circulation.[2] The accumulation of potentially toxic BAs leads to hepatocellular damage followed by inflammation and fibrosis, and, finally, depending on the disease severity and duration, may culminate in liver cirrhosis and hepatocellular or cholangiocellular cancer. To handle potentially toxic cholephils under physiologic and pathologic conditions, the liver possesses a complex network of nuclear receptor (NR)-regulated pathways that coordinate BA homeostasis and bile secretion to limit their concentrations and prevent hepatic as well as systemic accumulation. NRs are ligand-activated transcription factors that regulate a broad range of key hepatic processes[3] in addition to hepatobiliary excretory function, such as hepatic glucose and lipid metabolism, inflammation, regeneration, fibrosis, and tumorigenesis.[4] On activation by ligands, NRs change their conformation, which in turn facilitates the recruitment of coactivators and dissociation of corepressors and enables DNA binding and stimulation of gene transcription.[5] The recruitment of cofactors fine tunes the regulation of transcription by NRs.[6] The most relevant BA-activated NRs for regulation of hepatobiliary homeostasis, bile secretion, and, thereby understanding and treating cholestasis, include the farnesoid X receptor (FXR, NR1H4),[7] pregnane X receptor (PXR, NR1I2),[8,9] and vitamin D receptor (VDR, NR1I1).[10] Apart from BAs, other biliary constituents such as bilirubin can also activate NRs, such as the constitutive androstane receptor (CAR, NR1I3). Furthermore, other nuclear receptors such as glucocorticoid receptor (GR, NR3C1) and fatty acid-activated peroxisome proliferator-activated receptors (PPARs), in particular PPARα (NR1C1) and PPARγ (NR1C3) as regulators of inflammation, fibrosis, and energy homeostasis, may also impact on biliary homeostasis and cholestatic liver injury. Because of their capability to control hepatic metabolism, NRs have emerged as promising therapeutic targets in many liver diseases, including cholestatic disorders. In this article, the principal role of NRs in the pathogenesis of various cholestatic disorders and how they may serve as drug targets in the management of cholestatic patients are discussed.

NUCLEAR BA RECEPTOR FXR AND ITS BIOLOGY

FXR has been identified as a main nuclear BA receptor,[7,11,12] controlling synthesis and uptake of BAs as well as stimulating their elimination from liver. FXR is predominantly expressed in organs involved in BA transport and/or metabolism, such as liver, ileum, kidney, and adrenal glands.[13–15] As many other NRs, it exerts its transcriptional activity by heterodimer formation with another NR retinoid X receptor (RXR, NR2B1).[13,16] To initiate gene transcription, the FXR-RXR heterodimer binds to so-called inverted repeat 1 (IR-1) within the promoter sequence of target genes.[17] Four FXRα isoforms coded as FXRα1-4 have been described,[18] which have identical DNA-binding domain but may differ in gene regulation because of differences in ligand-dependent recruitment of coactivator/corepressor proteins, heterodimer formation with RXR, or DNA binding.[15,19,20]

The central role of FXR encompasses the regulation of the enterohepatic circulation and intracellular load of BAs (**Fig. 1**). By inhibition of the basolateral uptake transporter sodium/taurocholate cotransporting polypeptide, solute carrier family 10, member 1 (NTCP; SLC10A1) and upregulation of the canalicular export transporter bile salt export pump (BSEP; ABCB11) in hepatocytes, FXR reduces hepatocellular BA levels by limiting their uptake from the sinusoidal blood and promoting their biliary excretion (see **Fig. 1**).[21–24] In addition, FXR reduces endogenous BA synthesis via classical and alternative pathways through the inhibition of rate-limiting enzymes CYP7A1, CYP8B1, and CYP27A1 (reviewed in[25]) (see **Fig. 1**). The molecular mechanism underlying the inhibitory effects of FXR are linked to FXR-mediated induction of an atypical NR short heterodimer partner (SHP; NR0B2) and which acts as transcriptional repressor because of interference with other NRs such as liver X receptor (LXR, NR1H3), liver receptor homolog 1 (LRH-1, NR5A2), and hepatocyte nuclear factor 4α (HNF4α, NR2A1).[26–29] Additional important regulatory mechanisms for inhibition of BA synthesis include FXR-mediated induction of the intestinal hormonelike peptide fibroblast growth factor (FGF19; in rodents Fgf15), which reaches the liver via portal blood and binds to its specific receptor fibroblast growth factor receptor 4, resulting in activation of intracellular JNK pathway to inhibit CYP7A1 gene expression.[30–32] As a target of FXR, FGF19 (Fgf15) represents a hormone that signals after food intake via the gut liver axis, suppressing the BA synthesis, inducing gallbladder relaxation and refilling,[33] mediating (insulin-independent) insulin-mimetic effects such as stimulation of glycogen and protein synthesis and inhibition of gluconeogenesis,[34] while unlike insulin, suppressing the lipogenesis.[35] As such, FGF19 as an FXR target gene also represents an interesting target of anti-diabetic therapy.[36]

The role of FGF19 in cholestasis is yet to be elucidated. Although FGF19 is not expressed in hepatocytes and systemic FGF19 under physiologic conditions originate from the intestine, its hepatocellular expression is highly induced in cholestasis.[37] Furthermore, FGF19 is highly expressed by human gallbladder epithelium and is secreted to the bile especially after treatment with FXR ligands.[38] Because BAs may induce mucin production via FXR in gastric epithelial cells,[39] it is attractive to speculate that BA-FXR-FGF19 signaling cascade may protect biliary epithelia against detergent BAs via mucin secretion.

Apart from repression of BA synthesis, FXR is able to induce alternative basolateral BA transport through organic solute transporter α/β (OSTα/β)[40,41] and detoxification through transcriptional induction of hydroxylation enzyme CYP3A1, sulfoconjugation by sulfatation enzymes 2A1 (SULT2A1), and glucuronidation by glucuronidation enzyme (UGT2B4) as additional potent mechanisms protecting hepatocytes from BA toxicity (reviewed in[3,42]) (see **Fig. 1**).

Biliary BAs are normally present in the form of mixed micelles together with phospholipids and cholesterol. Importantly, hepatic FXR promotes bile secretion not only through regulation of BA export but also via induction of canalicular phopholipid floppase MDR3 (Mdr2 in rodents)[43] and human canalicular bilirubin conjugate export pump multidrug resistance protein 2 (MRP2; via a hormone response element ER-8) (see **Fig. 1**).[44] The regulatory role of FXR in secretion of biliary phospholipids (and perhaps even glutathione) may be critical for the protection of hepatocytes' canalicular membrane as well as the apical membrane of bile duct lining cells against the detergent proportion of excreted BAs.

In addition to BAs as principal endogenous FXR ligands, an intermediate product of BA synthesis oxysterol 22(R)-hydroxycholesterol and androsterone has been identified as endogenous FXR activators.[45,46] Furthermore, several other natural substances have been recognized to exert agonistic or antagonistic effects on FXR. For example, stigmasterol, a compound present in soy-derived lipid emulsions used for total parenteral nutrition, showed FXR antagonistic activity, probably contributing to the total parenteral nutrition–induced cholestasis by inhibiting its target genes BSEP, FGF19, and OSTα/β.[47]

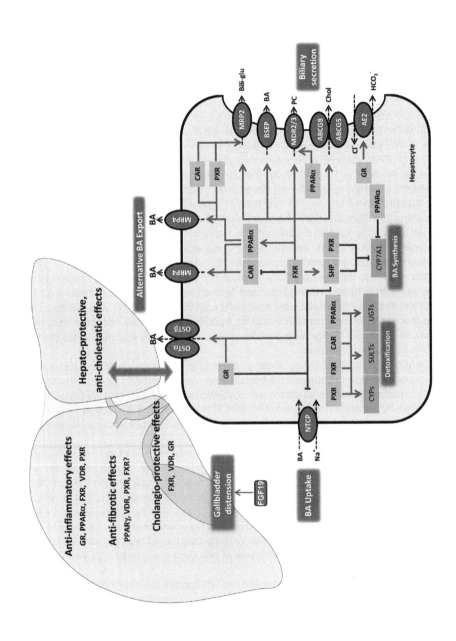

FXR IN CHOLESTATIC LIVER DISEASES

Because FXR is a central regulator of bile formation and BA homeostasis, one might expect that dysregulation or dysfunction of FXR may play a key role in the pathogenesis of cholestasis. However, FXR variants have been identified in only a few cholestatic syndromes[48–50] and FXR may rather orchestrate secondary adaptive responses to cholestasis. Among progressive familiar intrahepatic cholestasis (PFIC) syndromes, only PFIC1 patients showed reduced hepatic and ileal FXR levels.[49,50] Acquired cholestatic conditions, such as drug-induced liver injury and intrahepatic cholestasis of pregnancy (ICP), have also been associated with FXR dysfunction. In drug-induced liver injury and ICP, drug-mediated and hormone (metabolite)-mediated inhibition of hepatobiliary transporters may contribute to the pathogenesis.[51] A common FXR genetic variant FXR1*B was associated with reduced gene expression of hepatic target genes SHP and organic anion transporting polypeptide 1B3 (OATP1B3),[52] a sinusoidal transporter that mediates the uptake of several drugs and peptides such as cholecystokinin and digoxin.[53,54] These findings indicate that FXR dysfunction may largely influence the pharmacokinetics and pharmacodynamics of various drugs, thus significantly contributing to drug response as well as severity of potential side effects and therapeutic outcomes in affected patients.

FXR may play a role in gallstone disease because FXR knockout mice show biliary cholesterol supersaturation, formation of cholesterol crystals, and increased bile salt hydrophobicity, whereas synthetic FXR agonist GW4064 efficiently reduced gallstone formation in mice.[55] In contrast to these findings, no common polymorphism has been

---

Fig. 1. Role of nuclear receptors in maintaining hepatobiliary homeostasis. Activation of nuclear receptors (NRs) in hepatocytes ensures the balance between BA synthesis and detoxification, uptake, and excretion via regulation of expression of key hepatobiliary transporters. A network of negative feed-back and positive feed-forward mechanisms controls the intracellular load of biliary constituents, which may be hepatotoxic when they accumulate. BA-activated FXR is a central player in this network and represses (via GR in humans) hepatic BA uptake (NTCP) and (via SHP) BA synthesis (CYP7A1), promotes bile secretion via induction of canalicular transporters (BSEP, MRP2, ABCG5/8, MDR3), and induces BA elimination via alternative export systems at the hepatocellular basolateral (sinusoidal) membrane (OSTα/β). Several NR pathways converge at the level of CYP7A1 as a rate-limiting enzyme in BA synthesis. CAR and PXR facilitate adaptation to increased intracellular BA concentrations by upregulation of alternative hepatic export routes (MRP3 and MRP4) and induction of detoxification enzymes. PPARα regulates phospholipid secretion (via MDR3), but is also involved in detoxification pathways. Stimulation of AE2 expression by GR stimulates biliary bicarbonate secretion, thus reducing bile toxicity. Apart from regulating BA homeostasis, NRs have additional anti-inflammatory and anti-fibrotic effects. Their activation may result in induction of defensive mechanisms in bile duct epithelial cells. Green arrows indicate stimulatory effects and red lines indicate suppressive effects on target genes. AE, anion exchanger; BAs, bile acids; Bili-glu, bilirubin glucuronide; BSEP, bile salt export pump; CAR, constitutive androstane receptor; CYP7A1, cholesterol-7α hydroxylase; CYPs, cytochrome P450 enzymes; FGF, fibroblast growth factor; FXR, farnesoid X receptor; GR, glucocorticoid receptor; MDR3, multidrug resistance protein 3, phospholipid flippase; MRP2, multidrug resistance-associated protein 2; MRP3, multidrug resistance-associated protein 3; MRP4, multidrug resistance-associated protein 4; NTCP, sodium taurocholate cotransporting polypeptide; OSTα/β, organic solute transporter α and β; PC, phosphatidylcholine; PXR, pregnane X receptor; PPARα, peroxisome proliferator-activated receptor α; PPARγ, peroxisome proliferator-activated receptor γ; SHP, small heterodimer partner; SULTs, sulfatation enzymes; UGTs, glucuronidation enzymes; VDR, vitamin D receptor.

identified in patients with gallstone disease from different ethnic groups. However, an FXR variant was associated with gallstone prevalence in Mexican patients.[56] Interestingly, patients with gallstones showed repressed expression of PGC1α,[57] a transcriptional coactivator of FXR[58,59] that may additionally induce FXR gene transcription via PPARγ and HNF4α.[59] Thus, it is plausible to speculate that peroxisome proliferator-activated receptor gamma, coactivator 1 alpha (PGC1α)-associated reduction of FXR activity could contribute to altered bile composition and gallstone formation through inhibition of BSEP and MDR3. However, larger cohorts and more standardized sample analysis are required to draw conclusive statements regarding the role of FXR in human gallstone disease.

In chronic cholestatic liver diseases (eg, primary biliary cirrhosis [PBC] and primary sclerosing cholangitis [PSC]) prolonged duration of cholestasis may induce adaptive, secondary changes in transporter expression self-protective mechanisms of hepatocytes against retaining cholephils. For example, in PBC patients, repression of BA uptake systems (NTCP, OATP2) together with induction of basolateral efflux systems (MRP3, MRP4, and OSTα/β) support the elimination of retained BAs from the liver as cholestasis progresses with advanced disease.[41,60–65] Experimental studies in rodents have uncovered a complex interplay of several regulatory pathways under control of FXR and other NRs that are activated by accumulating biliary constituents mediating these transporter changes.[42] However, these intrinsic defense mechanisms are not sufficient to rescue the liver from cholestatic injury, because chronic cholestasis induces fibrosis and ultimately cirrhosis occurs, and additional pharmacologic activation may represent a mechanism of counteracting cholestasis by enhancing these intrinsic adaptive mechanisms as delineated below.[66]

An increasing body of evidence suggests that BA and FXR signaling regulates liver cell growth. Mice lacking FXR as well as mice lacking its downstream target SHP develop hepatocellular cancer (HCC).[67–69] Downregulation of SHP has also been observed in human HCC.[70] Notably, an increased risk for HCC has been observed in children with PFIC resulting from deficiency of the FXR target BSEP,[71] further underlining the carcinogenic potential of BAs in liver. A weakened defense against potential carcinogenic BAs, subsequent hepatic inflammation, together with the absence of direct regulatory effects on the cell cycle, may explain the carcinogenic potential resulting from loss of FXR and SHP.[69,72,73] A direct role of FXR on cell proliferation and apoptosis is underlined by the fact that not only does FXR play a crucial role in hepatocellular cancer, but also its alterations have also been implicated in colorectal and breast carcinogenesis.[74,75]

THERAPEUTIC POTENTIAL OF FXR IN CHOLESTASIS

In the last several years, various BA-derived or non-BA-based FXR activators have been developed as potential therapeutics against cholestasis. The protective effects of FXR were demonstrated in several animal models. A non-BA synthetic FXR agonist GW4064 and BA-derived 6α-ethyl derivative of chenodeoxycholic acid (6E-CDCA or INT-747 or obeticholic acid; OCA) have beneficial effects in mouse models of chemically induced liver injury (α-naphthylisothiocyanate (ANIT) and estradiol-induced) or in bile duct-ligation (BDL).[76,77]

Recently 3 BA-based therapeutic compounds were compared in Mdr2 (mouse ortholog of human phospholipid export pump MDR3) knockout mice, a model of bile duct injury and biliary fibrosis associated with the toxic bile composition caused by absent biliary phospholipids[78]: a selective FXR ligand (INT 747), a selective ligand (INT-777) for TGR5 (another G protein coupled BA receptor located at the plasma membrane), and dual ligand for FXR and TGR5, with strong FXR agonistic properties (INT-767). Only INT-767 with dual agonistic in vitro activity toward FXR and TGR5 improved serum liver tests, portal inflammation, and biliary fibrosis. This compound induced bile flow and biliary bicarbonate output with simultaneous reduction of biliary BA output in wild-type but not in FXR-deficient mice, emphasizing the role of FXR (but not TGR5) in mediating these effects. The underlying mechanisms seem to include FXR-dependent induction of carbonic anhydrase 14, a hepatocellular membrane-bound enzyme that may promote bicarbonate transport due to formation of a functional complex with bicarbonate transporter anion exchanger 2 (AE2).[79] These results uncovered an important role of FXR in regulation of biliary bicarbonate secretion protecting against intrinsic BA toxicity. Notably, the (weaker) selective FXR agonist INT-747 deteriorated liver injury in the Mdr2 knockout mice and the selective TGR5 agonist had no therapeutic effect, showing a minor role of biliary TGR5 for bile duct injury in this mouse model.

In addition to hepatocytes, cholangiocytes also play an important role in bile formation. Importantly, FXR is also expressed in human biliary epithelium, where it may play a critical role in ductular bile generation by alkalinization and fluidization through secretory mechanisms known to be predominantly regulated by complex neuroendocrine as well as local mechanisms.[80] The potential role of FXR in secretory function of biliary epithelium became apparent when endogenous FXR agonist CDCA as well as non-BA FXR agonist GW4064 induced gene expression of vasoactive intestinal polypeptide receptor 1 (VPAC-1),[80] a receptor of vasoactive intestinal polypeptide in human gallbladder. Because vasoactive intestinal polypeptide acts as a very potent secretagogue[81] in cholangiocytes, FXR-mediated VPAC-1 induction indicates a potential role for FXR in regulating the BA-independent bile flow in biliary epithelium.

In addition, CDCA (a potent endogenous FXR ligand) is able to induce expression of cathelecidin, the major anti-microbial peptide known to counteract the LPS, in human cholangiocytes, suggesting that BAs/FXR might play an important role in sterility of the biliary tree and protection against bile duct inflammation.[82] In fact, the observation that FXR-deficient mice showed increased baseline hepatic inflammation and are more prone to LPS-induced liver injury[67,83] suggests a direct anti-inflammatory role of FXR, which has been be explained via direct interference with the nuclear factor kappa-B (NF-κB).[83] Notably, this effect is not only hepatocyte-specific but also was reported in vascular smooth muscle cells.[84] The anti-inflammatory effects of FXR are further supported by induction of suppressor of cytokine signaling 3 that inhibits STAT3 signaling.[85] Notably the anti-inflammatory effects of FXR are not liver-specific, but were also demonstrated in intestine, where INT-747 reduced intestinal inflammation and permeability in experimental models of colitis.[86] Because bacterial overgrowth and increased intestinal permeability may play an important role in the pathogenesis of ascending biliary inflammation and cholestasis, a tight control of intestinal bacterial flora is likely to be protective in cholestasis. Bacterial overgrowth was successfully reversed by the oral BA supplementation in a rat model of intestinal BA depletion,[87,88] findings that together with prevention of postoperative endotoxemia by preoperative administration of sodium deoxycholate in patients with obstructive cholestasis[89] provide evidence for a role of intestinal BAs/FXR in maintaining the normal bacterial flora and gut integrity. Indeed, bacterial overgrowth and intestinal injury were decreased in the BDL model of obstructive cholestasis by GW4064 in an FXR-dependent manner[90] and selective intestinal FXR-overexpression reduced liver injury by decreasing the BA pool size and hydrophobicity as well as improving the intestinal permeability in BDL and ANIT-induced liver injury.[91] Moreover, FGF19 treatment protected mice from CBDL-induced liver injury, whereas selective intestinal

FXR overexpression decreased liver injury in the genetic Mdr2 knockout mouse model of cholestasis, confirming the importance of intestinal FXR for liver disease.[91] Taken together, FXR ligands counteract hepatic inflammation at several levels: directly via interaction with inflammatory pathways in hepatocytes as well as in non-parenchymal hepatic cells and by reducing release of inflammatory mediators from the intestine via a decrease in intestinal permeability and bacterial translocation. The latter may be of particular interest for the treatment of obstructive cholestasis with collapse of gut integrity and cholestatic liver disease associated with inflammatory bowel disease such as PSC.

Although many cholestatic liver diseases progress to liver fibrosis and finally cirrhosis, the question of whether FXR affects the fibrogenesis still remains unclear. Interestingly, FXR was also shown to have direct anti-fibrotic effects in hepatic stellate cells (HSCs) via activation of SHP.[92,93] However, another study showed very low or no FXR and SHP expression in human HSCs and murine periductal myofibroblasts,[94] suggesting indirect anti-fibrotic effects.

Collectively, FXR activation by endogenous or synthetic agonists represents an efficient mechanism to counteract cholestasis by a synchronized network of hepatoprotective mechanisms: (1) reducing intrahepatic BA load via repression of BA synthesis and an increase in BA export (via BSEP on the canalicular and $OST\alpha/\beta$ on the basolateral membrane); (2) changing bile composition at the hepatocellular level (by increasing relative phospholipid and bicarbonate secretion), ultimately resulting in a less toxic bile protecting hepatocytes and cholangiocytes; (3) impacting on ductular bicarbonate secretion (via induction of VPAC-1); (4) mediating direct anti-inflammatory effects in hepatocytes (via inhibition of NF-κB and STAT3) and non-parenchymal liver cells; (5) impacting on the gut-liver axis (by induction of FGF19, a suppressor of BA synthesis and by reducing a bacterial overgrowth and intestinal permeability in obstructive cholestasis).

Because targeted FXR activation has been recognized as a promising therapeutic option for patients with cholestasis, FXR agonists have already entered the clinical trials. Specifically, combination therapy of ursodeoxycholic acid (UDCA) with the INT-747 in phase II clinical trials in PBC patients not responding to UDCA showed substantial reduction of biochemical parameters of liver damage and cholestasis, such as ALT and ALP, after short-term and long-term administration.[95,96] In line with the results obtained with combination therapy, INT-747 monotherapy in PBC patients also achieved a significant reduction of serum markers of liver damage and cholestasis after 12 weeks of treatment.[97] Dose-dependent itching was reported to be the most common adverse event in patients receiving higher doses of INT-747. Because pruritus represents a common symptom of PBC that may lead to severe disability in suffering patients, subsequent clinical trials have excluded patients suffering from pruritus because of the disease. The results of a multicenter, placebo-controlled, randomized phase III clinical trial, testing INT-747 in PBC patients who have not non-responded to standard UDCA, are eagerly awaited.

NUCLEAR XENOBIOTIC RECEPTORS PXR AND CAR AND THEIR BIOLOGY

The primary function of PXR and CAR is to regulate genes responsible for the detoxification and elimination of a broad spectrum of potentially toxic endogenous and exogenous compounds.[98–100] To achieve their detoxifying function and to protect from various xenobiotics, both PXR and CAR act as low-affinity, broad-specificity xenosensors, which are activated by a broad range of structurally unrelated compounds (eg, rifampicin, clotrimazole, synthetic steroids such as 5β-pregnane-3,

20-dione, pregnenolone 16α-carbonitrile (PCN), dexamethasone, anti-depressant St. John's wort).[100–103] Apart from xenobiotics, also potentially toxic endogenous compounds such as BAs[8,9] and bilirubin[104] can activate PXR and CAR. After their activation, PXR and CAR coordinately induce a machinery of genes responsible for detoxification and elimination of their activating toxic ligands.

Various enzymes involved in phase I (catalyzing hydroxylation) and phase II (catalyzing glucuronidation and sulfatation) detoxification as well as many drug transporters are target genes of PXR and CAR, converting their substrates into more hydrophilic and therefore less toxic and easier cleared compounds (see **Fig. 1**).[98,100,105] In cholestatic condition, the activation of PXR and CAR may be beneficial because PXR, as a BA-activated receptor, is also responsible for basal repression of CYP7A1 as a rate-limiting enzyme for BA synthesis,[8] and both PXR and CAR are inducers of BA detoxification enzymes such as CYP3A4 (Cyp3a11 in mice), Cyp2b10, and SULT2A1 (see **Fig. 1**).[106] Furthermore, they activate the transcription of UGT1A1, a key enzyme for bilirubin glucuronidation (see **Fig. 1**).[9] Finally, PXR has been identified as an FXR target gene,[107] suggesting an evolutionary-based cross-talk between BA-activated NRs in the protection against BA toxicity.

PXR AND CAR IN CHOLESTATIC LIVER DISEASES

Altered function of PXR and CAR is involved in both pathogenesis and adaptation to cholestatic liver disease. Genetic variants of PXR are associated with increased susceptibility for ICP, as well as with lower neonatal weight and Apgar score in South American populations.[108] In contrast, PXR variants were not found to be associated with ICP in a Caucasian population, but it should be emphasized that this study considered only coding sequence and no regulatory promoter regions were examined.[109] Furthermore, PXR polymorphisms have been associated with the disease course in PSC.[110]

In patients with obstructive cholestasis, a pronounced increase in PXR and CAR expression is observed, followed by an increase in their target genes (MRP3 and MRP4),[111,112] consistent with activation of self-protective pathways in cholestatic hepatocytes (see **Fig. 1**). The role of PXR and CAR for limiting the progression of liver injury in cholestasis was confirmed by reduced expression of these NRs in late-stage cholestasis in children suffering from biliary atresia,[113] and low PXR and CAR expression were associated with poor prognosis in these patients. In PBC, a moderate reduction of PXR and CAR expression levels was observed.[66] The involvement of PXR and CAR in fibrogenic processes was further underlined by their low expression in hepatitis C patients with advanced fibrosis.[114] Of note, neonates have low hepatic expression of CAR, as the main NR coordinately regulating bilirubin clearance, thus providing a possible explanation for their higher susceptibility to (neonatal) jaundice.[104]

PXR AND CAR AS THERAPEUTIC TARGETS

Because of their central role in BA detoxification and transport, PXR and CAR represent attractive targets for drug therapy of cholestasis. Ligands for both receptors have already been used to treat cholestasis and pruritus, long before their mode of action has been fully understood. As such, rifampicin is a classic ligand for PXR and not only is effectively used to treat pruritus but also improves liver function tests in PBC, compatible with a direct anti-cholestatic effect.[115–117] In the otherwise healthy gallstone patients, rifampicin enhanced BA detoxification as well as bilirubin conjugation and excretion through induction of CYP3A4, UGT1A1, and MRP2, thereby decreasing bilirubin and deoxycholic acid concentrations in serum as well as lithocholic (LCA) and deoxycholic acid concentrations in bile.[118] The potential mechanisms by which rifampicin improves cholestatic pruritus have recently been further expanded by linking its action to the lysophospholipase autotaxin and its product, lysophosphatidic acid, as potential mediators of cholestatic pruritus.[119] Notably PXR inhibits autotaxin expression, which may add to the anti-pruritic action of rifampicin.[120]

Phenobarbital was also given to patients long before the identification of CAR as its molecular target.[115,121,122] Notably, 6,7-dimethylesculetin, a compound present in Yin Chin used in Asia to prevent and treat neonatal jaundice, accelerates bilirubin clearance by activation of CAR.[123] Activation of CAR increases hepatic expression of the bilirubin-clearance pathway, including the induction of bilirubin glucuronyl transferase, a key enzyme of bilirubin glucuronidation and canalicular bilirubin-glucuronide export pump MRP2.[104,123] In addition to CAR as prototypic bilirubin-activated receptor, PXR also promotes bilirubin detoxification and clearance via induction of its glucuronidation and export.[44,124]

In a rodent model, pharmacologic stimulation of PXR counteracted LCA-induced liver toxicity by induction of Cyp3a11 (CYP3A4 in human) and SULT2A1, both involved in BA detoxification.[8,9] Similarly, administration of PXR ligands reduced liver injury, bilirubin, and BA levels in CA-fed mice via induction of Cyp3a11 and MRP3.[125] LCA-induced hepatotoxicity was also diminished by pharmacologic activation of CAR, mediating a shift in BA biosynthesis toward the formation of less toxic BAs, as well as a decrease in hepatic bile acid concentrations.[126] In obstructive cholestasis (BDL) in mice, administration of PXR and CAR ligands reduced serum parameters of cholestasis (ie, bilirubin and serum BA levels) by induction of phases I and II detoxification and transport systems.[127] However, elevated liver enzymes in these animals point out potential hepatotoxic side effects of the used substances and concentrations, at least under conditions when bile flow is completely blocked.[127] However, pharmacologic stimulation of PXR and CAR could be therapeutically superior to activation of FXR in obstructive cholestasis, because stimulation of these xenobiotic sensors lacks potentially negative effects associated with stimulation of bile flow. This precaution is also underlined by the fact that FXR stimulation may lower the induction of MRP4 by CAR ligands, thereby limiting the main alternative BA export route from cholestatic hepatocytes.[128]

Apart from its anti-cholestatic effects, PXR also has anti-fibrotic and anti-inflammatory properties that may be beneficial in complex cholestatic liver diseases such as PSC and PBC. PXR stimulation in human HSC inhibits their transdifferentiation to fibrogenic myofibroblasts, inhibits expression of the major profibrogenic cytokine TGF-1β, and markedly slows proliferation.[129] In mice, PCN, a potent activator of rodent PXR, inhibited carbon tetrachloride–induced fibrosis in a PXR-dependent manner.[130] In addition, activation of PXR inhibited endotoxin-induced NF-κB activation and cytokine production, and mice lacking PXR have higher susceptibility to inflammatory agents.[131,132] Suppression of humoral and cellular immune response by rifampicin has been recognized 40 years ago[133] and may now at least in part be explained by ligand-induced SUMOylation of PXR subsequently repressing NF-κB target genes.[134]

Finally, PXR is essential for liver regeneration because mice lacking PXR have impaired hepatocyte proliferation.[135] Activation of CAR also induces a strong proliferative response in mouse liver by stimulating cyclin D1,[136] which is mandatory for cell-cycle progression in proliferating hepatocytes, suggesting that CAR agonists could also be potentially useful to stimulate hepatocyte proliferation after liver resection. However, CAR activation also plays a key role for liver tumor promotion in phenobarbital-treated mice.[137,138]

Collectively, pharmacologic stimulation of PXR and CAR in chronic cholestatic liver disease may improve the disease course via at least 4 potential beneficial mechanisms: (1) repression of BA synthesis and increase in BA and bilirubin detoxification and elimination pathways, which will enhance the ability of the liver to reduce levels of toxic cholephils; (2) suppression of inflammation and fibrosis; (3) promotion of hepatocellular regeneration; and (4) amelioration of pruritus. However, it must be emphasized that both PXR and CAR ligands are potentially hepatotoxic and carcinogenic; therefore, novel compounds targeting PXR and CAR with fewer side effects need to be developed.

VDR AND ITS BIOLOGY

The main function of VDR is to mediate the effects of its natural ligand calcitriol (1α, 25-dihydroxyvitamin D3 [1,25-VitD3]) on calcium homeostasis, but VDR also regulates cell proliferation and differentiation and has immunomodulatory as well as anti-microbial functions.[139] Importantly, VDR is also an intestinal sensor for secondary BAs and as such is activated by lithocholic acid.[10] In the liver, VDR is not expressed in hepatocytes, whereas other non-parenchymal liver cells such as Kupffer cells, endothelial cells, biliary epithelial cells, and HSCs show considerably high levels of expression.[140] In bile duct epithelial cells, activation of VDR by BAs or vitamin D induces cathelicidin expression, which is an anti-microbial peptide known to be protective against bacterial infection,[82] thus contributing to innate immunity in the biliary tract. In HSCs VDR is highly expressed in the quiescent state and its expression decreases during activation. Stimulation of VDR in activated HSCs inhibits their proliferation and suppresses collagen production, explaining the anti-fibrotic effects of vitamin D supplementation in the rat model for liver fibrosis.[141] In the intestine, stimulation of VDR increases the expression of human and rodent apical sodium/bile acid transporter (ASBT),[142] an ileal BA uptake transporter, and of MRP3, a basolateral BA export pump, in mouse colon.[143] In the liver, despite low expression of VDR in hepatocytes, treatment with VDR agonists stimulate BA detoxification enzymes (such as SULT2A1 and Cyp3a11, a mouse homolog of human CYP3A4).[10,144,145] Whether VDR may have beneficial effects on BA-induced hepatocellular injury is difficult to predict because of reported negative interactions of VDR with FXR and inhibition of FXR transactivation by 1,25-VitD3 in vitro.[146]

VDR AND CHOLESTATIC LIVER DISEASES

Multiple polymorphisms in the coding sequence and promoter region of VDR may alter the immune response and specific VDR variants are associated with several immune-mediated liver diseases. As such, VDR polymorphisms are associated with susceptibility and clinical appearance of PBC[147–151] and autoimmune hepatitis.[147,149]

Because impaired absorption of fat-soluble vitamins is a hallmark of cholestasis and severe liver dysfunction, low serum vitamin D levels are commonly observed in patients with cholestasis and may alter VDR activity with consequences beyond bone metabolism. Low 1,25-VitD3 levels impair fetal outcome (inversely correlating with meconium staining) in patients with ICP.[152] VDR expression in bile duct epithelial cells was inversely correlated with steatosis, lobular inflammation, and NAS score in patients with non-alcoholic fatty liver disease.[153] A growing body of evidence suggests that vitamin D signaling plays a role in the progression of fibrosis in various liver diseases, including fatty liver disease and hepatitis C,[141] and development of cancer,[154,155] including HCC,[156] but data for cholestatic liver diseases in this context are still limited. VDR expression in primary rat HSCs decreases on activation of these cells, whereas 1,25-VitD3 inhibits proliferation, decreases expression of profibrogenic, and increases expression of anti-fibrotic genes.[141]

Accumulation of LCA during cholestasis decreases the effects of vitamin D on human osteoblasts, acting as a competitive ligand for VDR[157] and thereby promoting osteoporosis in cholestatic patients. Interestingly, vitamin D supplementation was also associated with lower fatigue appearance in patients with PBC,[158] suggesting a potential link between vitamin D deficiency and this disabling symptom in cholestasis. Further studies will have to show whether this may be linked to muscular effects of vitamin D.

VDR AS THERAPEUTIC TARGET

According to the predominance of VDR in non-parenchymal liver cells, activation of VDR in the liver has mainly anti-inflammatory and anti-fibrotic effects that may be beneficial in chronic cholestatic liver disease (such as PBC and PSC). "Classical" targeting of VDR through vitamin D substitution improves bone density in patients where cholestasis leads to chronic vitamin D deficiency and increased rates of osteoporosis. The anti-fibrotic potential of VDR stimulation was confirmed by reduced fibrosis in a rat model of liver fibrosis.[141] Furthermore, treatment with 1,25-VitD3 suppressed the production of pro-inflammatory cytokines in the liver of BDL mice,[159] underlining the potential of VDR ligands to prevent cholestasis-induced inflammatory response. These anti-inflammatory and anti-fibrotic effects of vitamin D suggest that vitamin D supplementation could have additional therapeutic effects in patients with PBC and PSC beyond the rationale for preventing and treating hepatic osteodystrophy. However, the rather complex role of VDR in regulation of BA uptake in intestine and regulation of BA metabolism in liver as well as its negative effects on FXR must be considered also. Although the use of vitamin D or synthetic VDR agonist as disease-modifying agents represents an attractive therapeutic concept for cholestatic liver diseases, especially when vitamin D levels are already low because of cholestasis, data from controlled studies are lacking.

PPARS AND THEIR BIOLOGY

PPARα, PPARγ, and PPARδ are 3 structurally homologous receptors and are activated by endogenous fatty acids and their derivatives to control important metabolic pathways in lipid and energy homeostasis.[160–162] PPARα is highly expressed in tissues with active fatty acid catabolism, such as liver, heart, kidney, brown adipose tissue, muscle, small intestine, and large intestine; PPARγ is expressed mainly in adipose tissue and in the immune system and PPARδ is ubiquitously expressed.[163,164] PPARα controls energy expenditure and catabolic metabolism by inducing β-oxidation, whereas PPARγ is critical for adipocyte differentiation and energy storage by adipocytes mediating anabolic energy state.[165,166]

Besides its role in the regulation of fatty acid metabolism, PPARα is involved in BA homeostasis. Fibrates, which are PPARα activators, induce the expression of phase II enzymes SULT2A1, UGT2B4, and UGT1A3 as well as ASBT, BA uptake transporter, in cholangiocytes and enterocytes.[167–170] Furthermore, PPARα represses BA synthesis by reducing HNF4α binding to the CYP7A1 promoter (see **Fig. 1**).[171–174] PPAR ligands such as fibrates repress BA synthesis and promote phospholipid secretion into bile,[173,174] via induction of MDR3,[175] thus counteracting the aggressive biliary BA milieu (see **Fig. 1**).

In contrast to PPARα, a direct role for PPARγ in the regulation of BA metabolism has not yet been reported, probably because of a low expression pattern in hepatocytes.

Targeting PPARγ is of particular interest for inflammatory cholestasis because of its crucial role in attenuation of inflammation-mediated transporter and enzyme changes. In the LPS model of inflammatory cholestasis treatment with glitazones, as synthetic PPARγ ligands and accepted anti-diabetic drugs, attenuated repression of NTCP, BSEP, and Cyp3a11, without affecting cytokine levels via inhibition of RXRα, export from the nucleus.[176] In addition, PPARγ represses transcriptional activation of inflammatory response genes as a negative regulator of cellular toll-like receptor signaling in inflammatory cells as well as in cholangiocytes.[177] Moreover, in HSCs, PPARγ regulates their activation and has profound anti-fibrotic effects modulating the wound-healing process by amelioration of inflammation, oxidative stress, and matrix remolding in the injured liver.[178]

PPARS AND LIVER DISEASES

PPARγ is involved in inhibition of inflammation and production of pro-inflammatory cytokines. Because bile duct destruction in PBC is Th1 cytokine mediated, it may not be surprising that PPARγ expression, which is high in normal bile ducts, is reduced in damaged bile ducts and may be associated with the Th1-predominant milieu and favor the development of chronic cholangitis in PBC.[179] Immune modulation using PPARγ ligands may be of therapeutic benefit to attenuate biliary inflammation in PBC. In HSCs from BDL mice developing biliary cirrhosis, PPARγ expression and DNA binding was dramatically reduced, demonstrating that HSC activation is associated with the reductions in PPARγ expression.[180]

PPARS AS THERAPEUTIC TARGETS

The effects of PPARα on biliary phospholipid secretion, BA metabolism, and synthesis make PPARα an interesting therapeutic target in the treatment of cholestasis. One of the key rationales for a beneficial role of fibrates in cholangiopathies may be upregulation of MDR3[181] and its subcellular redistribution toward the canalicular membrane,[182] thereby increasing the biliary content of phosphatidylcholine and reducing the aggressive potential of BAs in bile, subsequently protecting the biliary tree. This concept is supported by findings in patients undergoing percutaneous transhepatic biliary drainage, who showed increased biliary phospholipid secretion after treatment with bezafibarte,[183] although the same study reported that patients with PBC had already increased MDR3 expression that was not further upregulated by bezafibrate treatment. Moreover, treatment with bezafibrate may have additional anti-cholestatic effects as supported by repression of BA synthesis (CYP7A1 and CYP27A1) and BA uptake (NTCP) and increased BA detoxification enzyme CYP3A4 in human hepatoma cell lines.[184] Repression of BA synthesis and increased detoxification of BA by fibrates were confirmed in early-stage PBC patients measuring reduction of 7α-hydroxy-4-cholesten-3-one (C4), a marker of BA synthesis, and an increase of 4β-hydroxycholesterol, a marker of CYP3A4/5 activity after bezafibrate and UDCA combination therapy in comparison to UDCA monotherapy.[191] Finally, the anti-inflammatory effects of PPARα could also add to potential beneficial effects in cholestasis.

Clinically the beneficial effects of PPAR ligands in cholestasis were recognized for more than a decade and multiple pilot studies have evaluated their therapeutic effectiveness in patients with PBC. More than a dozen uncontrolled pilot trials using bezafibrate and fenofibrate showed beneficial effects on biochemical parameters and in part also on histologic findings in patients with PBC.[184–200] Some of these studies have tested the fibrates as monotherapy in comparison to UDCA monotherapy, but most were designed to test their effects in patients with partial or absent UDCA response by add-on therapy with either fenofibrate or bezafibrate. All these pilot studies showed the benefit of combination therapy. However, no placebo-controlled randomized studies have been performed so far and such studies are urgently needed before implementing UDCA/fibrate combination therapy as standard for PBC patients with suboptimal response to UDCA. However, one should be aware that fibrates increase the risk for gallstone formation,[201] a side effect that could be linked to suppression of BA synthesis and that may represent a potential limitation for treatment in patients with biliary damage and an already increased susceptibility to gallstone formation such as PBC.

Moreover, PPARα ligands may also be beneficial in patients with chronic hepatic graft-versus-host disease of the liver. A combination of UDCA and bezafibrate therapy in this patient population significantly improved liver biochemistry after 1 month of treatment.[202] Long-term clinical trials are also needed.

Other hypolipidemic drugs, such as inhibitors of 3-hydroxy-3-methylglutaryl-coenzyme A reductase (statins), are indirect activators of PPAR, also have pleiotropic anti-inflammatory effects,[203] and stimulate phospholipid secretion by induction of Mdr2.[204,205] Statins have also been tested in the treatment of PBC. Although initial smaller studies suggested improvement of cholestasis under statin treatment,[206–208] a recent dose finding study was unable to demonstrate improvement of cholestasis in PBC patients with an incomplete response to UDCA.[209]

In addition to PPARα, PPARγ activation may also be effective in cholestatic diseases, in particular by ameliorating fibrosis and inflammation, thus limiting disease progression. The inhibitory effects of PPARγ ligands on collagen synthesis in HSCs[180] were also observed in a model of obstructive cholestasis (BDL) where treatment with troglitazone inhibited ductular reaction and fibrosis.[210] However, troglitazone, a PPARγ ligand, was meanwhile withdrawn from the market because of hepatotoxicity and no experimental or clinical data on other glitazones are available.[211,212] The plant extract curcumin, the yellow pigment of the spice turmeric, also targets PPARγ. Notably, natural compounds such as curcumin inhibited inflammatory activation of cholangiocytes and activation of portal myofibroblasts in a PPARγ-dependent manner, ameliorating biliary fibrosis in various animal models.[213,214]

GR AND ITS BIOLOGY

Glucocorticoids are natural ligands of GR. GR is expressed in most human cells and plays a role in numerous metabolic pathways including carbohydrate and protein homeostasis, mediates negative feedback on the hypothalamic–pituitary–adrenal axis, and has strong anti-inflammatory and immunosuppressive effects.[215] Apart from regulating systemic response to stress, GR and glucocorticoids also regulate BA homeostasis because GR regulates the expression of biliary transport systems including the human BA transporters NTCP, ASBT, and OSTα/β (see **Fig. 1**).[216–218] In addition, GR ligands may also modulate the function of other NRs including CAR, a primary GR response gene,[219] as well as PXR and RXRα.[219,220] On the other hand, GR activation promotes cholestasis in mice by repressing the beneficial transcriptional activity of FXR,[221] although such potentially negative effects have never been reported clinically in cholestatic patients. Nevertheless, serum BA levels are elevated in patients with increased serum glucocorticoid levels, such as Cushing disease or obesity, in comparison with healthy individuals, and correlate with elevated glucocorticoid levels. This induction of BA levels by GR ligands can also be explained by recruiting corepressor complexes to FXR and thereby blocking its transcriptional activity.[221]

GR AS THERAPEUTIC TARGET

Activation of GR by glucocorticoids is widely used to treat inflammatory and autoimmune diseases[222] and have also been tested for treatment of various cholestatic disorders including PBC.[223] Notably, in addition to their classic anti-inflammatory and immunomodulatory effects, GR ligands may also have anti-cholestatic effects through modulation of transporters. One of the most notable mechanisms of GR activation in chronic inflammatory bile duct disorders such as PBC may include stimulatory effects on AE2 expression, thus increasing cholangiocyte bicarbonate secretion[224,225] and stimulation/restoration of the biliary bicarbonate umbrella (see **Fig. 1**). This effect is especially interesting in the context of reduced AE2 expression and function in the liver and inflammatory cells of PBC patients,[226,227] which may be responsible for vulnerable cholangiocytes favoring an auto-immune hit on the bile ducts. Increased AE2 expression resulting in an increase of biliary bicarbonate secretion by UDCA and dexamethasone combination but not by UDCA or dexamethasone alone[225] could provide a potential explanation for the observed beneficial effects of the combination of glucocorticoids and UDCA. Of note, UDCA also activates GR[228,229] and promotes GR translocation in the nucleus in a ligand-independent manner,[230] favoring a combination therapy of glucocorticoids and UDCA in PBC patients from a mechanistic point of view.

Although (combination) therapy with steroids may be clinically beneficial, their use is limited by classic side effects including bone loss,[231] which outweigh the potential benefits. Moreover, it has been shown that patients receiving glucocorticoids have increased BA synthesis (see earlier discussion) and are prone to gallstone diseases.[232] Use of glucocorticoids is considered an independent risk factor for cholelithiasis.[233] Budesonide, a non-halogenated corticosteroid with a high GR-binding affinity and extensive hepatic first-pass metabolism-limiting (extrahepatic) side effects, may be an attractive alternative. Apart from GR-mediated effects, the induction of CYP3A4 via a PXR-dependent mechanism and thereby induction of BA detoxification, may also be an argument for the use of budesonide in inflammation-driven cholestatic diseases. Two randomized control trials have reported an additional benefit of budesonide and UDCA combination therapy on serum parameters of cholestasis and liver histology in PBC patients (stage I to III) in comparison to UDCA monotherapy.[234,235] However, in a study focusing on a subgroup of patients who did not respond to UDCA monotherapy (including patients with end-stage disease), significant increases in Mayo Risk Score were reported, despite beneficial effects on bilirubin and alkaline phosphatase levels with additional budesonide treatment.[236] The summary of reported data allows the conclusion that budesonide in combination with UDCA has favorable results on biochemical and histologic parameters in early-stage PBC, but not late-stage disease, where budesonide is contra-indicated (reports of severe side effects including portal vein thrombosis and death).[237]

URSODEOXYCHOLIC ACID — CURRENT ANTI-CHOLESTATIC DRUG STANDARD AND ITS EFFECTS ON NRS

UDCA is currently used as a therapeutic standard in cholestasis and has multiple beneficial mechanisms,[238] which may be mediated to at least in part by NRs. Although these various mechanisms of action of UDCA have been studied in detail in the last decades, the complete picture underlying the beneficial effects of UDCA remains to be determined. Notably, UDCA does not activate FXR[7,11,239] and has low affinity to GR,[228] but may activate PXR indirectly after its conversion to LCA by intestinal flora.[8,9] In addition, UDCA induced expression of protective cathelicidin via activation of VDR in cultured biliary epithelial cells and induced both VDR and cathelicidin gene expression in livers of PBC patients.[82] Furthermore, UDCA partially corrected calcium malabsorption in patients with PBC, who display low bone mass density and reduced fractional calcium malabsorption.[240] Of note, UDCA may indirectly even counteract FXR activation by decreasing the relative concentrations of endogenous BA as more efficient FXR ligands. These examples indicate that direct or potentially indirect interactions with several NRs or transcriptional factors may be responsible for beneficial effects of UDCA. Importantly, several UDCA derivatives have been synthesized to potentiate the UDCA actions. As such, a 24-norursodeoxycholic acid (norUDCA) showed beneficial effects in the Mdr2 knockout mouse model of biliary fibrosis.[241–243] Anti-cholestatic, anti-fibrotic, and anti-inflammatory effects of norUDCA were associated with induction of phase I and phase II detoxification enzymes with simultaneous induction of basolateral efflux systems, resulting in alternative renal BA excretion.[241,242] In addition, norUDCA induced induction of bicarbonate-rich bile flow. However, similar to its parent drug UDCA, no NR has been identified as a potential target for norUDCA and generation of bicarbonate-rich bile flow by norUDCA is thought to be mediated by the cholehepatic shunting of the compound.[242,244] Although no NRs have been identified so far as a target for norUDCA, a characteristic pattern of induction of CAR-regulated genes was observed in the gene expression array study, suggesting CAR involvement in the anti-cholestatic effect of this compound.[243] Furthermore, norUDCA has profound beneficial effects on lipoprotein composition, and hepatic lipid metabolism.[243,245] These properties make norUDCA a very attractive therapeutic candidate for cholestatic and metabolic liver diseases.

SUMMARY AND FUTURE PERSPECTIVES

NRs control several important hepatic functions involved in the pathophysiology of cholestatic liver disease such as BA homeostasis and enterohepatic circulation of BAs as well as hepatic inflammation and fibrosis. Novel concepts on NR (patho)physiology have successfully been integrated in the understanding of the development of cholestasis. At present, many drugs used as standard treatments for cholestasis act via NRs and stimulation of their target genes. A revolution of expanding use of NR targeting in the therapy for cholestatic diseases is being witnessed. The translation of expanding knowledge on NRs should result in optimizing the current standard therapy with careful selection of patients' subgroups benefiting from such novel NR-directed approaches.

REFERENCES

1. Erlinger S. What is cholestasis in 1985? J Hepatol 1985;1:687–93.
2. Trauner M, Meier PJ, Boyer JL. Molecular pathogenesis of cholestasis. N Engl J Med 1998;339:1217–27.
3. Wagner M, Zollner G, Trauner M. Nuclear receptors in liver disease. Hepatology 2011;53:1023–34.
4. Trauner M, Halilbasic E. Nuclear receptors as new perspective for the management of liver diseases. Gastroenterology 2011;140:1120–1125.e1–12.
5. McKenna NJ, Lanz RB, O'Malley BW. Nuclear receptor coregulators: cellular and molecular biology. Endocr Rev 1999;20:321–44.
6. Perissi V, Rosenfeld MG. Controlling nuclear receptors: the circular logic of cofactor cycles. Nat Rev Mol Cell Biol 2005;6:542–54.
7. Makishima M, Okamoto AY, Repa JJ, et al. Identification of a nuclear receptor for bile acids. Science 1999;284:1362–5.

8. Staudinger JL, Goodwin B, Jones SA, et al. The nuclear receptor PXR is a litho-cholic acid sensor that protects against liver toxicity. Proc Natl Acad Sci U S A 2001;98:3369–74.

9. Xie W, Radominska-Pandya A, Shi Y, et al. An essential role for nuclear receptors SXR/PXR in detoxification of cholestatic bile acids. Proc Natl Acad Sci U S A 2001;98:3375–80.

10. Makishima M, Lu TT, Xie W, et al. Vitamin D receptor as an intestinal bile acid sensor. Science 2002;296:1313–6.

11. Parks DJ, Blanchard SG, Bledsoe RK, et al. Bile acids: natural ligands for an orphan nuclear receptor. Science 1999;284:1365–8.

12. Wang H, Chen J, Hollister K, et al. Endogenous bile acids are ligands for the nuclear receptor FXR/BAR. Mol Cell 1999;3:543–53.

13. Forman BM, Goode E, Chen J, et al. Identification of a nuclear receptor that is activated by farnesol metabolites. Cell 1995;81:687–93.

14. Lu TT, Repa JJ, Mangelsdorf DJ. Orphan nuclear receptors as eLiXiRs and FiXeRs of sterol metabolism. J Biol Chem 2001;276:37735–8.

15. Zhang Y, Kast-Woelbern HR, Edwards PA. Natural structural variants of the nuclear receptor farnesoid X receptor affect transcriptional activation. J Biol Chem 2003;278:104–10.

16. Seol W, Choi HS, Moore DD. Isolation of proteins that interact specifically with the retinoid X receptor: two novel orphan receptors. Mol Endocrinol 1995;9:72–85.

17. Laffitte BA, Kast HR, Nguyen CM, et al. Identification of the DNA binding spec-ificity and potential target genes for the farnesoid X-activated receptor. J Biol Chem 2000;275:10638–47.

18. Huber RM, Murphy K, Miao B, et al. Generation of multiple farnesoid-X-receptor isoforms through the use of alternative promoters. Gene 2002;290:35–43.

19. Downes M, Verdecia MA, Roecker AJ, et al. A chemical, genetic, and structural analysis of the nuclear bile acid receptor FXR. Mol Cell 2003;11:1079–92.

20. Anisfeld AM, Kast-Woelbern HR, Meyer ME, et al. Syndecan-1 expression is regulated in an isoform specific manner by the farnesoid-X receptor. J Biol Chem 2003;26:26.

21. Denson LA, Sturm E, Echevarria W, et al. The orphan nuclear receptor, shp, mediates bile acid-induced inhibition of the rat bile acid transporter, ntcp. Gastroenterology 2001;121:140–7.

22. Ananthanarayanan M, Balasubramanian N, Makishima M, et al. Human bile salt export pump promotor is transactivated by the farnesoid X receptor/bile acid receptor. J Biol Chem 2001;276:28857–65.

23. Gerloff T, Geier A, Roots I, et al. Functional analysis of the rat bile salt export pump gene promoter. Eur J Biochem 2002;269:3495–503.

24. Plass JR, Mol O, Heegsma J, et al. Farnesoid X receptor and bile salts are involved in transcriptional regulation of the gene encoding the human bile salt export pump. Hepatology 2002;35:589–96.

25. Floranta JJ, Kullak-Ublick GA. Coordinate transcriptional regulation of bile acid homeostasis and drug metabolism. Arch Biochem Biophys 2005;433:397–412.

26. Gupta S, Pandak WM, Hylemon PB. LXR alpha is the dominant regulator of CYP7A1 transcription. Biochem Biophys Res Commun 2002;293:338–43.

27. Brendel C, Schoonjans K, Botrugno OA, et al. The small heterodimer partner interacts with the liver X receptor alpha and represses its transcriptional activity. Mol Endocrinol 2002;16:2065–76.

28. Kir S, Zhang Y, Gerard RD, et al. Nuclear receptors HNF4-alpha and LRH-1 cooperate in regulating Cyp7a1 in Vivo. J Biol Chem 2012;287(49):41334–41.

29. Abrahamsson A, Gustafsson U, Ellis E, et al. Feedback regulation of bile acid synthesis in human liver: importance of HNF-4alpha for regulation of CYP7A1. Biochem Biophys Res Commun 2005;330:395–9.

30. Holt JA, Luo G, Billin AN, et al. Definition of a novel growth factor-dependent signal cascade for the suppression of bile acid biosynthesis. Genes Dev 2003;17:1581–91.

31. Inagaki T, Choi M, Moschetta A, et al. Fibroblast growth factor 15 functions as an enterohepatic signal to regulate bile acid homeostasis. Cell Metab 2005;2:217–25.

32. Kim I, Ahn SH, Inagaki T, et al. Differential regulation of bile acid homeostasis by the farnesoid X receptor in liver and intestine. J Lipid Res 2007;48:2664–72.

33. Choi M, Moschetta A, Bookout AL, et al. Identification of a hormonal basis for gallbladder filling. Nat Med 2006;12:1253–5.

34. Kir S, Beddow SA, Samuel VT, et al. FGF19 as a postprandial, insulin-independent activator of hepatic protein and glycogen synthesis. Science 2011;331:1621–4.

35. Tomlinson E, Fu L, John L, et al. Transgenic mice expressing human fibroblast growth factor-19 display increased metabolic rate and decreased adiposity. Endocrinology 2002;143:1741–7.

36. Fu L, John LM, Adams SH, et al. Fibroblast growth factor 19 increases metabolic rate and reverses dietary and leptin-deficient diabetes. Endocrinology 2004;145:2594–603.

37. Schaap FG, van der Gaag NA, Gouma DJ, et al. High expression of the bile salt-homeostatic hormone fibroblast growth factor 19 in the liver of patients with extrahepatic cholestasis. Hepatology 2009;49:1228–35.

38. Zweers SJ, Booij KA, Komuta M, et al. The human gallbladder secretes fibroblast growth factor 19 into bile: towards defining the role of fibroblast growth factor 19 in the enterobiliary tract. Hepatology 2012;55:575–83.

39. Xu Y, Watanabe T, Tanigawa T, et al. Bile acids induce cdx2 expression through the farnesoid x receptor in gastric epithelial cells. J Clin Biochem Nutr 2010;46:81–6.

40. Dawson PA, Hubbert M, Haywood J, et al. The heteromeric organic solute transporter alpha-beta, Ostalpha-Ostbeta, is an ileal basolateral bile acid transporter. J Biol Chem 2005;280:6960–8.

41. Boyer JL, Trauner M, Mennone A, et al. Upregulation of a basolateral FXR-dependent bile acid efflux transporter OSTalpha-OSTbeta in cholestasis in humans and rodents. Am J Physiol Gastrointest Liver Physiol 2006;290:G1124–30.

42. Zollner G, Marschall HU, Wagner M, et al. Role of nuclear receptors in the adaptive response to bile acids and cholestasis: pathogenetic and therapeutic considerations. Mol Pharm 2006;3:231–51.

43. Huang L, Zhao A, Lew JL, et al. Farnesoid X-receptor activates transcription of the phospholipid pump MDR3. J Biol Chem 2003;278:51085–90.

44. Kast HR, Goodwin B, Tarr PT, et al. Regulation of multidrug resistance-associated protein 2 (ABCC2) by the nuclear receptors pregnane X receptor, farnesoid X-activated receptor, and constitutive androstane receptor. J Biol Chem 2002;277:2908–15.

45. Deng R, Yang D, Yang J, et al. Oxysterol 22(R)-hydroxycholesterol induces the expression of the bile salt export pump through nuclear receptor farsenoid X receptor but not liver X receptor. J Pharmacol Exp Ther 2006;317:317–25.

46. Wang S, Lai K, Moy FJ, et al. The nuclear hormone receptor farnesoid X receptor (FXR) is activated by androsterone. Endocrinology 2006;147:4025–33.

47. Carter BA, Prendergast DR, Taylor OA, et al. Stigmasterol, a soy lipid-derived phytosterol, is an antagonist of the bile acid nuclear receptor FXR. Pediatr Res 2007;62(3):301–6.
48. Van Mil SW, Milona A, Dixon PH, et al. Functional variants of the central bile acid sensor FXR identified in intrahepatic cholestasis of pregnancy. Gastroenterology 2007;133:507–16.
49. Alvarez L, Jara P, Sanchez-Sabate E, et al. Reduced hepatic expression of farnesoid X receptor in hereditary cholestasis associated to mutation in ATP8B1. Hum Mol Genet 2004;13:2451–60.
50. Chen F, Ananthanarayanan M, Emre S, et al. Progressive familial intrahepatic cholestasis, type 1, is associated with decreased farnesoid X receptor activity. Gastroenterology 2004;126:756–64.
51. Pauli-Magnus C, Meier PJ. Hepatobiliary transporters and drug-induced cholestasis. Hepatology 2006;44:778–87.
52. Marzolini C, Tirona RG, Gervasini G, et al. A common polymorphism in the bile acid receptor farnesoid x receptor is associated with decreased hepatic target gene expression. Mol Endocrinol 2007;21:1769–80.
53. Ismair MG, Stieger B, Cattori V, et al. Hepatic uptake of cholecystokinin octapeptide by organic anion-transporting polypeptides OATP4 and OATP8 of rat and human liver. Gastroenterology 2001;121:1185–90.
54. Kullak-Ublick GA, Ismair MG, Stieger B, et al. Organic anion-transporting polypeptide B (OATP-B) and its functional comparison with three other OATPs of human liver. Gastroenterology 2001;120:525–33.
55. Moschetta A, Bookout AL, Mangelsdorf DJ. Prevention of cholesterol gallstone disease by FXR agonists in a mouse model. Nat Med 2004;10:1352–8.
56. Kovacs P, Kress R, Rocha J, et al. Variation of the gene encoding the nuclear bile salt receptor FXR and gallstone susceptibility in mice and humans. J Hepatol 2008;48(1):116–24.
57. Bertolotti M, Gabbi C, Anzivino C, et al. Decreased hepatic expression of PPAR-gamma coactivator-1 in cholesterol cholelithiasis. Eur J Clin Invest 2006;36:170–5.
58. Kanaya E, Shiraki T, Jingami H. The nuclear bile acid receptor FXR is activated by PGC-1alpha in a ligand-dependent manner. Biochem J 2004;382:913–21.
59. Zhang Y, Castellani LW, Sinal CJ, et al. Peroxisome proliferator-activated receptor-gamma coactivator 1alpha (PGC-1alpha) regulates triglyceride metabolism by activation of the nuclear receptor FXR. Genes Dev 2004;18:157–69.
60. Zollner G, Fickert P, Silbert D, et al. Adaptive changes in hepatobiliary transporter expression in primary biliary cirrhosis. J Hepatol 2003;38:717–27.
61. Zollner G, Wagner M, Moustafa T, et al. Coordinated induction of bile acid detoxification and alternative elimination in mice: role of FXR-regulated organic solute transporter-alpha/beta in the adaptive response to bile acids. Am J Physiol Gastrointest Liver Physiol 2006;290:G923–32.
62. Donner MG, Keppler D. Up regulation of basolateral multidrug resistance protein 3 (Mrp3) in cholestatic rat liver. Hepatology 2001;34:351–9.
63. Shoda J, Kano M, Oda K, et al. The expression levels of plasma membrane transporters in the cholestatic liver of patients undergoing biliary drainage and their association with the impairment of biliary secretory function. Am J Gastroenterol 2001;96:3368–78.
64. Ogawa K, Suzuki H, Hirohashi T, et al. Characterization of inducible nature of MRP3 in rat liver. Am J Physiol Gastrointest Liver Physiol 2000;278:G438–46.

65. Keitel V, Burdelski M, Warskulat U, et al. Expression and localization of hepato-biliary transport proteins in progressive familial intrahepatic cholestasis. Hepatology 2005;41:1160–72.
66. Zollner G, Wagner M, Fickert P, et al. Expression of bile acid synthesis and detoxification enzymes and the alternative bile acid efflux pump MRP4 in patients with primary biliary cirrhosis. Liver Int 2007;27:920–9.
67. Kim I, Morimura K, Shah Y, et al. Spontaneous hepatocarcinogenesis in farne-soid X receptor-null mice. Carcinogenesis 2007;28:940–6.
68. Yang F, Huang X, Yi T, et al. Spontaneous development of liver tumors in the absence of the bile acid receptor farnesoid X receptor. Cancer Res 2007;67:863–7.
69. Zhang Y, Xu P, Park K, et al. Orphan receptor small heterodimer partner suppresses tumorigenesis by modulating cyclin D1 expression and cellular proliferation. Hepatology 2008;48:289–98.
70. He N, Park K, Zhang Y, et al. Epigenetic inhibition of nuclear receptor small het-erodimer partner is associated with and regulates hepatocellular carcinoma growth. Gastroenterology 2008;134:793–802.
71. Knisely AS, Strautnieks SS, Meier Y, et al. Hepatocellular carcinoma in ten chil-dren under five years of age with bile salt export pump deficiency. Hepatology 2006;44:478–86.
72. Zhang Y, Soto J, Park K, et al. Nuclear receptor SHP, a death receptor that targets mitochondria, induces apoptosis and inhibits tumor growth. Mol Cell Biol 2010;30:1341–56.
73. Chen WD, Wang YD, Zhang L, et al. Farnesoid X receptor alleviates age-related proliferation defects in regenerating mouse livers by activating forkhead box m1b transcription. Hepatology 2010;51:953–62.
74. De Gottardi A, Touri F, Maurer CA, et al. The bile acid nuclear receptor FXR and the bile acid binding protein IBABP are differently expressed in colon cancer. Dig Dis Sci 2004;49:982–9.
75. Journe F, Durbecq V, Chaboteaux C, et al. Association between farnesoid X receptor expression and cell proliferation in estrogen receptor-positive luminal-like breast cancer from postmenopausal patients. Breast Cancer Res Treat 2009;115:523–35.
76. Liu Y, Binz J, Numerick MJ, et al. Hepatoprotection by the farnesoid X receptor agonist GW4064 in rat models of intra- and extrahepatic cholestasis. J Clin Invest 2003;112:1678–87.
77. Fiorucci S, Clerici C, Antonelli E, et al. Protective effects of 6-ethyl chenodeox-ycholic acid, a farnesoid X receptor ligand, in estrogen-induced cholestasis. J Pharmacol Exp Ther 2005;313:604–12.
78. Baghdasaryan A, Claudel T, Gumhold J, et al. Dual FXR/TGR5 agonist INT-767 reduces liver injury in the Mdr2−/−(Abcb4−/−) mouse cholangiopathy model by promoting biliary HCO3− output. Hepatology 2011;54(4):1303–12.
79. McMurtrie HL, Cleary HJ, Alvarez BV, et al. The bicarbonate transport metabo-lon. J Enzyme Inhib Med Chem 2004;19:231–6.
80. Chignard N, Mergey M, Barbu V, et al. VPAC1 expression is regulated by FXR agonists in the human gallbladder epithelium. Hepatology 2005;42:549–57.
81. Cho WK, Boyer JL. Vasoactive intestinal polypeptide is a potent regulator of bile secretion from rat cholangiocytes. Gastroenterology 1999;117:420–8.
82. D'Aldebert E, Biyeyeme Bi Mve MJ, Mergey M, et al. Bile salts control the anti-microbial peptide cathelicidin through nuclear receptors in the human biliary epithelium. Gastroenterology 2009;136:1435–43.

83. Wang YD, Chen WD, Wang M, et al. Farnesoid X receptor antagonizes nuclear factor kappaB in hepatic inflammatory response. Hepatology 2008;48:1632–43.
84. Li YT, Swales KE, Thomas GJ, et al. Farnesoid X receptor ligands inhibit vascular smooth muscle cell inflammation and migration. Arterioscler Thromb Vasc Biol 2007;27:2606–11.
85. Xu Z, Huang G, Gong W, et al. FXR ligands protect against hepatocellular inflammation via SOCS3 induction. Cell Signal 2012;24:1658–64.
86. Gadaleta RM, van Erpecum KJ, Oldenburg B, et al. Farnesoid X receptor activation inhibits inflammation and preserves the intestinal barrier in inflammatory bowel disease. Gut 2011;60:463–72.
87. Ding JW, Andersson R, Soltesz V, et al. The role of bile and bile acids in bacterial translocation in obstructive jaundice in rats. Eur Surg Res 1993;25:11–9.
88. Lorenzo-Zuniga V, Bartoli R, Planas R, et al. Oral bile acids reduce bacterial overgrowth, bacterial translocation, and endotoxemia in cirrhotic rats. Hepatology 2003;37:551–7.
89. Cahill CJ. Prevention of postoperative renal failure in patients with obstructive jaundice–the role of bile salts. Br J Surg 1983;70:590–5.
90. Inagaki T, Moschetta A, Lee YK, et al. Regulation of antibacterial defense in the small intestine by the nuclear bile acid receptor. Proc Natl Acad Sci U S A 2006; 103:3920–5.
91. Modica S, Petruzzelli M, Bellafante E, et al. Selective activation of nuclear bile acid receptor FXR in the intestine protects mice against cholestasis. Gastroenterology 2012;142(2):355–365.e1-4.
92. Fiorucci S, Antonelli E, Rizzo G, et al. The nuclear receptor SHP mediates inhibition of hepatic stellate cells by FXR and protects against liver fibrosis. Gastroenterology 2004;127:1497–512.
93. Fiorucci S, Rizzo G, Antonelli E, et al. A FXR-SHP regulatory cascade modulates TIMP-1 and MMPs expression in HSCs and promotes resolution of liver fibrosis. J Pharmacol Exp Ther 2005;314(2):584–95.
94. Fickert P, Fuchsbichler A, Wagner M, et al. The role of the hepatocyte cytokeratin network in bile formation and resistance to bile acid challenge and cholestasis in mice. Hepatology 2009;50:893–9.
95. Mason A, Luketic V, Lindor K, et al. Farnesoid-X Receptor agonists: a new class of drugs for the treatment of PBC? An international study evaluating the addition of obeticholic acid (INT-747) to ursodeoxycholic acid. Hepatology 2010;52: 357A.
96. Hirschfield G, Mason A, Gordon S, et al. A long term safty extenion trial of the farnesoid X receptor (FXR) agonist obeticholic acid (OCA) and UDCA in pimary biliary cirrhosis (PBC). Hepatology 2011;54:429A.
97. Kowdley KV, Jones D, Luketic V, et al, The OCA PBC Study Group. An international study evaluating the farnesoid X receptor agonist obeticholic acid as monotherapy in PBC. J Hepatol 2012;54:S13.
98. Kliewer SA, Goodwin B, Willson TM. The nuclear pregnane X receptor: a key regulator of xenobiotic metabolism. Endocr Rev 2002;23:687–702.
99. Blumberg B, Sabbagh W Jr, Juguilon H, et al. SXR, a novel steroid and xenobiotic-sensing nuclear receptor. Genes Dev 1998;12:3195–205.
100. Kliewer SA, Moore JT, Wade L, et al. An orphan nuclear receptor activated by pregnanes defines a novel steroid signaling pathway. Cell 1998;92:73–82.
101. Lehmann JM, McKee DD, Watson MA, et al. The human orphan nuclear receptor PXR is activated by compounds that regulate CYP3A4 gene expression and cause drug interactions. J Clin Invest 1998;102:1016–23.

102. Moore LB, Parks DJ, Jones SA, et al. Orphan nuclear receptors constitutive androstane receptor and pregnane X receptor share xenobiotic and steroid ligands. J Biol Chem 2000;275:15122–7.
103. Wentworth JM, Agostini M, Love J, et al. St John's wort, a herbal antidepressant, activates the steroid X receptor. J Endocrinol 2000;166:R11–6.
104. Huang W, Zhang J, Chua SS, et al. Induction of bilirubin clearance by the constitutive androstane receptor (CAR). Proc Natl Acad Sci U S A 2003;100:4156–61.
105. Wada T, Gao J, Xie W. PXR and CAR in energy metabolism. Trends Endocrinol Metab 2009;20:273–9.
106. Xie W, Barwick JL, Simon CM, et al. Reciprocal activation of xenobiotic response genes by nuclear receptors SXR/PXR and CAR. Genes Dev 2000;14:3014–23.
107. Jung D, Mangelsdorf DJ, Meyer UA. Pregnane X receptor is a target of farnesoid X receptor. J Biol Chem 2006;281:19081–91.
108. Castano G, Burgueno A, Fernandez Gianotti T, et al. The influence of common gene variants of the xenobiotic receptor (PXR) in genetic susceptibility to intrahepatic cholestasis of pregnancy. Aliment Pharmacol Ther 2010;31:583–92.
109. Owen BM, Van Mil SW, Boudjelal M, et al. Sequencing and functional assessment of hPXR (NR1I2) variants in intrahepatic cholestasis of pregnancy. Xenobiotica 2008;38:1289–97.
110. Karlsen TH, Lie BA, Frey Froslie K, et al. Polymorphisms in the steroid and xenobiotic receptor gene influence survival in primary sclerosing cholangitis. Gastroenterology 2006;131:781–7.
111. Chai J, He Y, Cai SY, et al. Elevated hepatic multidrug resistance-associated protein 3/ATP-binding cassette subfamily C 3 expression in human obstructive cholestasis is mediated through tumor necrosis factor alpha and c-Jun NH2-terminal kinase/stress-activated protein kinase-signaling pathway. Hepatology 2012;55:1485–94.
112. Chai J, Luo D, Wu X, et al. Changes of organic anion transporter MRP4 and related nuclear receptors in human obstructive cholestasis. J Gastrointest Surg 2011;15:996–1004.
113. Chen HL, Liu YJ, Wu SH, et al. Expression of hepatocyte transporters and nuclear receptors in children with early and late-stage biliary atresia. Pediatr Res 2008;63:667–73.
114. Hanada K, Nakai K, Tanaka H, et al. Effect of nuclear receptor downregulation on hepatic expression of cytochrome P450 and transporters in chronic hepatitis C in association with fibrosis development. Drug Metab Pharmacokinet 2012;27:301–6.
115. Bachs L, Pares A, Elena M, et al. Comparison of rifampicin with phenobarbitone for treatment of pruritus in biliary cirrhosis. Lancet 1989;1:574–6.
116. Cancado EL, Leitao RM, Carrilho FJ, et al. Unexpected clinical remission of cholestasis after rifampicin therapy in patients with normal or slightly increased levels of gamma-glutamyl transpeptidase. Am J Gastroenterol 1998;93:1510–7.
117. Yerushalmi B, Sokol RJ, Narkewicz MR, et al. Use of rifampin for severe pruritus in children with chronic cholestasis. J Pediatr Gastroenterol Nutr 1999;29:442–7.
118. Marschall HU, Wagner M, Zollner G, et al. Complementary stimulation of hepatobiliary transport and detoxification systems by rifampicin and ursodeoxycholic acid in humans. Gastroenterology 2005;129:476–85.
119. Kremer AE, Martens JJ, Kulik W, et al. Lysophosphatidic acid is a potential mediator of cholestatic pruritus. Gastroenterology 2010;139:1008–18.

120. Kremer AE, van Dijk R, Leckie P, et al. Serum autotaxin is increased in pruritus of cholestasis, but not of other origin, and responds to therapeutic interventions. Hepatology 2012;56:1391–400.
121. Stiehl A, Thaler MM, Admirand WH. The effects of phenobarbital on bile salts and bilirubin in patients with intrahepatic and extrahepatic cholestasis. N Engl J Med 1972;286:858–61.
122. Bloomer JR, Boyer JL. Phenobarbital effects in cholestatic liver diseases. Ann Intern Med 1975;82:310–7.
123. Huang W, Zhang J, Moore DD. A traditional herbal medicine enhances bilirubin clearance by activating the nuclear receptor CAR. J Clin Invest 2004;113:137–43.
124. Chen C, Staudinger JL, Klaassen CD. Nuclear receptor, pregname X receptor, is required for induction of UDP-glucuronosyltranferases in mouse liver by pregnenolone-16 alpha-carbonitrile. Drug Metab Dispos 2003;31:908–15.
125. Teng S, Piquette-Miller M. Hepatoprotective role of PXR activation and MRP3 in cholic acid-induced cholestasis. Br J Pharmacol 2007;151:367–76.
126. Beilke LD, Aleksunes L, Holland R, et al. Car-mediated changes in bile acid composition contributes to hepatoprotection from lca-induced liver injury in mice. Drug Metab Dispos 2009;37(5):1035–45.
127. Wagner M, Halilbasic E, Marschall HU, et al. CAR and PXR agonists stimulate hepatic bile acid and bilirubin detoxification and elimination pathways in mice. Hepatology 2005;42:420–30.
128. Renga B, Migliorati M, Mencarelli A, et al. Farnesoid X receptor suppresses constitutive androstane receptor activity at the multidrug resistance protein-4 promoter. Biochim Biophys Acta 2011;1809:157–65.
129. Haughton EL, Tucker SJ, Marek CJ, et al. Pregnane X receptor activators inhibit human hepatic stellate cell transdifferentiation in vitro. Gastroenterology 2006; 131:194–209.
130. Marek CJ, Tucker SJ, Konstantinou DK, et al. Pregnenolone-16alpha-carbonitrile inhibits rodent liver fibrogenesis via PXR (pregnane X receptor)-dependent and PXR-independent mechanisms. Biochem J 2005;387:601–8.
131. Wallace K, Cowie DE, Konstantinou DK, et al. The PXR is a drug target for chronic inflammatory liver disease. J Steroid Biochem Mol Biol 2010;120:137–48.
132. Zhou C, Tabb MM, Nelson EL, et al. Mutual repression between steroid and xenobiotic receptor and NF-kappaB signaling pathways links xenobiotic metabolism and inflammation. J Clin Invest 2006;116:2280–9.
133. Paunescu E. In vivo and in vitro suppression of humoral and cellular immunological response by rifampicin. Nature 1970;228:1188–90.
134. Hu G, Xu C, Staudinger JL. Pregnane X receptor is SUMOylated to repress the inflammatory response. J Pharmacol Exp Ther 2010;335:342–50.
135. Dai G, He L, Bu P, et al. Pregnane X receptor is essential for normal progression of liver regeneration. Hepatology 2008;47:1277–87.
136. Columbano A, Ledda-Columbano GM, Pibiri M, et al. Gadd45beta is induced through a CAR dependent, TNF independent pathway in murine liver hyperplasia. Hepatology 2005;42:1118–26.
137. Huang W, Zhang J, Washington M, et al. Xenobiotic stress induces hepatomegaly and liver tumors via the nuclear receptor constitutive androstane receptor. Mol Endocrinol 2005;19:1646–53.
138. Yamamoto Y, Moore R, Goldsworthy TL, et al. The orphan nuclear receptor constitutive active/androstane receptor is essential for liver tumor promotion by phenobarbital in mice. Cancer Res 2004;64:7197–200.

139. Campbell MJ, Adorini L. The vitamin D receptor as a therapeutic target. Expert Opin Ther Targets 2006;10:735 48.
140. Gascon-Barre M, Demers C, Mirshahi A, et al. The normal liver harbors the vitamin D nuclear receptor in nonparenchymal and biliary epithelial cells. Hepatology 2003;37:1034–42.
141. Abramovitch S, Dahan-Bachar L, Sharvit E, et al. Vitamin D inhibits proliferation and profibrotic marker expression in hepatic stellate cells and decreases thioacetamide-induced liver fibrosis in rats. Gut 2011;60(12):1728–37.
142. Chen X, Chen F, Liu S, et al. Transactivation of rat apical sodium-dependent bile acid transporter and increased bile acid transport by 1alpha, 25-dihydroxyvitamin D3 via the vitamin D receptor. Mol Pharmacol 2006;69:1913–23.
143. McCarthy TC, Li X, Sinal CJ. Vitamin D receptor-dependent regulation of colon multidrug resistance-associated protein 3 gene expression by bile acids. J Biol Chem 2005;280:23232–42.
144. Echchgadda I, Song CS, Roy AK, et al. Dehydroepiandrosterone sulfotransferase is a target for transcriptional induction by the vitamin D receptor. Mol Pharmacol 2004;65:720–9.
145. Chatterjee B, Echchgadda I, Song CS. Vitamin D receptor regulation of the steroid/bile acid sulfotransferase SULT2A1. Methods Enzymol 2005;400: 165–91.
146. Honjo Y, Sasaki S, Kobayashi Y, et al. 1,25-dihydroxyvitamin D3 and its receptor inhibit the chenodeoxycholic acid-dependent transactivation by farnesoid X receptor. J Endocrinol 2006;188:635–43.
147. Vogel A, Strassburg CP, Manns MP. Genetic association of vitamin D receptor polymorphisms with primary biliary cirrhosis and autoimmune hepatitis. Hepatology 2002;35:126–31.
148. Tanaka A, Nezu S, Uegaki S, et al. Vitamin D receptor polymorphisms are associated with increased susceptibility to primary biliary cirrhosis in Japanese and Italian populations. J Hepatol 2009;50:1202–9.
149. Fan L, Tu X, Zhu Y, et al. Genetic association of vitamin D receptor polymorphisms with autoimmune hepatitis and primary biliary cirrhosis in the Chinese. J Gastroenterol Hepatol 2005;20:249–55.
150. Halmos B, Szalay F, Cserniczky T, et al. Association of primary biliary cirrhosis with vitamin D receptor BsmI genotype polymorphism in a Hungarian population. Dig Dis Sci 2000;45:1091–5.
151. Kempinska-Podhorecka A, Wunsch E, Jarowicz T, et al. Vitamin D receptor polymorphisms predispose to primary biliary cirrhosis and severity of the disease in polish population. Gastroenterol Res Pract 2012;2012:408723.
152. Wikstrom Shemer E, Marschall HU. Decreased 1,25-dihydroxy vitamin D levels in women with intrahepatic cholestasis of pregnancy. Acta Obstet Gynecol Scand 2010;89:1420–3.
153. Barchetta I, Carotti S, Labbadia G, et al. Liver VDR, CYP2R1 and CYP27A1 expression: relationship with liver histology and vitamin D3 levels in patients with NASH or HCV hepatitis. Hepatology 2012;56(6):2180–7.
154. Spina CS, Ton L, Yao M, et al. Selective vitamin D receptor modulators and their effects on colorectal tumor growth. J Steroid Biochem Mol Biol 2007;103: 757–62.
155. de Lyra EC, da Silva IA, Katayama ML, et al. 25(OH)D3 and 1,25(OH)2D3 serum concentration and breast tissue expression of 1alpha-hydroxylase, 24-hydroxylase and Vitamin D receptor in women with and without breast cancer. J Steroid Biochem Mol Biol 2006;100:184–92.

156. Li Q, Gao Y, Jia Z, et al. Dysregulated Kruppel-like factor 4 and vitamin D receptor signaling contribute to progression of hepatocellular carcinoma. Gastroenterology 2012;143:799–810.e1–2.

157. Ruiz-Gaspa S, Guanabens N, Enjuanes A, et al. Lithocholic acid downregulates vitamin D effects in human osteoblasts. Eur J Clin Invest 2010;40:25–34.

158. Al-Harthy N, Kumagi T, Coltescu C, et al. The specificity of fatigue in primary biliary cirrhosis: evaluation of a large clinic practice. Hepatology 2010;52: 562–70.

159. Ogura M, Nishida S, Ishizawa M, et al. Vitamin D3 modulates the expression of bile acid regulatory genes and represses inflammation in bile duct-ligated mice. J Pharmacol Exp Ther 2009;328:564–70.

160. Chawla A, Repa JJ, Evans RM, et al. Nuclear receptors and lipid physiology: opening the X-files. Science 2001;294:1866–70.

161. Krey G, Braissant O, L'Horset F, et al. Fatty acids, eicosanoids, and hypolipidemic agents identified as ligands of peroxisome proliferator-activated receptors by coactivator-dependent receptor ligand assay. Mol Endocrinol 1997;11: 779–91.

162. Kota BP, Huang TH, Roufogalis BD. An overview on biological mechanisms of PPARs. Pharmacol Res 2005;51:85–94.

163. Bookout AL, Jeong Y, Downes M, et al. Anatomical profiling of nuclear receptor expression reveals a hierarchical transcriptional network. Cell 2006;126: 789–99.

164. Braissant O, Foufelle F, Scotto C, et al. Differential expression of peroxisome proliferator-activated receptors (PPARs): tissue distribution of PPAR-alpha, -beta, and -gamma in the adult rat. Endocrinology 1996;137:354–66.

165. Kliewer SA, Xu HE, Lambert MH, et al. Peroxisome proliferator-activated receptors: from genes to physiology. Recent Prog Horm Res 2001;56:239–63.

166. Tontonoz P, Hu E, Spiegelman BM. Stimulation of adipogenesis in fibroblasts by PPAR gamma 2, a lipid-activated transcription factor. Cell 1994;79:1147–56.

167. Fang HL, Strom SC, Cai H, et al. Regulation of human hepatic hydroxysteroid sulfotransferase gene expression by the peroxisome proliferator-activated receptor alpha transcription factor. Mol Pharmacol 2005;67:1257–67.

168. Barbier O, Duran-Sandoval D, Pineda-Torra I, et al. Peroxisome proliferator-activated receptor alpha induces hepatic expression of the human bile acid glucuronidating UDP-glucuronosyltransferase 2B4 enzyme. J Biol Chem 2003; 278.32852–60.

169. Jung D, Fried M, Kullak-Ublick GA. Human apical sodium-dependent bile salt transporter gene (SLC10A2) is regulated by the peroxisome proliferator-activated receptor alpha. J Biol Chem 2002;277:30559–66.

170. Barbier O, Trottier J, Kaeding J, et al. Lipid-activated transcription factors control bile acid glucuronidation. Mol Cell Biochem 2009;326(1–2):3–8.

171. Marrapodi M, Chiang JY. Peroxisome proliferator-activated receptor alpha (PPARalpha) and agonist inhibit cholesterol 7alpha-hydroxylase gene (CYP7A1) transcription. J Lipid Res 2000;41:514–20.

172. Patel DD, Knight BL, Soutar AK, et al. The effect of peroxisome-proliferator-activated receptor-alpha on the activity of the cholesterol 7 alpha-hydroxylase gene. Biochem J 2000;351(Pt 3):747–53.

173. Post SM, Duez H, Gervois PP, et al. Fibrates suppress bile acid synthesis via peroxisome proliferator-activated receptor-alpha-mediated downregulation of cholesterol 7alpha-hydroxylase and sterol 27-hydroxylase expression. Arterioscler Thromb Vasc Biol 2001;21:1840–5.

174. Roglans N, Vazquez-Carrera M, Alegret M, et al. Fibrates modify the expression of key factors involved in bile-acid synthesis and biliary-lipid secretion in gallstone patients. Eur J Clin Pharmacol 2004;59:855–61.
175. Ghonem N, Ananthanarayanan M, Soroka CJ, et al. Fenofibrate, a specific peroxisome proliferator-activated receptor alpha (PPARα) agonist, up-regulates MDR3/ABCB4 expression in human hepatocytes. Hepatology 2012;56(S1):541A.
176. Ghose R, Mulder J, von Furstenberg RJ, et al. Rosiglitazone attenuates suppression of RXRalpha-dependent gene expression in inflamed liver. J Hepatol 2007; 46:115–23.
177. Harada K, Nakanuma Y. Biliary innate immunity: function and modulation. Mediators Inflamm 2010;2010.
178. Zhang F, Lu Y, Zheng S. Peroxisome proliferator-activated receptor-gamma cross-regulation of signaling events implicated in liver fibrogenesis. Cell Signal 2012;24:596–605.
179. Harada K, Isse K, Kamihira T, et al. Th1 cytokine-induced downregulation of PPARgamma in human biliary cells relates to cholangitis in primary biliary cirrhosis. Hepatology 2005;41:1329–38.
180. Miyahara T, Schrum L, Rippe R, et al. Peroxisome proliferator-activated receptors and hepatic stellate cell activation. J Biol Chem 2000;275:35715–22.
181. Matsumoto T, Miyazaki H, Nakahashi Y, et al. Multidrug resistance3 is in situ detected in the liver of patients with primary biliary cirrhosis, and induced in human hepatoma cells by bezafibrate. Hepatol Res 2004;30:125–36.
182. Shoda J, Inada Y, Tsuji A, et al. Bezafibrate stimulates canalicular localization of NBD-labeled PC in HepG2 cells by PPARalpha-mediated redistribution of ABCB4. J Lipid Res 2004;45:1813–25.
183. Nakamuta M, Fujino T, Yada R, et al. Therapeutic effect of bezafibrate against biliary damage: a study of phospholipid secretion via the PPARalpha-MDR3 pathway. Int J Clin Pharmacol Ther 2010;48:22–8.
184. Honda A, Ikegami T, Nakamuta M, et al. Anticholestatic effects of bezafibrate in patients with primary biliary cirrhosis treated with ursodeoxycholic acid. Hepatology 2012. [Epub ahead of print].
185. Ohmoto K, Mitsui Y, Yamamoto S. Effect of bezafibrate in primary biliary cirrhosis: a pilot study. Liver 2001;21:223–4.
186. Yano K, Kato H, Morita S, et al. Is bezafibrate histologically effective for primary biliary cirrhosis? Am J Gastroenterol 2002;97:1075–7.
187. Kanda T, Yokosuka O, Imazeki F, et al. Bezafibrate treatment: a new medical approach for PBC patients? J Gastroenterol 2003;38:573–8.
188. Kurihara T, Maeda A, Shigemoto M, et al. Investigation into the efficacy of bezafibrate against primary biliary cirrhosis, with histological references from cases receiving long term monotherapy. Am J Gastroenterol 2002;97:212–4.
189. Kurihara T, Niimi A, Maeda A, et al. Bezafibrate in the treatment of primary biliary cirrhosis: comparison with ursodeoxycholic acid. Am J Gastroenterol 2000;95: 2990–2.
190. Nakai S, Masaki T, Kurokohchi K, et al. Combination therapy of bezafibrate and ursodeoxycholic acid in primary biliary cirrhosis: a preliminary study. Am J Gastroenterol 2000;95:326–7.
191. Han XF, Wang QX, Liu Y, et al. Efficacy of fenofibrate in Chinese patients with primary biliary cirrhosis partially responding to ursodeoxycholic acid therapy. J Dig Dis 2012;13:219–24.
192. Liberopoulos EN, Florentin M, Elisaf MS, et al. Fenofibrate in primary biliary cirrhosis: a pilot study. Open Cardiovasc Med J 2010;4:120–6.

193. Levy C, Peter JA, Nelson DR, et al. Pilot study: fenofibrate for patients with primary biliary cirrhosis and an incomplete response to ursodeoxycholic acid. Aliment Pharmacol Ther 2011;33:235–42.

194. Dohmen K, Mizuta T, Nakamuta M, et al. Fenofibrate for patients with asymptomatic primary biliary cirrhosis. World J Gastroenterol 2004;10:894–8.

195. Itakura J, Izumi N, Nishimura Y, et al. Prospective randomized crossover trial of combination therapy with bezafibrate and UDCA for primary biliary cirrhosis. Hepatol Res 2004;29:216–22.

196. Miyaguchi S, Ebinuma H, Imaeda H, et al. A novel treatment for refractory primary biliary cirrhosis? Hepatogastroenterology 2000;47:1518–21.

197. Hazzan R, Tur-Kaspa R. Bezafibrate treatment of primary biliary cirrhosis following incomplete response to ursodeoxycholic acid. J Clin Gastroenterol 2010;44:371–3.

198. Iwasaki S, Akisawa N, Saibara T, et al. Fibrate for treatment of primary biliary cirrhosis. Hepatol Res 2007;37(Suppl 3):S515–7.

199. Takeuchi Y, Ikeda F, Fujioka S, et al. Additive improvement induced by bezafibrate in patients with primary biliary cirrhosis showing refractory response to ursodeoxycholic acid. J Gastroenterol Hepatol 2011;26:1395–401.

200. Akbar SM, Furukawa S, Nakanishi S, et al. Therapeutic efficacy of decreased nitrite production by bezafibrate in patients with primary biliary cirrhosis. J Gastroenterol 2005;40:157–63.

201. Caroli-Bosc FX, Le Gall P, Pugliese P, et al. Role of fibrates and HMG-CoA reductase inhibitors in gallstone formation: epidemiological study in an unselected population. Dig Dis Sci 2001;46:540–4.

202. Hidaka M, Iwasaki S, Matsui T, et al. Efficacy of bezafibrate for chronic GVHD of the liver after allogeneic hematopoietic stem cell transplantation. Bone Marrow Transplant 2010;45(5):912–8.

203. Landrier JF, Thomas C, Grober J, et al. Statin induction of liver fatty acid-binding protein (L-FABP) gene expression is peroxisome proliferator-activated receptor-alpha-dependent. J Biol Chem 2004;279:45512–8.

204. Carrella M, Feldman D, Cogoi S, et al. Enhancement of mdr2 gene transcription mediates the biliary transfer of phosphatidylcholine supplied by an increased biosynthesis in the pravastatin-treated rat. Hepatology 1999;29:1825–32.

205. Hooiveld GJ, Vos TA, Scheffer GL, et al. 3-Hydroxy-3-methylglutaryl-coenzyme A reductase inhibitors (statins) induce hepatic expression of the phospholipid translocase mdr2 in rats. Gastroenterology 1999;117:678–87.

206. Kurihara T, Akimoto M, Abe K, et al. Experimental use of pravastatin in patients with primary biliary cirrhosis associated with hypercholesterolemia. Clin Ther 1993;15:890–8.

207. Kamisako T, Adachi Y. Marked improvement in cholestasis and hypercholesterolemia with simvastatin in a patient with primary biliary cirrhosis. Am J Gastroenterol 1995;90:1187–8.

208. Ritzel U, Leonhardt U, Nather M, et al. Simvastatin in primary biliary cirrhosis: effects on serum lipids and distinct disease markers. J Hepatol 2002;36:454–8.

209. Stojakovic T, Putz-Bankuti C, Fauler G, et al. Atorvastatin in patients with primary biliary cirrhosis and incomplete biochemical response to ursodeoxycholic acid. Hepatology 2007;46:776–84.

210. Marra F, DeFranco R, Robino G, et al. Thiazolidinedione treatment inhibits bile duct proliferation and fibrosis in a rat model of chronic cholestasis. World J Gastroenterol 2005;11:4931–8.

211. Snow KL, Moseley RH. Effect of thiazolidinediones on bile acid transport in rat liver. Life Sci 2007;80:732–40.

212. Funk C, Ponelle C, Scheuermann G, et al. Cholestatic potential of troglitazone as a possible factor contributing to troglitazone-induced hepatotoxicity: in vivo and in vitro interaction at the canalicular bile salt export pump (Bsep) in the rat. Mol Pharmacol 2001;59:627–35.

213. Baghdasaryan A, Claudel T, Kosters A, et al. Curcumin improves sclerosing cholangitis in Mdr2−/− mice by inhibition of cholangiocyte inflammatory response and portal myofibroblast proliferation. Gut 2010;59:521–30.

214. Rivera-Espinoza Y, Muriel P. Pharmacological actions of curcumin in liver diseases or damage. Liver Int 2009;29:1457–66.

215. Rose AJ, Vegiopoulos A, Herzig S. Role of glucocorticoids and the glucocorticoid receptor in metabolism: insights from genetic manipulations. J Steroid Biochem Mol Biol 2010;122:10–20.

216. Jung D, Fantin AC, Scheurer U, et al. Human ileal bile acid transporter gene ASBT (SLC10A2) is transactivated by the glucocorticoid receptor. Gut 2004; 53:78–84.

217. Eloranta JJ, Jung D, Kullak-Ublick GA. The human Na+-taurocholate cotransporting polypeptide gene is activated by glucocorticoid receptor and peroxisome proliferator-activated receptor-gamma coactivator-1alpha, and suppressed by bile acids via a small heterodimer partner-dependent mechanism. Mol Endocrinol 2006;20:65–79.

218. Khan AA, Chow EC, Porte RJ, et al. Expression and regulation of the bile acid transporter, OSTalpha-OSTbeta in rat and human intestine and liver. Biopharm Drug Dispos 2009;30:241–58.

219. Pascussi JM, Gerbal-Chaloin S, Fabre JM, et al. Dexamethasone enhances constitutive androstane receptor expression in human hepatocytes: consequences on cytochrome P450 gene regulation. Mol Pharmacol 2000;58:1441–50.

220. Pascussi JM, Gerbal-Chaloin S, Drocourt L, et al. The expression of CYP2B6, CYP2C9 and CYP3A4 genes: a tangle of networks of nuclear and steroid receptors. Biochim Biophys Acta 2003;1619:243–53.

221. Lu Y, Zhang Z, Xiong X, et al. Glucocorticoids promote hepatic cholestasis in mice by inhibiting the transcriptional activity of the farnesoid x receptor. Gastroenterology 2012;143:1630–1640.e8.

222. Gossard AA, Lindor KD. Autoimmune hepatitis: a review. J Gastroenterol 2012; 47:498–503.

223. Poupon R. Treatment of primary biliary cirrhosis with ursodeoxycholic acid, budesonide and fibrates. Dig Dis 2011;29:85–8.

224. Alvaro D, Gigliozzi A, Marucci L, et al. Corticosteroids modulate the secretory processes of the rat intrahepatic biliary epithelium. Gastroenterology 2002; 122:1058–69.

225. Arenas F, Hervias I, Uriz M, et al. Combination of ursodeoxycholic acid and glucocorticoids upregulates the AE2 alternate promoter in human liver cells. J Clin Invest 2008;118:695–709.

226. Prieto J, Qian C, Garcia N, et al. Abnormal expression of anion exchanger genes in primary biliary cirrhosis. Gastroenterology 1993;105:572–8.

227. Medina JF. Role of the anion exchanger 2 in the pathogenesis and treatment of primary biliary cirrhosis. Dig Dis 2011;29:103–12.

228. Tanaka H, Makino I. Ursodeoxycholic acid-dependent activation of the glucocorticoid receptor. Biochem Biophys Res Commun 1992;188:942–8.

229. Miura T, Ouchida R, Yoshikawa N, et al. Functional modulation of the glucocorticoid receptor and suppression of NF-kappaB-dependent transcription by ursodeoxycholic acid. J Biol Chem 2001;276:47371–8.

230. Tanaka H, Makino Y, Miura T, et al. Ligand-independent activation of the glucocorticoid receptor by ursodeoxycholic acid. Repression of IFN-gamma-induced MHC class II gene expression via a glucocorticoid receptor-dependent pathway. J Immunol 1996;156:1601–8.

231. Mitchison HC, Bassendine MF, Malcolm AJ, et al. A pilot, double-blind, controlled 1-year trial of prednisolone treatment in primary biliary cirrhosis: hepatic improvement but greater bone loss. Hepatology 1989;10:420–9.

232. Yamanishi Y, Nosaka Y, Kawasaki H, et al. Sterol and bile acid metabolism after short-term prednisolone treatment in patients with chronic active hepatitis. Gastroenterol Jpn 1985;20:246–51.

233. Volzke H, Baumeister SE, Alte D, et al. Independent risk factors for gallstone formation in a region with high cholelithiasis prevalence. Digestion 2005;71: 97–105.

234. Leuschner M, Maier KP, Schlichting J, et al. Oral budesonide and ursodeoxycholic acid for treatment of primary biliary cirrhosis: results of a prospective double-blind trial. Gastroenterology 1999;117:918–25.

235. Rautiainen H, Karkkainen P, Karvonen AL, et al. Budesonide combined with UDCA to improve liver histology in primary biliary cirrhosis: a three-year randomized trial. Hepatology 2005;41:747–52.

236. Angulo P, Jorgensen RA, Keach JC, et al. Oral budesonide in the treatment of patients with primary biliary cirrhosis with a suboptimal response to ursodeoxycholic acid. Hepatology 2000;31:318–23.

237. Hempfling W, Grunhage F, Dilger K, et al. Pharmacokinetics and pharmacodynamic action of budesonide in early- and late-stage primary biliary cirrhosis. Hepatology 2003;38:196–202.

238. Poupon R. Ursodeoxycholic acid and bile-acid mimetics as therapeutic agents for cholestatic liver diseases: an overview of their mechanisms of action. Clin Res Hepatol Gastroenterol 2012;36(Suppl 1):S3–12.

239. Sato H, Macchiarulo A, Thomas C, et al. Novel potent and selective bile acid derivatives as TGR5 agonists: biological screening, structure-activity relationships, and molecular modeling studies. J Med Chem 2008;51(6):1831–41.

240. Verma A, Maxwell JD, Ang L, et al. Ursodeoxycholic acid enhances fractional calcium absorption in primary biliary cirrhosis. Osteoporos Int 2002;13:677–82.

241. Fickert P, Wagner M, Marschall HU, et al. 24-norUrsodeoxycholic acid is superior to ursodeoxycholic acid in the treatment of sclerosing cholangitis in Mdr2 (Abcb4) knockout mice. Gastroenterology 2006;130:465–81.

242. Halilbasic E, Fiorotto R, Fickert P, et al. Side chain structure determines unique physiologic and therapeutic properties of norursodeoxycholic acid in Mdr2–/– mice. Hepatology 2009;49:1972–81.

243. Moustafa T, Fickert P, Magnes C, et al. Alterations in lipid metabolism mediate inflammation, fibrosis, and proliferation in a mouse model of chronic cholestatic liver injury. Gastroenterology 2012;142:140–151.e12.

244. Yoon YB, Hagey LR, Hofmann AF, et al. Effect of side-chain shortening on the physiologic properties of bile acids: hepatic transport and effect on biliary secretion of 23-nor-ursodeoxycholate in rodents. Gastroenterology 1986;90:837–52.

245. Trauner M, Claudel T, Fickert P, et al. Bile acids as regulators of hepatic lipid and glucose metabolism. Dig Dis 2010;28:220–4.

Drug-Induced Cholestasis

Einar S. Bjornsson, MD, PhD[a],*, Jon Gunnlaugur Jonasson, MD[b]

KEYWORDS

- Drugs • Drug-induced liver Injury • Cholestasis • Liver disease • Pathology

KEY POINTS

- Cholestasis caused by drugs is an important liver disease in patients with a biochemical cholestatic pattern and normal hepatobiliary imaging.
- Cholestatic drug-induced liver injury (DILI) is more common than hepatocellular DILI among the elderly.
- Most cases of cholestatic DILI are mild but in rare cases, ductopenia and cholestatic cirrhosis can develop.
- Approximately 10% of patients with cholestatic jaundice caused by drugs develop liver failure.

INTRODUCTION

In general, drugs are involved in the differential diagnoses in a patient with cholestasis and normal hepatobiliary imaging. When a drug-induced liver injury (DILI) is suspected, cholestasis is defined as an increase in alkaline phosphatase (ALP) greater than 2 N and/or an ALT/ALP ratio less than 2.[1,2] Mixed liver injury is the intermediate between cholestatic and hepatocellular injury with an ALT/ALP ratio greater than 2 and less than 5. Mixed injury is considered to have more in common with cholestatic than hepatocellular injury and cholestatic and mixed patterns are sometimes taken together as 1 condition. Before a drug can be deemed responsible for cholestatic liver injury, a reasonable diagnostic work-up has to be undertaken. Cholestasis has traditionally been classified as acute or prolonged (**Box 1**). Pure or bland cholestasis is defined histologically to have features of cholestasis such as hepatocyte cholestasis and canalicular dilatation, often with bile plugs, without significant inflammation.[3] Cholestatic hepatitis is the most commonly observed cholestatic liver injury associated with drugs.[3,4] The consequences of cholestatic injury caused by drugs are mild in most cases and liver test abnormalities reverse with the cessation of the offending drug.[5] In the worst case scenario, this can lead to vanishing bile duct

[a] Division of Gastroenterology and Hepatology, The National University Hospital of Iceland, Hringbraut 101, Reykjavik, Iceland; [b] Department of Pathology, The National University Hospital of Iceland, Hringbraut 101, Reykjavik, Iceland
* Corresponding author.
E-mail address: einarsb@landspitali.is

Clin Liver Dis 17 (2013) 191–209
http://dx.doi.org/10.1016/j.cld.2012.11.002
1089-3261/13/$ – see front matter © 2013 Elsevier Inc. All rights reserved.

Box 1
Mechanisms of drug-induced cholestatic injury

1. Hepatocellular
   a. Pure cholestasis or canalicular cholestasis
   b. Cholestatic hepatitis or hepatocanalicular hepatitis
2. Ductular or ductal
   a. Acute
   b. Prolonged with ductopenia

---

syndrome, a condition that may or may not be reversible, and may lead to biliary fibrosis and cirrhosis with decompensated liver disease.[6]

APPROACH TO THE PATIENT WITH SUSPECTED DRUG-INDUCED CHOLESTATIC LIVER INJURY

The clinical presentation of cholestatic liver disease is variable. Asymptomatic increase in liver enzymes can be observed, particularly increased ALP, but jaundice with or without pruritus is a common presentation. Some patients present with fever and abdominal pain that can simulate gallstone disease. Because some patients can have stones in the gallbladder, this can lead to unnecessary cholecystectomies. Unfortunately, there is no marker of hepatotoxicity that is completely reliable and specific for DILI. Thus, there is often guilt by association and thorough exclusion of other potential causes must be done to make a diagnosis of DILI. In clinical research on DILI, the most common causality assessment method that has been used is the Roussel Uclaf Assessment model (RUCAM).[1,2] This model is based on the important factors that must be taken into consideration when assessing the history of a patient with suspected DILI. These factors are the time from initial drug intake until the start of the reaction, the course of the liver injury after termination of the suspected drug, risk factors for DILI, concomitant drugs, exclusion of other causes, documented hepatotoxicity of this particular drug, and, if available, the results of rechallenge. With regard to the evaluation of the dechallenge, that is, the course of liver enzymes after discontinuation of the drug, it is well known that the regression of cholestasis is slower than in those with hepatocellular injury and the RUCAM instrument takes that into account. The RUCAM method is far from perfect and its reliability has been put into question.[7] Expert opinion has been used in clinical research on DILI as well but this is obviously not standardized and suffers from lack of reproducibility and subjectivity.[8,9] Some drugs have a signature pattern, that is, they tend to give a similar type of liver injury and liver injury develops following a similar duration of drug intake.

Clinical information about the patient is also important to establish the diagnosis of a cholestatic reaction. Abdominal pain can occur as part of cholestatic hepatitis caused by drugs but abdominal discomfort is probably more prevalent; painless jaundice is also a frequent presentation of DILI. If abdominal pain predominates, a drug is unlikely to be the cause. In these cases, even though suspicion of a drug has been raised, it may be necessary to do a cholangiography with magnetic resonance cholangiopancreatography or endoscopic retrograde choledochopancreatography despite a normal abdominal ultrasonograph. In some cases, a stone can be observed in the intrahepatic biliary tract. In all types of alcoholic liver disease, cholestasis can be a prominent feature both biochemically and histologically, and alcohol abuse needs to be ruled out in the work-up of suspected cholestatic injury caused by drugs.

Pure cholestasis can occur in association with sepsis and cardiac failure, and clinical judgment is of great importance to distinguish these conditions from a suspected cholestatic DILI. Although infectious hepatitis presents most often with a hepatocellular pattern, a biochemical cholestatic pattern can occur in infectious hepatitis such as hepatitis A and Epstein-Barr virus[10] and in other infections such as typhoid fever[11] and acute Q fever caused by *Coxiella burnetii*.[12] Thus, in the appropriate setting, rare infectious disease have to be ruled out before the suspected drug can be established as the cause. Cases with jaundice and histologic cholestatic hepatitis caused by hyperthyroidism have been reported.[13] Thus, in some patients, the differential diagnosis can be complicated and the number of conditions with associated cholestatic features is beyond the scope of this article. The number of serologic tests and the extent of radiological imaging to exclude other competing causes rely entirely on the clinical context. The management of patients with cholestatic DILI consists mainly of discontinuing the suspected drug after careful consideration of the relationship between the drug and the reaction and exclusion of competing causes. In well-controlled studies, no therapy has been shown to be capable of changing the course of the liver injury. Patients with jaundice and impaired liver function should be considered for liver transplantation.

INCIDENCE OF CHOLESTATIC LIVER INJURY CAUSED BY DRUGS

Limited data exist on the incidence of DILI with cholestatic reactions included in the general population. A landmark population-based study on the incidence of DILI in society was undertaken in France in a defined population and revealed an incidence of 13.9 cases per 100,000 per year.[14] Thirty-three percent of cases had a cholestatic or mixed pattern.[14] In the largest series, cholestatic pattern was present in 20% to 40%, mixed pattern in 12% to 20% and hepatocellular pattern in 48% to 58% (**Table 1**).

RISK FACTORS
Chemical Properties of Drugs

For most drugs, little is known about the risk of DILI for the individual patient. The chemical properties of some drugs have indicated that some have hepatotoxic potential. Temafloxacin and trovafloxacin have a unique difluorinated side chain that does not occur in other quinolones. This makes these drugs extra lipophilic and they are associated with cholestatic liver disease.[15] Drugs given orally in a daily dose of more than 50 mg are much more likely to lead to DILI than those with a lower daily dose.[16] Data from 2 pharmaceutical databases were used to examine the relationship between daily dose of commonly prescribed oral medicines in the United States and their reported frequency of hepatotoxicity. Among US prescription medicines, a higher daily doses of oral medications were associated significantly with liver failure, liver

Table 1 Type of liver injury in the largest DILI series			
	Cholestatic (%)	Mixed (%)	Hepatocellular (%)
Bjornsson and Olsson,[5] 2005	26	22	52
Andrade et al,[20] 2005	20	22	58
Chalasani et al,[68] 2008	23	20	56
De Valle et al,[70] 2006	40	12	48

transplantation, and death from DILI. In approximately one-third of cases, the observed pattern was of cholestatic type.[16] These results were reproduced in a study of approximately 600 cases of DILI from the Spanish Hepatotoxicity Registry, demonstrating that 77% of patients with DILI received medications with daily doses greater than 50 mg,[17] 50% having cholestatic or mixed pattern.[17]

It has recently been shown that drugs with 50% or greater hepatic metabolism caused a significantly higher frequency (compared with drugs with less hepatic metabolism) of hepatic adverse events.[18] Compared with medications without biliary excretion, compounds with biliary excretion significantly increased the incidence of jaundice (74% vs 40%; $P<.0001$).[18] However, the drug-induced cholestasis per se was not further analyzed and warrants further study.

Little data are available to support the notion that a previous episode of cholestasis due to drugs predisposes to a risk of DILI in the future. Data from the Spanish Hepatotoxicity Registry suggest that multiple episodes of DILI associated with different drugs are rare[19]; 9/742 (1.2%) cases were caused by different type of drugs but all except 1 were of hepatocellular type, with mostly autoimmune hepatitis-like patterns.[19]

Effect of Age

The cholestatic type of DILI is more common among the elderly, whereas hepatocellular DILI seems to be more common in younger individuals.[17,20] Overall, cholestatic presentation occurred in 61% of patients aged 60 years and older versus 39% in younger patients, and mixed pattern was also significantly more common in older patients than younger patients. Older age was independently associated with cholestatic-type injury. Advancing age has been shown to be a risk factor for the development of amoxicillin/clavulanate cholestatic-type injury.[17] The reason for this age-related susceptibility to cholestatic liver injury is unclear. It can be speculated that expression of hepatocellular transporters could be related to age. In a recent study, a significant interindividual variability was demonstrated.[21] A total of 15% to 20% of individuals were classified as low or very low expressers of at least 1 of the proteins investigated. However, this variability could not be related to age or sex.[21] Thus, differences in the susceptibility to develop drug-induced cholestasis were not related to age differences in baseline expression levels of canalicular transporter proteins.[21]

Disease States

Susceptibility to oral contraceptives or postmenopausal hormone replacement therapy seems to be increased in patients with intrahepatic cholestasis of pregnancy.[22,23] These observations support the concept that a genetically determined canalicular transporter deficiency is the common denominator. In general, it is controversial whether preexisting liver disease is a risk factor the development of DILI. However, rifampicin seems to be associated with an increased risk for hepatotoxicity in patients with primary biliary cirrhosis. In 2 studies that tested rifampicin for the treatment pruritus in patients with primary biliary cirrhosis, a high frequency of hepatotoxicity was observed.[24,25]

Genetic Determinants

One of the most common drug combinations leading to DILI in many large series is amoxicillin/clavulanate, which is mostly associated with cholestatic or mixed injury. One of the first HLA haplotypes associated with DILI, HLA B1*1501-DRB5*0101-DQB1*0602,149 was observed in 57% of patients with amoxicillin/clavulanate-induced DILI, but in only 12% of controls.[26] Another study from England confirmed the association between HLA DRB1*15 and liver injury caused by amoxicillin/clavulanate.[27] A more recent study based on data from the Spanish Registry did not confirm this association, but patients with amoxicillin/clavulanate-associated DILI had a significantly higher prevalence of HLA-DQR1*06 than controls.[28] Those with cholestatic/mixed DILI had a significantly higher frequency of HLA-DRB1*15 and HLADQB1*06 alleles and a lower frequency of DRB1*07 and DQB1*02 alleles.[28]

In a landmark study, Daly and colleagues[29] recently reported the results of their genome-wide association studies of flucloxacillin-induced liver injury, a drug mostly associated with cholestasis. This study showed an association peak in the major histocompatibility complex region with the strongest association observed for rs2395029, a marker in complete linkage disequilibrium with HLA-B*5701.[29] Direct genotyping for HLA-B*5701 in 51 cases and 63 drug-exposed controls revealed a strong relationship between this allele and flucloxacillin-induced liver injury (odds ratio 80.6). There were additional significant single nucleotide polymorphisms (HLA-DRB1*0701, tumor necrosis factor rs361525, tumor necrosis factor rs1799964, HSPAIL rs2227956), but their significance was deemed not independent of HLA-B*5701. Increased susceptibility of cholestatic injury caused by contraceptives has been reported to be associated with bile salt export pump (BSEP) 1331 T to C polymorphism.[30]

VANISHING BILE DUCT SYNDROME

Chronic intrahepatic cholestatic patterns are rarely associated with DILI. The liver histology can mimic that of primary biliary cirrhosis with granulomatous duct injury.[31] Vanishing bile duct syndrome is a rare syndrome and has been considered to occur in only 0.5% of cases of small duct biliary disease.[32] In a minority of patients, progressive ductopenia occurs, which can lead to near complete absence of ducts with variable amount of inflammation.[33] This is diagnosed mainly in patients with prolonged cholestasis for many months or several years, often with jaundice. In rare cases, this can lead to cirrhosis.[6,33–35] The list of drugs reported to be associated with vanishing bile duct syndrome is long and this review cannot cover all these reports. The prototype of drugs leading to this syndrome is chlorpromazine.[6] Many other drugs have been implicated such as amoxicillin,[36] carbamazepine,[37,38] and flucloxacillin,[34,36] and ductopenia has been associated with more than 40 drugs.[35,39] Ductopenia can also be progressive, without resolution of jaundice and lead to fibrosis and biliary cirrhosis.[6,34,35,40–42] This has been associated with inability of bile duct ductular proliferation leading to prolonged and occasionally irreversible changes resulting in death from cholestatic cirrhosis.[43] In some cases, the vanishing bile duct syndrome seems to reverse with disappearance of jaundice during long-term follow-up.[38,44] Based on animal experiments, improved biliary drainage has been associated with neoductular proliferation.[45] The basis for the reversibility of the vanishing bile duct syndrome caused by drugs has been reported.[44] A sequence of changes documented with repeated liver biopsies demonstrating restoration of bile ducts was nicely illustrated.[44] This is probably caused by regeneration of the terminal branches of the biliary tree from a progenitor cell compartment located at the interface of bile ducts with hepatic parenchyma.[44]

THE PATHOLOGY OF DRUG-INDUCED CHOLESTASIS

For almost 2 centuries, pathologists have recognized morphologic changes in the liver in jaundiced patients,[46,47] although the molecular basis for cholestasis has only been revealed in the last 2 to 3 decades.[48] There is a long tradition in pathology to use the term cholestasis in pathology reports on liver tissue. This morphologic cholestasis refers to the deposition of bile in hepatocytes and/or the biliary passages of the liver tissue, which can be detected under the microscope.[49] The conventional separation of cholestasis into extrahepatic and intrahepatic in the minds of most people refers to intrahepatic cholestasis when no mechanical obstruction can be demonstrated. Numerous diseases and other causative factors are responsible for cholestasis. Drugs do have a diverse effect on the morphology of the liver tissue and it is claimed that they should be included the differential diagnosis for any morphologic pattern recognized in this organ.[49] The evaluation of a liver biopsy in a suspected liver injury caused by drugs is 1 of the most challenging in liver pathology.[3] In the interpretation of such a biopsy, it is imperative that a clinicopathologic approach is undertaken to accomplish an educated interpretation of the biopsy and the disease in general. Of the various different patterns of drug-induced liver damage,[3] cholestatic liver injury is the most common. The cholestatic pattern of DILI is present in up to two-thirds of all DILIs.[50] Histologically, a cholestatic pattern of liver injury can be separated into acute and chronic injury, of which acute cholestasis is much more common.

Acute Cholestasis in DILI

The acute intrahepatic cholestasis accounted for by drugs can be separated into pure (bland) cholestasis and cholestasis accompanied by inflammatory cell infiltrate, degenerative changes, especially bile duct degeneration and/or necrosis of liver tissue, referred to as cholestatic hepatitis, hypersensitivity cholestasis, or cholangiolitic cholestasis.

In pure cholestasis, bile plugs are detected in canaliculi and/or hepatocytes and this is, in general, most prominent in zone 3 of the liver parenchyma (**Fig. 1**). No inflammation, hepatocytic degeneration, or necrosis is present and no bile duct damage can be seen. Such a pattern is common and has been associated with oral contraceptives, anabolic steroids, warfarin, prochlorperazine, and thiabendazole to name a few examples. Differential diagnosis of pure cholestasis would include sepsis, shock, and cardiac failure, as well as postoperative cholestasis and intrahepatic cholestasis of pregnancy in the relevant clinical settings.

In cholestatic hepatitis (hypersensitivity cholestasis), accumulation of bile in the liver tissue is accompanied by inflammation and hepatocellular injury. Eosinophils may be present and if present the prognosis seems to be better (**Fig. 2**).[51] Bile ductular reaction/proliferation can be present to some extent. This histologic pattern is generally manifested as mixed cholestatic and parenchymal liver injury on biochemical tests.

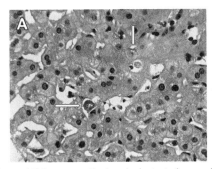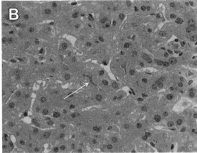

Fig. 1. (*A*) Pure canalicular cholestasis (*arrows*). (*B*) Pure canalicular cholestasis. Arrow highlights cholestasis.

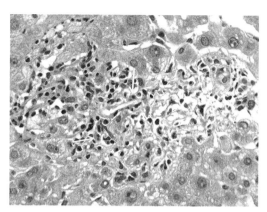

Fig. 2. Mixed inflammatory infiltrate in a portal tract, including several eosinophils (*arrow*).

Various drugs have been associated with such a liver injury, for example, erythromycin and chlorpromazine. In the differential diagnosis, acute viral hepatitis, autoimmune hepatitis, and acute large duct obstruction must be considered.[52]

In general, it can be claimed that acute cholestatic liver injury, with or without accompanying liver cell damage and inflammation, predominantly located in the centrilobular area/zone 3 of the liver parenchyma is most likely caused by drug injury.[48,49,52]

Chronic Cholestasis in DILI

Drugs accounting for cholestasis for more than 3 months are referred to as being responsible for chronic cholestatic DILI.[52] Most commonly, cholestasis caused by drugs resolves without significant consequences after termination of drug intake. In some instances, liver injury caused by drugs does persist and becomes chronic. Drugs such as amoxicillin/calvulanic acid, flucloxacillin, amiodarone, some antifungal agents, and rarely some oral contraceptives have been associated with chronic cholestatic DILI.[34,50,53,54]

Cholestasis with varying degree of necroinflammatory response of liver tissue persisting for more than several months does affect the histology of the liver tissue. This leads to duct sclerosis and loss, periportal cholate stasis, portal fibrosis, and copper accumulation. Eventually this leads to loss of bile ducts and can evolve to the syndrome of vanishing bile ducts. Paucity of bile ducts should be diagnosed if more than 50% of portal tracts are lacking bile ducts in a representative liver biopsy.[3] This can be the result of anticonvulsants such as carbamazepine,[38] zonisamide[44] as well as chlorpromazine,[6] ibuprofen,[36] and other drugs. Persistent inflammation and ductular reaction can be present. In chronic DILI, cholate stasis can be seen. This histologic feature shows clear cytoplasmic changes in periportal hepatocytes or hepatocytes accounting for maximal bile acid transport, also located at the periphery of regenerative nodules in cirrhosis. These cells often contain copper and its binding protein. This can be demonstrated with Shikata orcein stain as black/brown granules and CK7 and 19 stains of the hepatocytes. In severe chronic DILI, a variable amount of fibrosis of the liver can be seen and, eventually, established cirrhosis.

When 1 diagnostic disease pattern is noticed in a liver biopsy, it should not prevent the pathologist from looking thoroughly through the biopsy for another different pathologic condition, suggesting a second disease. **Fig. 3** is an example of such a case

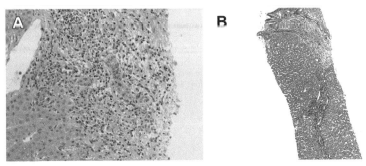

Fig. 3. (*A*) A portal tract showing considerable inflammation and some degree of bile duct degeneration. (*B*) Masson Trichrome stain of a core biopsy of liver illustrating considerable fibrosis (blue stain indicates fibrosis).

where the patient became acutely jaundiced after taking oral contraceptives. A liver biopsy illustrated acute canalicular cholestasis consistent with acute DILI, but, in addition, there was considerable fibrosis present as well as bile duct lesions, suggestive of primary biliary cirrhosis. Blood tests revealed significant increase of antimitochondrial antibodies (AMA) and subsequently the diagnosis of acute cholestatic DILI on top of primary biliary cirrhosis was made. The patient recovered from jaundice but still has somewhat increased ALP and high titers of AMA.

THE PATHOPHYSIOLOGY OF DRUG-INDUCED CHOLESTASIS

Hepatic detoxification of xenobiotics involves either phase I reactions followed by phase II reactions or phase I alone or rarely only phase II.[55] Phase II reactions result in anionic conjugates with sulfate, glucuronate, or glutathione. These drug metabolites are transported across hepatocyte membranes by transporters (uptake or efflux transporters) on the apical or the canalicular membranes.[56] This hepatic drug transport has been shown to be involved in the pathophysiology of cholestatic adverse effects caused by drugs.[56,57] In the liver, transport at the apical membrane into hepatocytes involves the organic anion transporting polypeptide.[56] Little data exist on defects in these uptake transporters and the risk for cholestatic liver injury.[56] Basolateral transport processes probably determine hepatic exposure to drugs and their metabolites that reach the canalicular membrane.[58] Inhibition of this basolateral transport does not seem to increase the risk of cholestasis caused by drugs.[59] In contrast, inhibition of efflux proteins can lead to cholestatic liver injury caused by certain compounds or their metabolites.[57] The efflux of drugs into bile involves canalicular transporters of the MRP family, which includes the glycoproteins MDR1 (ABCB1), MDR3 (ABCB4), MRP2 (ABCC2), and BSEP (ABCB11).[57] The BSEP has been shown to be a major transporter of bile salts and drug metabolites from hepatocytes into bile.[57] Drugs that inhibit export on the canalicular side through inhibition of BSEP can lead to cholestasis in susceptible individuals.[57]

Data are accumulating to suggest that cholestatic forms of drug-induced liver damage result from a drug-mediated or metabolite-mediated inhibition of hepatobiliary transporter systems.[57] Rifampin, troglitazone, glibenclamide, and bosentan can lead to cholestatic liver disease, and this has been shown to be related to inhibition of bile salt export pump function in animal experiments.[57] Cholestasis caused by flucloxacillin, terbinafine, sulindac, and bosentan has been associated with inhibition of the canalicular BSEP.[60–62] Bosentan, which has a well-documented hepatotoxicity, has been shown to inhibit BSEP, leading to accumulation of toxic bile acids within the hepatocytes.[63,64] Mutations that disturb BSEP function have been identified in patients with a history of cholestasis caused by drugs.[65] Patients with mutations in genes that encode BSEP or MDR3 have a 3-fold increased risk of cholestatic DILI from oral contraceptives, psychotropic drugs, proton pump inhibitors, and certain antibiotics.[65] Other molecular mechanisms of cholestasis have been reported, including destruction of the cytoskeleton, impaired trafficking and disruption of the tight junction network, inhibition of ATP-dependent transporters, and modulation of fluidity of the canalicular membrane.[66]

MOST IMPORTANT DRUGS LEADING TO CHOLESTATIC LIVER INJURY

The list of drugs associated with cholestatic injury is long. A comprehensive list of drugs reported to have induced hepatotoxicity has been published.[67] This article focuses on the most common types of drugs and new observations in this context.

Antibiotics and Antifungals

In all large series published on DILI, antibiotics are the most common type of drugs involved.[5,20,60–71]

Amoxicillin/clavulanate
This particular combination of drugs is widely used in some countries and, in most DILI series, it is among the most common antibiotics leading to DILI.[20,68] In a recent study from the United Kingdom, one-third of drug-induced jaundice was associated with amoxicillin/clavulanate.[71] In the Spanish Hepatotoxicity Registry, amoxicillin/clavulanate was the most common cause of DILI, with 59/461 (13%) of all DILIs related to amoxicillin/clavulanate[20]; in the United States amoxicillin/clavulanate was the most common antibiotic associated with DILI.[68] Liver injury can develop early in the course of treatment but also late in the course of prolonged treatment and even after discontinuation of therapy.[72] Most cases of amoxicillin/clavulanate-induced liver injury have a cholestatic or mixed pattern. Liver injury is mainly related to the clavulanic acid component, as the incidence of DILI with amoxicillin/clavulanate is markedly higher than that of amoxicillin alone.[73] Risk factors for hepatotoxicity are age greater than 65 years, female sex, and repeated courses of the antibiotic.[71–73] Most cases are mild but a protracted course is also possible and in rare cases can lead to acute liver failure or require transplantation.[72,74]

Penicillinase-resistant penicillins and other penicillins
Flucloxacillin-induced cholestasis is well documented.[34,36,75,76] Flucloxacillin is commonly prescribed in the United Kingdom, Sweden, and Australia, and is the most common reason for idiosyncratic liver injury in Sweden (16% of all DILI cases)[5] and the second most common cause of drug-induced jaundice in the United Kingdom.[71] Incidence of reactions reported to Swedish authorities was 1 of 11,000 to 1 of 30,000 prescriptions[34] but this is probably an underestimation as it is based on spontaneous reporting. Female sex, age, and high daily doses have been shown to be associated with higher risk of liver injury caused by flucloxacillin.[34,76] A total of 7/129 (5%) patients died due to reported flucloxacillin liver injury in Sweden from 1970 to 2004.[5] Ductopenia[36] and cholestatic cirrhosis leading to liver transplantation have been reported.[34,75] Other semisynthetic penicillinase-resistant penicillins such as cloxacillin, dicloxacillins, and oxacillins have been shown to induce cholestatic hepatitis.[34,68,75] Treatment with penicillinase-sensitive penicillins rarely causes liver

damage.[77] However, prolonged and severe cholestasis has been reported for benzylpenicillin.[78]

Macrolides

Erythromycin may cause a cholestatic liver injury.[77] Erythromycin was the second most commonly reported antibiotic to the Swedish authorities in 1 study.[5] In a collection of case reports from the literature, cholestatic injury was observed in 69% and immunoallergic features in one-third of cases.[51] The prognosis is generally favorable and reports of acute liver failure and death are rare.[5,51] Clarithromycin and azithromycin have both been associated with cholestatic liver injury.[79,80]

Trimethoprim/sulfamethoxazole

In most recent series on DILI, this drug combination is high on the list of drugs associated with DILI.[5,51,68,69] After amoxicillin/clavulanate, nitrofurantoin, and isoniazid, trimethoprim/sulfamethoxazole was the fourth most common antibiotic inducing DILI in the North American DILIN study.[68] The sulfonamide component is considered to be responsible and sulfonamides mostly lead to cholestatic patterns.[81] Almost 60% of reactions are of cholestatic nature[51] and in 1 study, 2/21 (9.5%) of patients with jaundice caused by trimethoprim/sulfamethoxazole either died or underwent liver transplantation.[5]

Tetracyclines

In the past, tetracycline hepatotoxicity was associated with large doses that were often given intravenously and in pregnancy.[82] However, with normal low-dose tetracyclines such as doxycycline, the incidence seems to be lower than most reported antibiotics leading to DILI and with a generally favorable prognosis.[83,84] Liver injury was designated as cholestatic, hepatocellular, and mixed, with similar frequencies.[83] No deaths caused by tetracyclines have been reported to the Swedish authorities by spontaneous reporting.[5,83]

Other antibiotics

The antifungal terbinafine has been shown to induce cholestatic injury that can be severe and lead to acute liver failure requiring liver transplantation.[85,86] Terbinafine-induced hepatotoxicity has been reported in several patients from large series from Sweden and the United States.[5,68] Other antibiotics in common use and shown to lead to cholestatic hepatitis are ciprofloxacin[87,88] and cephalosporins.[89] DILI caused by cephalosporins has previously been considered to be extremely rare. However, a recent study from the DILIN network in the United States described 32 cases of a total of 655 (5%) enrolled between 2004 and 2010.[90] Most demonstrated a cholestatic pattern and in several cases the toxicity occurred after therapy had been stopped; at least 1 fatal outcome was attributed to cephalosporin-induced hepatotoxicity.[90]

Psychotropic Drugs

Cholestatic-type injury caused by chlorpromazine is a well-documented, and leads to cholestatic hepatitis, ductopenia, and cholestatic cirrhosis.[6] Chlorpromazine has been replaced by other antipsychotic drugs such as risperidone.[91,92] Cholestasis due to both drugs has been reported to occur in the same patient at times.[92] Cholestatic hepatitis has also been reported after tricyclic antidepressants such as imipramine and amitryptiline.[4] Duloxetine, a commonly used antidepressant, has recently been associated with cholestatic hepatitis.[93] This reaction has been found to be dose related.[16,93]

Antiinflammatory Drugs

Azathioprine, an important and commonly used drug in patients with inflammatory bowel disease (IBD) has been associated with DILI. Several cases of severe cholestatic hepatitis have been reported in the literature.[94–96] Nodular regenerative liver hyperplasia is a rare but potentially serious complication of treatment with azathioprine.[97]

Most patients develop liver injury during the first 3 months of therapy.[97] The frequency of DILI associated with azathioprine is unclear. According to a systematic review, the mean prevalence of liver injury induced by azathioprine or 6-mercaptopurine in IBD was approximately 3%, and the mean annual drug-induced liver disorder rate was only 1.4%.[98] This low figure was based on retrospective studies and contrasts with approximately 10% incidence reported by a prospective study.[97] In the prospective study, hepatotoxicity occurred in 16/161 (10%) after a median of 85 days, but azathioprine therapy had to be discontinued only in approximately one-third of cases.[97]

Diclofenac, a commonly used nonsteroidal antiinflammatory drug (NSAID) with a well-known, although rare, potential to cause liver injury, is mostly associated with a hepatocellular pattern.[99] However, cholestatic reactions associated with diclofenac have been reported.[100,101] Hepatotoxicity caused by ibuprofen is much less well documented than for diclofenac, but cases of ibuprofen hepatotoxicity have been included in some series on DILI.[5,20] Ibuprofen-induced vanishing bile duct syndrome leading to cirrhosis has been reported in a previously healthy child.[102] Other NSAIDs associated with occasional cholestatic injury include sulindac and nimesulide.[103]

Drugs Against Human Immunodeficiency Virus

Liver injury has been attributed to highly active antiretroviral therapy (HAART) but causality assessment is often difficult as some patients have concomitant hepatitis C, other comorbidities, and medications.[104] In a large group of patients with AIDS and jaundice, it was reported that DILI was the most likely cause in one-third of patients.[105] The largest series on DILI have not included many cases with drugs against human immunodeficiency virus (HIV).[5,20,68] However, among cases of DILI reported to the WHO monitoring center, drugs against HIV such as stavudine, didanosine, and nevirapine were among the top 10 most common causes of fatal liver injury caused by drugs.[106] Recently, noncirrhotic portal hypertension (NCPH) in persons infected with HIV has been associated with antiretroviral therapy, particularly the drug didanosine.[107–111] Most patients develop cholestatic liver disease before signs and symptoms of portal hypertension, such as variceal bleeding and ascites, became apparent.[107,109] The prognosis seems to be favorable until portal hypertension becomes clinically apparent.[110] However, in 4/15 (26%) patients with NCPH and esophageal varices, the cause of death was liver related.[109] In multivariate analysis, the only independent predictor of NCPH was didanosine exposure.[110]

Other Types of Drugs Associated with Cholestatic Liver Injury

The long-term use of oral contraceptives has been associated with an increased risk of certain types of liver disease: acute intrahepatic canalicular cholestasis, benign hepatic tumors such as hepatic adenoma, and focal nodular hyperplasia as well as hepatic vein thrombosis and portal vein thrombosis.[23,111] Although cholestatic liver disease has been associated with oral contraceptives for many decades, oral contraceptives have rarely been reported in the large series on DILI; less than 1% of cases in Sweden,[5] Spain[20] and the United States[68] were attributed to oral contraceptives. In a survey of adverse liver reactions to oral contraceptives in Sweden from 1966 to 1989, there was a sharp decline in the number of reports during the study period, suggesting changes in reporting habits.[112] However, there was also a significantly lower incidence of reports for oral contraceptives with medium compared with high levels of estrogen, and a further decrease in incidence with oral contraceptives with a low level of estrogen. Cholestatic and hepatocellular liver enzyme patterns were equally frequent in patients with adverse reactions from low-dose estrogen oral contraceptives. Interval between treatment and reported hepatic reaction ranged from 3 to 360 days (median 60 days). There was no report of liver tumors related to use of low-dose estrogen oral contraceptives.[112] Thus, it seems that the lower doses of estrogens and gestagens are associated with a decrease in the incidence of adverse liver reactions. Liver injury associated with oral contraceptives generally has a favorable prognosis. Hepatotoxicity due to anabolic steroids is well-documented, mainly in the form of intrahepatic cholestasis.[113] Hepatotoxicity associated with dietary supplements containing anabolic steroids has been increasingly recognized in the United States.[114,115] Several other dietary supplements have been associated with cholestasis, although for some reason a hepatocellular pattern is more frequently found to be associated with dietary supplements.[115] Many other drugs and types of drugs can lead to cholestatic liver injury.

THE PROGNOSIS OF PATIENTS WITH CHOLESTASIS CAUSED BY DRUGS

Drug-induced jaundice has been associated with a poor prognosis[4] and a severe drug reaction on the liver was found by Hy Zimmerman to lead to at least 10% mortality.[4] This has been named Hy's law and was later validated in a large series of patients with DILI; the mortality/liver transplantation rate was 9% to 12%.[5,20,68] Originally, this association was believed to be true only for hepatocellular jaundice, and the prognosis of those with cholestatic injury was mainly related to comorbidities and age.[4] In recent series, cholestatic DILI has also been associated with mortality of 5% to 14%.[5,20,68] In the DILIN study, not all these patients died from a liver-related cause.[68] However, in a prospective study on serious liver disease caused by drugs, the case fatality rate was not significantly different between those with hepatocellular and cholestatic liver injury.[116] Mortality and liver transplantation among patients with different patterns of liver injury are shown in **Table 2**.

A prospective follow-up of the patients in the Spanish Registry revealed development of chronic liver injury in 28/493 (5.7%) of patients followed for a mean of 20 months.[117] In this study, the definition of chronic liver injury was as follows: hepatocellular pattern of damage defined as chronic if liver tests showed persistent abnormality

Table 2
Biochemical patterns and mortality rates in the most recent series on DILI

	Cholestatic Pattern (%)	Mixed Pattern (%)	Hepatocellular Pattern (%)
Ibanez et al,[116] 2002	12.9	5	17.8
Andrade et al,[20] 2005	5	2	7
Bjornsson and Olsson,[5] 2005	7.8	2.4	12.7
Chalasani et al,[68] 2008	14.3	2.1	7.5

more than 3 months after stopping the drug therapy; in cholestatic/mixed type of injury, the abnormality was considered chronic if it was present for more than 6 months after drug discontinuation.[117] The most frequent drug associated with chronicity was amoxicillin/clavulanate. Patients with cholestatic liver injury were more likely to develop chronic liver injury.[117] Ductal lesions developed in 3 patients in the cholestatic/mixed group.[117]

Results from a single-center study from Sweden were similar in terms of the proportion of patients with DILI with chronic evolution. Three of 50 (6%) patients diagnosed with DILI had persistently abnormal liver biochemistries after a median follow-up of 48 months.[118] Among the first 300 cases enrolled in the DILIN study, the rate of chronic liver injury at 6 months was 13.6%.[68] Features of the implicated agent, pattern of DILI, or patient age were not associated with chronicity.[68] However, the long-term outcome of these patients is unknown.

A 10-year follow-up study of patients with DILI who originally all had DILI and concomitant jaundice[119] revealed that development of a clinically important liver disease after severe DILI was rare. A total of 23/685 (3.4%) DILI patients who had survived acute DILI were hospitalized for liver disease during the study period and 5 died from liver-related causes.[119] Among these patients, 5 of 8 with cirrhosis did not have an identifiable cause of cirrhosis; DILI may have played a role in this development and 2 of these patients had cholestatic liver injury. A significantly longer duration of drug therapy before the detection of DILI was observed in those who developed liver-related morbidity and mortality during follow-up.[119] The most common cause of hospitalization for DILI during follow-up was a protracted course of the DILI. Most patients with protracted courses (86%) were of cholestatic/mixed type and had a mean follow-up of 13 years. In this subgroup of patients, liver tests were normal for all patients except 1 (with 6 years follow-up) at last follow-up and they remained free of liver morbidity thereafter.[119]

REFERENCES

1. Benichou C, Danan G, Flahault A. Causality assessment of adverse reactions to drugs–II. An original model for validation of drug causality assessment methods: case reports with positive rechallenge. J Clin Epidemiol 1993;46:1331–6.
2. Danan G, Benichou C. Causality assessment of adverse reactions to drugs–I. A novel method based on the conclusions of international consensus meetings: application to drug-induced liver injuries. J Clin Epidemiol 1993;46:1323–30.
3. Kleiner DE. The pathology of drug-induced liver injury. Semin Liver Dis 2009;29: 364–72.
4. Zimmerman H. Hepatotoxicity: the adverse effects of drugs and other chemicals on the liver. Philadelphia: Lippincott Williams & Wilkins; 1999.
5. Bjornsson E, Olsson R. Outcome and prognostic markers in severe drug-induced liver disease. Hepatology 2005;42:481–9.
6. Moradpour D, Altorfer J, Flury R, et al. Chlorpromazine-induced vanishing bile duct syndrome leading to biliary cirrhosis. Hepatology 1994;20:1437–41.
7. Rochon J, Protiva P, Seeff LB, et al. Reliability of the Roussel Uclaf Causality Assessment Method for assessing causality in drug-induced liver injury. Hepatology 2008;48:1175–83.
8. Rockey DC, Seeff LB, Rochon J, et al. Causality assessment in drug-induced liver injury using a structured expert opinion process: comparison to the Roussel-Uclaf causality assessment method. Hepatology 2010;51: 2117–26.

9. Hayashi PH. Causality assessment in drug-induced liver injury. Semin Liver Dis 2009;29:340–56.
10. Maggio MC, Liotta A, Cardella F, et al. Stevens-Johnson syndrome and cholestatic hepatitis induced by acute Epstein-Barr virus infection. Eur J Gastroenterol Hepatol 2011;23:289.
11. Ratnayake EC, Shivanthan C, Wijesiriwardena BC. Cholestatic hepatitis in a patient with typhoid fever - a case report. Ann Clin Microbiol Antimicrob 2011;10:35.
12. Choi HC, Lee SH, Kim J, et al. A case of acute q Fever with severe acute cholestatic hepatitis. Gut Liver 2009;3:141–4.
13. Breidert M, Offensperger S, Blum HE, et al. Weight loss and severe jaundice in a patient with hyperthyroidism. Z Gastroenterol 2011;49:1267–9.
14. Sgro C, Clinard F, Ouazir K, et al. Incidence of drug-induced hepatic injuries: a French population-based study. Hepatology 2002;36:451–5.
15. Lucena MI, Andrade RJ, Rodrigo L, et al. Trovafloxacin-induced acute hepatitis. Clin Infect Dis 2000;30:400–1.
16. Lammert C, Einarsson S, Niklasson A, et al. Relationship between daily dose of oral medications and idiosyncratic drug-induced liver injury (DILI). Search for signals. Hepatology 2008;47:2003–9.
17. Lucena MI, Andrade RJ, Kaplowitz N, et al. Phenotypic characterization of idiosyncratic drug-induced liver injury: the influence of age and gender. Hepatology 2009;49:2001–9.
18. Lammert C, Bjornsson E, Niklasson A, et al. Oral medications with significant hepatic metabolism at higher risk for hepatic adverse events. Hepatology 2010;51:615–20.
19. Lucena MI, Kaplowitz N, Hallal H, et al. Recurrent drug-induced liver injury (DILI) with different drugs in the Spanish Registry: the dilemma of the relationship to autoimmune hepatitis. J Hepatol 2011;55:820–7.
20. Andrade RJ, Lucena MI, Fernandez MC, et al. Drug-induced liver injury: an analysis of 461 incidences submitted to the Spanish Registry over a 10-year period. Gastroenterology 2005;129:512–21.
21. Meier Y, Pauli-Magnus C, Zanger UM, et al. Interindividual variability of canalicular ATP-binding-cassette (ABC)-transporter expression in human liver. Hepatology 2006;44:62–74.
22. Leevy CB, Koneru B, Klein KM. Recurrent familial prolonged intrahepatic cholestasis of pregnancy associated with chronic liver disease. Gastroenterology 1997;113:966–72.
23. Lindberg MC. Hepatobiliary complications of oral contraceptives. J Gen Intern Med 1992;7:199–209.
24. Bachs L, Pares A, Elena M, et al. Effects of long-term rifampicin administration in primary biliary cirrhosis. Gastroenterology 1992;102:2077–80.
25. Prince MI, Burt AD, Jones DE. Hepatitis and liver dysfunction with rifampicin therapy for pruritus in primary biliary cirrhosis. Gut 2002;50:436–9.
26. Hautekeete ML, Horsmans Y, Van Waeyenberge C, et al. HLA association of amoxicillin-clavulanate–induced hepatitis. Gastroenterology 1999;117:1181–6.
27. O'Donohue J, Oien KA, Donaldson P, et al. Co-amoxiclav jaundice: clinical and histological features and HLA class II association. Gut 2000;47:717–20.
28. Andrade RJ, Lucena MI, Alonso A, et al. HLA class II genotype influences the type of liver injury in drug-induced idiosyncratic liver disease. Hepatology 2004;39:1603–12.

29. Daly AK, Donaldson PT, Bhatnagar P, et al. HLA-B*5701 genotype is a major determinant of drug-induced liver injury due to flucloxacillin. Nat Genet 2009; 41:816–21.
30. Meier Y, Zodan T, Lang C, et al. Increased susceptibility for intrahepatic cholestasis of pregnancy and contraceptive-induced cholestasis in carriers of the 1331T>C polymorphism in the bile salt export pump. World J Gastroenterol 2008;14:38–45.
31. Brown PJ, Lesna M, Hamlyn AM, et al. Primary biliary cirrhosis after long-term practolol administration. Br Med J 1978;1(6127):1591.
32. Ludwig J. Idiopathic adulthood ductopenia: an update. Mayo Clin Proc 1998;73: 193–9.
33. Degott C, Feldmann G, Larrey D, et al. Drug-induced prolonged cholestasis in adults: a histological semiquantitative study demonstrating progressive ductopenia. Hepatology 1992;15:244–51.
34. Olsson R, Wiholm BE, Sand C, et al. Liver damage from flucloxacillin, cloxacillin and dicloxacillin. J Hepatol 1992;15:154–61.
35. Desmet V. Vanishing bile duct syndrome in drug-induced liver disease. J Hepatol 1997;26:31–5.
36. Davies MH, Harrison RF, Elias E, et al. Antibiotic-associated acute vanishing bile duct syndrome: a pattern associated with severe, prolonged, intrahepatic cholestasis. J Hepatol 1994;20:112–6.
37. Forbes GM, Jeffrey GP, Shilkin KB, et al. Carbamazepine hepatotoxicity: another cause of the vanishing bile duct syndrome. Gastroenterology 1992;102:1385–8.
38. Ramos AM, Gayotto LC, Clemente CM, et al. Reversible vanishing bile duct syndrome induced by carbamazepine. Eur J Gastroenterol Hepatol 2002;14: 1019–22.
39. Padda MS, Sanchez M, Akhtar AJ, et al. Drug-induced cholestasis. Hepatology 2011;53:1377–87.
40. Gregory DH, Zaki GF, Sarcosi GA, et al. Chronic cholestasis following prolonged tolbutamide administration. Arch Pathol 1967;84:194–201.
41. Glober GA, Wilkenson JA. Biliary cirrhosis following administration of methyltestosterone. JAMA 1968;204:170–3.
42. Ishii M, Miyazaki Y, Yamamoto T, et al. A case of drug-induced ductopenia resulting in fatal biliary cirrhosis. Liver 1993;13:227–31.
43. Eckstein RP, Dowsett JF, Lunzer MR. Flucloxacillin induced liver disease: histopathological findings at biopsy and autopsy. Pathology 1993;25:223–38.
44. Vuppalanchi R, Chalasani N, Saxena R. Restoration of bile ducts in drug-induced vanishing bile duct syndrome due to zonisamide. Am J Surg Pathol 2006;30:1619–23.
45. Alpini G, Lenzi R, Sarkozi L, et al. Biliary physiology in rats with bile ductular cell hyperplasia. Evidence for a secretory function of proliferated bile ductules. J Clin Invest 1988;81:569–78.
46. Anderson J. On hemorrhage from the umbilicus after the separation of the fetus. Boston Med Surg J 1850;41:440–2.
47. Crawford JM. Basic mechanisms in hepatopathology. In: Burt AD, Portmann BC, Ferrell LD, editors. MacSween's pathology of the liver. 5th edition. Philadelphia: Churchill Livingstone Elsevier; 2007. p. 75–117.
48. Trauner M, Boyer JL. Bile salt transporters: molecular characterization, function, and regulation. Physiol Rev 2003;83:633–71.
49. Geller SA, Petrovic LM, editors. Biopsy interpretation of the liver. 2nd edition. Philadelphia: Lippincott Williams & Wilkins; 2009.

50. Friis H, Andreasen PB. Drug induced hepatic injury: an analysis of 1100 cases reported to the Danish Committee on adverse drug reactions between 1978 and 1987. J Intern Med 1992;232:133–8.
51. Björnsson E, Kalaitzakis E, Olsson R. The impact of eosinophilia and hepatic necrosis on prognosis in patients with drug-induced liver injury. Aliment Pharmacol Ther 2007;25:1411–21.
52. Ramanchandran R, Kakar S. Histological patterns in drug-induced liver disease. J Clin Pathol 2009;62:481–92.
53. Larrey D, Vial T, Micaleff A, et al. Hepatitis associated with amoxicillin-clavulanic acid combination: report of 15 cases. Gut 1992;33:368–71.
54. Chang CC, Petrelli M, Thomashefski JF Jr, et al. Severe intrahepatic cholestasis caused by amiodarone toxicity after withdrawal of the drug: a case report and review of the literature. Arch Pathol Lab Med 1999;123:251–6.
55. Gibson GG, Skett P. Introduction to drug metabolism. 3rd edition. Cheltenham (United Kingdom): Nelson Thornes; 2001.
56. Ho RH, Kim RB. Transporters and drug therapy: implications for drug disposition and disease. Clin Pharmacol Ther 2005;78:260–77.
57. Pauli-Magnus C, Meier PJ. Hepatobiliary transporters and drug-induced cholestasis. Hepatology 2006;44:778–87.
58. Pauli-Magnus C, Stieger B, Meier Y, et al. Enterohepatic transport of bile salts and genetics of cholestasis. J Hepatol 2005;43:342–57.
59. Vavricka SR, Van Montfoort J, Ha HR, et al. Interactions of rifamycin SV and rifampicin with organic anion uptake systems of human liver. Hepatology 2002;36:164–72.
60. Lakehal F, Dansette PM, Becquemont L, et al. Indirect cytotoxicity of flucloxacillin toward human biliary epithelium via metabolite formation in hepatocytes. Chem Res Toxicol 2001;14:694–701.
61. Iverson SL, Uetrecht JP. Identification of a reactive metabolite of terbinafine: insights into terbinafine-induced hepatotoxicity. Chem Res Toxicol 2001;14: 175–81.
62. Bolder U, Trang NV, Hagey LR, et al. Sulindac is excreted into bile by a canalicular bile salt pump and undergoes a cholehepatic circulation in rats. Gastroenterology 1999;117:962–71.
63. Fattinger K, Funk C, Pantze M, et al. The endothelin antagonist bosentan inhibits the canalicular bile salt export pump: a potential mechanism for hepatic adverse reactions. Clin Pharmacol Ther 2001;69:223–31.
64. Leslie EM, Watkins PB, Kim RB, et al. Differential inhibition of rat and human Na$^+$-dependent taurocholate cotransporting polypeptide (NTCP/SLC10A1) by bosentan: a mechanism for species differences in hepatotoxicity. J Pharmacol Exp Ther 2007;321:1170–8.
65. Lang C, Meier Y, Stieger B, et al. Mutations and polymorphisms in the bile salt export pump and the multidrug resistance protein 3 associated with drug-induced liver injury. Pharmacogenet Genomics 2007;17:47–60.
66. Trauner M, Meier PJ, Boyer JL. Molecular pathogenesis of cholestasis. N Engl J Med 1998;339:1217–27.
67. Biour M, Ben Salem C, Chazouilleres O, et al. Drug-induced liver injury; fourteenth updated edition of the bibliographic database of liver injuries and related drugs. Gastroenterol Clin Biol 2004;28:720–59.
68. Chalasani N, Fontana RJ, Bonkovsky HL, et al. Causes, clinical features, and outcomes from a prospective study of drug-induced liver injury in the United States. Gastroenterology 2008;135:1924–34, 1934.e1–4.

69. Björnsson E, Jerlstad P, Bergqvist A, et al. Fulminant drug-induced hepatic failure leading to death or liver transplantation in Sweden. Scand J Gastroenterol 2005;40:1095–101.
70. De Valle MB, Av Klinteberg V, Alem N, et al. Drug-induced liver injury in a Swedish University hospital out-patient hepatology clinic. Aliment Pharmacol Ther 2006;24:1187–95.
71. Hussaini SH, O'Brien CS, Despott EJ, et al. Antibiotic therapy: a major cause of drug-induced jaundice in southwest England. Eur J Gastroenterol Hepatol 2007; 19:15–20.
72. Lucena MI, Andrade RJ, Fernández MC, et al. Determinants of the clinical expression of amoxicillin-clavulanate hepatotoxicity: a prospective series from Spain. Hepatology 2006;44:850–6.
73. García Rodríguez LA, Stricker BH, Zimmerman HJ. Risk of acute liver injury associated with the combination of amoxicillin and clavulanic acid. Arch Intern Med 1996;156:1327–32.
74. Fontana RJ, Shakil AO, Greenson JK, et al. Acute liver failure due to amoxicillin and amoxicillin/clavulanate. Dig Dis Sci 2005;50:1785–90.
75. Turner IB, Eckstein RP, Riley JW, et al. Prolonged hepatic cholestasis after flucloxacillin therapy. Med J Aust 1989;151:701–5.
76. Fairley CK, McNeil JJ, Desmond P, et al. Risk factors for development of flucloxacillin associated jaundice. BMJ 1993;306:233–5.
77. Polson JE. Hepatotoxicity due to antibiotics. Clin Liver Dis 2007;11:549–61.
78. Andrade RJ, Guilarte J, Salmerón FJ, et al. Benzylpenicillin-induced prolonged cholestasis. Ann Pharmacother 2001;35:783–4.
79. Brown BA, Wallace RJ Jr, Griffith DE, et al. Clarithromycin-induced hepatotoxicity. Clin Infect Dis 1995;20:1073–4.
80. Lockwood AM, Cole S, Rabinovich M. Azithromycin-induced liver injury. Am J Health Syst Pharm 2010;67:810–4.
81. Mainra RR, Card SE. Trimethoprim-sulfamethoxazole-associated hepatotoxicity - part of a hypersensitivity syndrome. Can J Clin Pharmacol 2003;10:175–8.
82. Anon. Tetracycline hepatotoxicity. Br Med J 1964;2(5424):1545–6.
83. Björnsson E, Lindberg J, Olsson R. Liver reactions to oral low-dose tetracyclines. Scand J Gastroenterol 1997;32:390–5.
84. Heaton PC, Fenwick SR, Brewer DE. Association between tetracycline or doxycycline and hepatotoxicity: a population based case-control study. J Clin Pharm Ther 2007;32:483–7.
85. Zapata Garrido AJ, Romo AC, Padilla FB. Terbinafine hepatotoxicity. A case report and review of literature. Ann Hepatol 2003;2:47–51.
86. Agarwal K, Manas DM, Hudson M. Terbinafine and fulminant hepatic failure. N Engl J Med 1999;340:1292–3.
87. Hautekeete ML, Kockx MM, Naegels S, et al. Cholestatic hepatitis related to quinolones: a report of two cases. J Hepatol 1995;23:759–60.
88. Bataille L, Rahier J, Geubel A. Delayed and prolonged cholestatic hepatitis with ductopenia after long-term ciprofloxacin therapy for Crohn's disease. J Hepatol 2002;37:696–9.
89. Skoog SM, Smyrk TC, Talwalkar JA. Cephalexin-induced cholestatic hepatitis. J Clin Gastroenterol 2004;38:833.
90. Alqahtani S, Hoofnagle JH, Ghabril M, et al. Cephalosporin induced liver injury: clinical and biochemical features. Hepatology 2011;54:516A.
91. Krebs S, Dormann H, Muth-Selbach U, et al. Risperidone-induced cholestatic hepatitis. Eur J Gastroenterol Hepatol 2001;13:67–9.

92. Wright TM, Vandenberg AM. Risperidone- and quetiapine-induced cholestasis. Ann Pharmacother 2007;41:1518 23.

93. Vuppalanchi R, Hayashi PH, Chalasani N, et al. Duloxetine hepatotoxicity: a case-series from the drug-induced liver injury network. Aliment Pharmacol Ther 2010;32:1174–83.

94. Romagnuolo J, Sadowski DC, Lalor E, et al. Cholestatic hepatocellular injury with azathioprine: a case report and review of the mechanisms of hepatotoxicity. Can J Gastroenterol 1998;12:479–83.

95. Ben Salem C, Ben Salah L, Belajouza C, et al. Azathioprine-induced severe cholestatic hepatitis in patient carrying TPMT*3C polymorphism. Pharm World Sci 2010;32:701–3.

96. Roda G, Caponi A, Belluzzi A, et al. Severe cholestatic acute hepatitis following azathioprine therapy in a patient with ulcerative pancolitis. Dig Liver Dis 2009; 41:914–5.

97. Bastida G, Nos P, Aguas M, et al. Incidence, risk factors and clinical course of thiopurine-induced liver injury in patients with inflammatory bowel disease. Aliment Pharmacol Ther 2005;22:775–82.

98. Gisbert JP, González-Lama Y, Maté J. Thiopurine-induced liver injury in patients with inflammatory bowel disease: a systematic review. Am J Gastroenterol 2007; 102:1518–27.

99. Aithal GP. Diclofenac-induced liver injury: a paradigm of idiosyncratic drug toxicity. Expert Opin Drug Saf 2004;3:519–23.

100. Watanabe N, Takashimizu S, Kojima S, et al. Clinical and pathological features of a prolonged type of acute intrahepatic cholestasis. Hepatol Res 2007;37:598–607.

101. Hackstein H, Mohl W, Püschel W, et al. Diclofenac-associated acute cholestatis hepatitis. Z Gastroenterol 1998;36:385–9 [in German].

102. Srivastava M, Perez-Atayde A, Jonas MM. Drug-associated acute-onset vanishing bile duct and Stevens-Johnson syndromes in a child. Gastroenterology 1998;115:743–6.

103. Levy C, Lindor KD. Drug-induced cholestasis. Clin Liver Dis 2003;7:311–30.

104. Servoss JC, Kitch DW, Andersen JW, et al. Predictors of antiretroviral-related hepatotoxicity in the adult AIDS Clinical Trial Group (1989-1999). J Acquir Immune Defic Syndr 2006;43:320–3.

105. Akhtar AJ, Shaheen M. Jaundice in African-American and Hispanic patients with AIDS. J Natl Med Assoc 2007;99:825–9.

106. Björnsson E, Olsson R. Suspected drug-induced liver fatalities reported to the WHO database. Dig Liver Dis 2006;38:33–8.

107. Schiano TD, Kotler DP, Ferran E, et al. Hepatoportal sclerosis as a cause of noncirrhotic portal hypertension in patients with HIV. Am J Gastroenterol 2007;102: 2536–40.

108. Saifee S, Joelson D, Braude J, et al. Noncirrhotic portal hypertension in patients with human immunodeficiency virus-1 infection. Clin Gastroenterol Hepatol 2008;6:1167–9.

109. Kovari H, Ledergerber B, Peter U, et al. Association of noncirrhotic portal hypertension in HIV-infected persons and antiretroviral therapy with didanosine: a nested case-control study. Clin Infect Dis 2009;49:626–35.

110. Cachay ER, Peterson MR, Goicoechea M, et al. Didanosine exposure and noncirrhotic portal hypertension in a HIV Clinic in North America: a follow-up study. Br J Med Med Res 2011;1:346–55.

111. Dourakis SP, Tolis G. Sex hormonal preparations and the liver. Eur J Contracept Reprod Health Care 1998;3:7–16.

112. Lindgren A, Olsson R. Liver damage from low-dose oral contraceptives. J Intern Med 1993;234:287–92.
113. Erlinger S. Drug-induced cholestasis. J Hepatol 1997;26(Suppl 1):1–4.
114. Kafrouni MI, Anders RA, Verma S. Hepatotoxicity associated with dietary supplements containing anabolic steroids. Clin Gastroenterol Hepatol 2007;5: 809–12.
115. Navarro VJ. Herbal and dietary supplement hepatotoxicity. Semin Liver Dis 2009;29:373–82.
116. Ibáñez L, Pérez E, Vidal X, et al. Prospective surveillance of acute serious liver disease unrelated to infectious, obstructive, or metabolic diseases: epidemiological and clinical features, and exposure to drugs. J Hepatol 2002;37: 592–600.
117. Andrade RJ, Lucena MI, Kaplowitz N, et al. Outcome of acute idiosyncratic drug-induced liver injury: long-term follow-up in a hepatotoxicity registry. Hepatology 2006;44:1581–8.
118. Björnsson E, Kalaitzakis E, Av Klinteberg V, et al. Long-term follow-up of patients with mild to moderate drug-induced liver injury. Aliment Pharmacol Ther 2007; 26:79–85.
119. Bjornsson E, Davidsdottir L. The long-term follow-up after idiosyncratic drug-induced liver injury with jaundice. J Hepatol 2009;50:511.

Primary Sclerosing Cholangitis

Claudia O. Zein, MD, MSc

KEYWORDS

- Sclerosing cholangitis • Cholestatic liver disease • Cholangiography
- Biliary stricture • Cholangiocarcinoma

KEY POINTS

- Primary sclerosing cholangitis (PSC) is a chronic cholestatic liver disease characterized by diffuse inflammation, fibrosis, and strictures of intra and extrahepatic bile ducts.
- PSC is progressive and can lead to liver cirrhosis, portal hypertension, and liver failure.
- The key diagnostic test in PSC is cholangiography. Endoscopic retrograde cholangiography remains the classic gold standard test, but magnetic resonance cholangiography is favored as a less invasive option.
- There is no effective medical therapy for PSC.
- Endoscopic therapy is the mainstay management of dominant strictures.
- Liver transplantation is the only curative option.
- Cholangiocarcinoma may occur in patients with PSC; therefore patients should be closely monitored for this potential complication.

ETIOPATHOGENESIS OF PRIMARY SCLEROSING CHOLANGITIS

Although the exact etiopathogenetic mechanisms are still unclear, it is thought that primary sclerosing cholangitis (PSC) results from the combination of genetic predisposition and immune-mediated events that lead to ongoing biliary duct damage. It has been postulated that the initial insult leading to the sustained immune-mediated injury in genetically susceptible individuals might be triggered by bacteria-related injury.

Evidence of a genetic susceptibility to PSC was initially suggested by reports of familial occurrence of PSC[1] and further supported by data demonstrating an increased risk of PSC, up to 100-fold, among siblings of PSC patients compared with the general population.[2] Specific genetic loci, including human leukocyte antigen (HLA) class I, HLA class II, as well as non-HLA loci have been associated with PSC.[3–8] The strongest genetic associations recognized have been localized in the major histocompatibility complex in chromosome 6.[4,5] Although several haplotypes have been

Disclosures: No competing interests to disclose.
Dr Claudia Zein is supported by Grant Number KL2 RR024990 from the National Center for Research Resources (NCRR), a component of the NIH and NIH Roadmap for Medical research.
Department of Gastroenterology and Hepatology, Digestive Disease Institute, Cleveland Clinic, 9500 Euclid Avenue, A31, Cleveland, OH 44195, USA
E-mail address: zeinc@ccf.org

Clin Liver Dis 17 (2013) 211–227
http://dx.doi.org/10.1016/j.cld.2012.11.003
1089-3261/13/$ – see front matter © 2013 Elsevier Inc. All rights reserved.

associated with an increased risk of disease, some haplotypes have been linked with a protective effect.[3,5] Genome-wide association studies have demonstrated several genetic associations, including potential disease genes.[5,6] Recently, potential functional implications of PSC genetic associations have been proposed, suggesting that specific genetic associations may relate to different pathogenetic features of PSC, including inflammation, cholangiocyte function, fibrosis, and carcinogenesis.[5,9] Future studies might possibly elucidate if genetic predisposition may in fact define different subgroups of PSC patients at higher risk of specific complications.[9]

There is substantial data supportive of the immune nature of the injury in PSC. The biliary duct injury in PSC is characterized by infiltrating immune cells including T-cells, natural killer cells, B-cells, macrophages, and biliary epithelial cells (BECs).[10,11] BECs of PSC patients differ from normal BECs in that they express HLA class II molecules,[12] and although they lack the classical costimulatory molecules, they express molecules of the B7 family and thus may possibly act as antigen-presenting cells in PSC.[9]

PSC is also associated with presence of multiple autoantibodies including antineutrophil cytoplasmic antibody (ANCA), antinuclear antibody (ANA), antismooth muscle antibody (ASMA), perinuclear ANCA (pANCA), and others. Although these autoantibodies are frequently found in patients with PSC, with one study reporting that 81% of patients with PSC are positive for 3 or more autoantibodies,[13] there is no evidence that they play a direct role in the pathogenesis of the disease. However, it has been shown that pANCAs in PSC and ulcerative colitis (UC) are directed against human tubulin beta isoform 5 and cross-react with a bacterial cell division protein, indicating that there might be an altered immune response to intestinal bacteria in these patients.[14]

Several additional features further support that PSC is an immune-mediated disease. A high rate of concurrent autoimmune disorders has been reported in patients with PSC.[15] In addition, patients with PSC have elevated gamma globulin levels, decreased number of circulatory T-cells, increased levels of circulating immune complexes,[16] and activation of the complement system.[17]

A potential role has been proposed for bacteria or bacterial products originated in the inflamed colonic mucosa in triggering the initial insult in PSC. Based on this hypothesis, bacterial products, such as endotoxin, enter the portal circulation through a permeable colon and evoke an immune response in genetically susceptible individuals.[18] Although some data, such as the presence of bacterial endotoxin in BECs of patients with PSC by immunostaining,[19] are compatible with this hypothesis, the evidence supporting it is still insufficient. The role of exogenous factors in PSC remains mostly undefined. The geographic variation in the prevalence of PSC[20,21] is in great part attributable to different HLA susceptibility across ethnic groups causing population differences,[22] but a role of yet undefined environmental factors may exist. Nonsmoking seems to be a risk factor for PSC based on some studies.[23–25]

EPIDEMIOLOGY AND NATURAL HISTORY

Only a handful of population-based studies looking at the epidemiology of PSC have been done, based mainly in North America and Europe. Overall, the incidence of PSC ranges between 0 to 1.3 per 100,000 inhabitants per year and a prevalence of 0 to 16.2 per 100,000 inhabitants.[26–30] Wide variation in the geographic distribution of PSC has been reported, with the highest frequency of PSC reported in Northern Europe, New Zealand, and North America. Although further studies are needed, this variation seems to be in great part because of differences in genetic susceptibility to the disease among different ethnic groups.[22,26] Although some studies have suggested a trend toward increase in the incidence and prevalence of PSC over time,[20,30,31] it is likely that improved diagnostic awareness and diagnostic techniques have played a role in this.

PSC predominantly affects men, with a 2:1 male to female ratio, and although it can occur at any age, most cases are diagnosed around a median age of 40 years.[27–31] There is a strong association between PSC and inflammatory bowel disease (IBD). Most patients with PSC have concurrent IBD. The proportion of concurrent IBD in patients with PSC is of approximately 70%,[27,28,30] most commonly UC.

Although the natural history of PSC can vary significantly in individual patients, it follows a progressive course that affects survival.[27,32] The mean survival from the time of diagnosis to death free of liver transplantation in patients with PSC ranges between 7 and 18 years.[27,30,32,33] Patients who are asymptomatic at the time of diagnosis may have better survival compared with those with symptoms.[34] Although several prognostic models have been proposed in an attempt to predict clinical outcome in patients with PSC, the highly variable course of this disease limits their applicability in the clinical setting. Variables that have been identified as predictors in prognostic models have included age, liver tests results, cholangiographic findings, histologic stage, and clinical manifestations of advanced disease.

CLINICAL PRESENTATION

It has been reported that around 44% of patients with PSC are asymptomatic at the time of diagnosis.[34] This may be the case in patients with known IBD in whom a cholestatic biochemical profile is found incidentally. Eventually, symptoms may develop, with one study reporting that approximately 22% of patients who were asymptomatic at diagnosis developed symptoms within 5 years.[34,35]

The most common symptoms in patients with PSC are fatigue and pruritus. Patients may also present with complaints of abdominal discomfort, jaundice, and weight loss.[34] Less commonly, frank bacterial cholangitis may be the presenting clinical picture.[35] The clinical course of patients with PSC may be complicated by the development of dominant biliary strictures. Complications associated with chronic cholestatic liver disease may occur including fat-soluble vitamin deficiencies and metabolic bone disease. Complications of advanced liver disease including portal hypertension, coagulopathy, and liver failure eventually occur. Patients with PSC are also at high risk of developing hepatobiliary and other gastrointestinal malignancies.

DIAGNOSIS
Laboratory Findings

Laboratory tests typically demonstrate a cholestatic biochemical profile with predominant elevation of alkaline phosphatase and lesser elevation of transaminases.[34–36] However, normal liver enzymes do not rule out PSC. Bilirubin levels are typically within the normal range early in the disease, but higher levels are present in advanced disease. Hypergammaglobulinemia is present in most patients with PSC.[37] In addition, as mentioned earlier, most patients with PSC have autoantibodies present in serum.[13,38] The most common serum autoantibody found in PSC is the ANCA autoantibody, but other autoantibodies can be found including, among others, ANA, ASMA, antiendothelial cell antibody, and anticardiolipin antibody.[13,38] Unfortunately, although commonly found, these autoantibodies lack specificity in PSC and are not useful for diagnostic purposes.

Liver Ultrasound and Computed Tomography Findings

Liver ultrasound (US) and computed tomography (CT) do not typically provide useful diagnostic information in patients with PSC. However, it is important to be aware that nonspecific abnormal biliary and gallbladder findings may be noted on US or CT in patients with PSC. In some cases, bile duct wall thickening or dilatation may be evident on US or CT. Gallbladder abnormalities including gallbladder enlargement and wall thickening are found in patients with PSC compared with subjects with other causes of chronic liver disease and normal controls.[39] Said and colleagues[40] reported one or more gallbladder abnormalities in 41% of PSC patients undergoing US including gallbladder wall thickening and gallbladder mass lesions, among others. Another radiological finding often noted in patients with PSC is intra-abdominal lymphadenopathy, but this finding is most frequently nonspecific and not necessarily an indication of underlying malignancy.[41]

Cholangiography

Adequate assessment of the biliary tree is central to establish the diagnosis of PSC. This assessment can be accomplished by endoscopic retrograde cholangiography (ERC) (**Fig. 1**) or magnetic resonance cholangiography (MRC) (**Fig. 2**) imaging. The typical diagnostic finding is cholangiographic evidence of multifocal short biliary strictures interspersed with normal or dilated segments, involving the intra and extrahepatic biliary ducts.[35,42] These strictures may in some cases also involve the cystic duct and in a small proportion of patients ($\sim$3%) the pancreatic duct.[42] The multifocal strictures may produce the classic "beaded" appearance of the bile ducts on cholangiography. In the most patients, both intra and extrahepatic ducts are involved, but some cases may present with disease limited to intrahepatic ($\sim$27%) or extrahepatic ($\sim$6%) ducts alone.[34]

Now MRC is the initial diagnostic test of choice for PSC.[43] MRC is noninvasive and safe and has been found to have sensitivity (85%–88%) and specificity (92%–97%) comparable to ERC for the diagnosis of PSC and with good interobserver

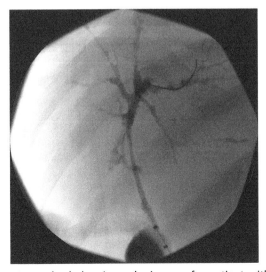

Fig. 1. Endoscopic retrograde cholangiography image of a patient with PSC. There is an intrahepatic ductal narrowing and dilatation characteristic of PSC.

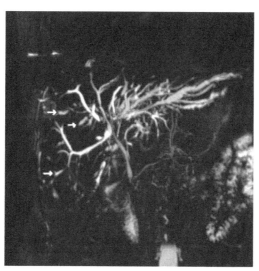

Fig. 2. MRC of a patient with PSC. There is dilatation of intrahepatic biliary ducts. Peripheral discontinuous segmental dilatation, characteristic of PSC, is seen (*arrows*). There is evidence of hilar stricture with dilated intrahepatic biliary ducts tapering at the confluence of the right and left hepatic ducts.

agreement.[44–46] Although up until recently ERC was the preferred diagnostic test for PSC, it is invasive and can lead to complications including cholangitis and pancreatitis. Therefore, today, ERC is most often reserved for cases with a high likelihood of needing a biliary intervention. ERC also remains useful as an initial diagnostic test in patients with suspected PSC in whom MRC is nondiagnostic.[43]

Liver Biopsy

Most often the changes found on liver biopsy in PSC patients are not specific; however, in some patients the classic histopathologic appearance of concentric periductal "onion skinning" fibrosis (**Fig. 3**) is seen. Although a liver biopsy may support the

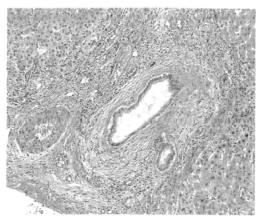

Fig. 3. Hematoxylin and eosin stain. Injured bile duct with periductal fibrosis characteristic of PSC.

diagnosis of PSC, it is not necessary for PSC diagnosis in patients with typical MRC or ERC findings.[47] However, a liver biopsy should be done in patients in whom PSC is suspected but cholangiographic images are nondiagnostic or those who have disproportionately elevated transaminases or other findings suggesting possible overlap with autoimmune hepatitis.[43] Findings characteristic of PSC on liver biopsy in the setting of nondiagnostic cholangiography are diagnostic of "small duct PSC."

Diagnostic Considerations

When evaluating a patient with a suspected diagnosis of PSC, it is important to keep in mind other potential causes of sclerosing cholangitis (**Box 1**). Small duct PSC, as mentioned earlier, is diagnosed when findings of PSC are found on liver biopsy in the setting of normal cholangiography. Patients with small duct PSC have a better prognosis than large duct PSC, with longer survival and no development of cholangiocarcinoma (CCA).[48] However, approximately a fourth of patients with small duct PSC progresses to large duct PSC.[48,49] Other "variant" forms of primary sclerosing cholangitis including overlap of PSC and autoimmune hepatitis and IgG4-associated sclerosing cholangitis should also be kept in mind. These conditions are discussed in separate sections. Secondary sclerosing cholangitis, important to consider in the differential diagnosis, is also discussed in a separate section.

MANAGEMENT OF PATIENTS WITH PSC

As stated earlier, PSC is a progressive condition with mean survival without liver transplantation ranging between 7 and 18 years from the time of diagnosis.[27,30,32,33]

Box 1
Diagnostic considerations in patients with PSC

IgG4-associated cholangitis
- Serum IgG4 should be measured in all PSC patients
- IgG4 levels are elevated in approximately 10% of PSC patients
- Associated with more severe clinical course
- May have clinical response to steroid therapy

Small-duct PSC
- Biochemical and histology findings of PSC
- Normal cholangiogram
- Milder clinical course, longer survival
- Twenty-five percent of cases progress to classic PSC

Autoimmune hepatitis-PSC overlap
- Should be suspected in
  - PSC patients with ANA or ASMA
  - PSC patients with AIH findings on histology
  - AIH patients with IBD
  - AIH patients with IBD and cholestatic profile
- Suboptimal response to steroid therapy

Abbreviation: AIH, autoimmune hepatitis.

Unfortunately, to date there is no medical therapy proved to cure or delay the progression of PSC. Liver transplantation is the only available curative therapy for PSC. Otherwise, the management of patients with PSC is centered on monitoring for and managing associated conditions, symptoms, and potential complications (**Box 2, Fig. 4**).

Primary Pharmacologic Therapy

To date, no medical therapy has been shown to be beneficial in PSC. Ursodeoxycholic acid (UDCA) has been the most investigated pharmacologic agent in PSC. In the 1990s, a randomized controlled trial of UDCA at a dose of 12 to 15 mg/kg/d in patients with PSC was associated with improved liver tests; however no beneficial effects on survival were demonstrated.[50] Subsequently, a placebo controlled trial of 219 patients testing a higher UCDA dose (17–23 mg/kg/d) suggested a trend toward improved survival, but statistical significance was not reached.[51] Recently, in a large 5-year randomized controlled trial of UCDA at 28 to 30 mg/kg/d, high dose UDCA was associated with improved liver enzymes but did not improve survival and was associated with a higher likelihood of undesirable endpoints including death and liver transplantation and higher rates of serious adverse events.[52] Based on this, high dose UDCA

Box 2
Special considerations in the clinical course of patients with PSC

Strong association with IBD

- Approximately 80% of patients with PSC have or will develop UC
- Up to 10% of patients with PSC have Crohn disease
- Approximately 5% of patients with IBD have or will develop PSC
- The course of IBD in the setting of PSC has unique features:
  - Higher prevalence of pancolitis
  - PSC is an added risk factor for colorectal cancer (CRC) in IBD
  - IBD may worsen or develop de novo after OLT

High risk of hepatobiliary malignancies

- High risk of CCA
  - High index of clinical suspicion warranted
  - Suspect if any clinical or laboratory deterioration occurs
  - Annual imaging and Ca19-9 recommended
- High risk of gallbladder cancer
  - Annual US to screen for gallbladder polyps
  - Cholecystectomy recommended regardless of polyp size
- High risk of CRC
  - Higher risk of CRC in patients with IBD-PSC
  - Colonoscopy at PSC diagnosis and every 1 year
- Risk of hepatocellular carcinoma (HCC)
  - Patients with cirrhosis due to PSC are at risk for HCC
  - Imaging every 6 months for surveillance in patients with cirrhosis

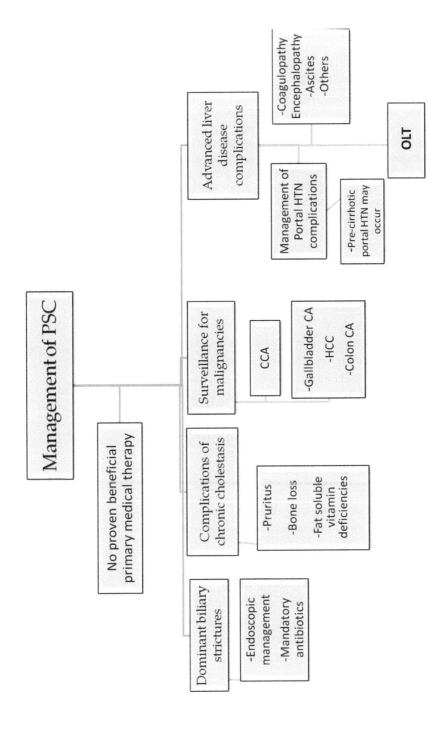

Fig. 4. Diagram summarizing the key aspects in the clinical management of PSC patients.

(28–30 mg/kg/d) should not be used in patients with PSC because it may be harm-ful,[43,52] and UDCA at the lower doses of 12 to 15 mg/kg/d should not be used either because there is clear evidence that it provides no survival benefit in PSC.[50] The avail-able data regarding "mid-dose" UDCA (17–23 mg/kg/d) are still unclear, and although it does not allow for any specific recommendations,[51,53] the possibility of future research trials reevaluating the potential role of "mid-dose" UDCA in PSC should not be ruled out. Current evidence does not support the recommendation of UDCA at any dose for the treatment of PSC.

Many other agents have been evaluated in small studies in PSC patients. No clear benefits of these agents in patients with PSC have been demonstrated in several small uncontrolled and some placebo controlled studies, including penicillamine, metho-trexate, colchicine, nicotine, budesonide, and others. Corticosteroids and other immunosuppressants are not recommended for use in PSC, except in specific cases of overlap with autoimmune hepatitis. Unfortunately, there is no pharmacologic therapy that is recommended at this time in PSC.

Dominant Biliary Strictures

Most patients with PSC (~50%) will develop dominant strictures during the course of their disease[36,54] and present with deterioration of liver tests, jaundice, worsening pruritus, bacterial cholangitis, or signs of decompensation. A dominant stricture is defined as a total or subtotal stenosis of the common duct (<1.5 mm) or of the left or right hepatic duct (<1 mm) close to the bifurcation.[55,56] Therapy to relieve the obstruction is indicated, and a prompt endoscopic approach is preferred when possible.[56] Repeated interventions are often needed. Balloon dilatation alone is preferred to dilatation with stent placement because a higher rate of complications is associated with stents in PSC patients.[43,56,57] High-grade stenoses greater than 2 cm above the bifurcation may not be amenable to endoscopic therapy. In those cases, if endoscopic therapy fails, percutaneous cholangiography, with or without stent placement, may be considered.[43,56,57] Successful dilatation of dominant biliary stric-tures results in rapid biochemical and clinical improvement. Furthermore, successful endoscopic therapy of biliary strictures also appears to be associated with improved survival as predicted by the Mayo Risk Score.[58–60]

Because of the risk of bacterial cholangitis, antibiotic therapy is mandatory at the time of any biliary intervention in patients with PSC. In addition, although most domi-nant strictures in patients with PSC are of benign nature, the possibility of CCA should be kept in mind; thus, brush cytology and biopsy to exclude malignancy should always be done before dilatation.

Patients who fail endoscopic and percutaneous treatment might be candidates, if noncirrhotic, to surgical management of dominant strictures with biliary bypass or resection of extrahepatic strictures with Roux-en-Y anastomosis.[61,62] However, thanks to advancement of endoscopic techniques, surgical management is now rarely required.

Complications Associated with Chronic Cholestasis

Pruritus

Pruritus is frequent in PSC, with approximately 30% of patients reporting pruritus at the time of PSC diagnosis.[34] Worsening of pruritus may be an indicator of a dominant stric-ture; therefore, this possibility should be excluded. If there is no dominant stricture, medical management of pruritus is indicated. Cholestyramine is the first choice of therapy,[53] at a dose of up to 12 g/d in 3 divided doses. Rifampin (150 to 300 mg by mouth twice per day) and opiate antagonists (eg, naltrexone, starting at 12.5 mg/d and increasing up to 50 mg/d) are alternative options in cases where cholestyramine fails or is not tolerated.

Metabolic bone disease

Bone loss is common in patients with PSC. Among patients with PSC, the prevalence of osteoporosis is 15%, and the prevalence of osteopenia without osteoporosis is 41%.[63] Nonpharmacologic interventions recommended in all PSC patients with osteopenia include weight bearing exercises and calcium and vitamin D supplementation. Bone mineral density screening should be done at diagnosis and subsequently every 2 to 3 years.[43] Bisphosphonates should be considered in PSC patients with proven osteoporosis, given the evidence of improved bone mineral density in patients with osteoporosis and primary biliary cirrhosis.[64]

Fat-soluble vitamin deficiencies

Fat-soluble vitamin deficiencies are common among patients with PSC, and the prevalence increases among patients with advanced disease.[65] Levels should be measured, particularly in patients with advanced disease, and replacement should be done as required.

Portal Hypertension

Portal hypertension may develop in patients with PSC as the disease progresses, and manifestations of portal hypertension complications may occur, including splenomegaly and associated cytopenias, portal hypertensive gastropathy, esophageal varices, gastric varices, ascites, peripheral edema, and portosystemic encephalopathy. A study of 283 patients with PSC reported a 36% prevalence of esophageal varices at endoscopy.[66] Low platelet count (150×10^3/dL or less) indicates a higher likelihood of esophageal varices.[66]

Although most patients with PSC with portal hypertension have established cirrhosis, noncirrhotic portal hypertension may occur in a small minority of cases, mostly related to nodular regenerative hyperplasia or obliterative portal venopathy.[67] Complications of noncirrhotic portal hypertension in patients with PSC should be managed in similar fashion to those of cirrhotic portal hypertension.

Cholangiocarcinoma

The development of CCA is one of the gravest complications of PSC. The annual rate of development of CCA in patients with PSC is 0.5% to 1%, and a 10-year cumulative risk of 7% to 10% has been reported.[68–70] In a significant proportion (up to 50%) of patients with CCA, the diagnosis is made within the first year of PSC diagnosis.[43,70,71]

A high index of suspicion is required for diagnosis, and CCA development should be suspected with patients with deterioration of clinical status, worsening liver tests, or elevated CA19-9 levels (>129) in the absence of bacterial cholangitis.[72] Patients in whom CCA is suspected should undergo imaging evaluation with MRI and ERC with biopsies and brushings for conventional cytology as well as fluorescence in situ hybridization and digital image analysis, if available.[43] The diagnosis of CCA is very difficult, partly because of the limited ability of imaging and cholangiographic studies to detect early stage CCA and also because of the limited sensitivity of conventional brush cytology studies.

The lack of highly sensitive and cost-effective diagnostic tests for CCA has limited the ability of issuing surveillance guidelines for CCA in patients with PSC. Expert opinion–based recommendations include maintaining a high index of suspicion for CCA and considering annual imaging and CA 19-9 in patients with PSC.[43]

Unfortunately, the survival of patients with PSC diagnosed with CCA is poor with overall mortality rate greater than 90% at 2 years.[68,73] This poor prognosis is partly because at the time of diagnosis most patients have multifocal or advanced stage disease. Chemotherapy options have shown limited effectiveness and are further limited by the advanced liver disease in PSC patients. The only potentially curative therapy approach for CCA, with reported survival up to 70% at 5 years, is an aggressive multimodal treatment approach of neoadjuvant chemoradiation followed by liver transplantation.[74] However, only a minority of patients with early stage CCA (<3 cm) and no evidence of metastatic disease are candidates for this therapy.

Other Malignancies

In addition to CCA, patients with PSC are at increased risk of developing additional hepatic and extrahepatic malignancies. A study of a cohort of 604 patients with PSC reported a frequency of 28.6% for all gastrointestinal cancers and 13.3% for hepatobiliary malignancies.[69]

Gallbladder cancer

The risk of gallbladder cancer is increased in patients with PSC.[68] Gallbladder abnormalities are common in PSC patients,[40] with approximately 6% of patients having gallbladder mass lesions on US[75] and 3% having gallbladder epithelial dysplasia in the absence of mass. The likelihood of malignancy in gallbladder polyps in PSC has been reported to be as high as 57%.[75] Because of this high risk of gallbladder malignancies, patients with PSC should undergo annual US to screen for mass lesions, and if these are identified, cholecystectomy is recommended independently of lesion size.[43]

Hepatocellular carcinoma

Patients with cirrhosis due to PSC are at risk for Hepatocellular carcinoma (HCC), with frequencies of 2% and 4% reported in 2 series.[69,76] Established guidelines for imaging surveillance and therapy of HCC should be followed.

Colorectal cancer

Patients with PSC and UC are at higher risk (odds ratio 4.79) of colorectal cancer (CRC) compared with UC patients without PSC[77,78] and appear to develop CRC at a younger age.[79] An increased risk for CRC has also been reported for PSC patients with Crohn disease.[80] A colonoscopy with biopsies should be done in all patients newly diagnosed with PSC even if there are no previous symptoms or history of IBD. Surveillance colonoscopy with biopsies should be done at 1 to 2-year intervals in patients with PSC and IBD (UC or Crohn disease) from the time of diagnosis of PSC.[43,53]

Liver Transplantation

Liver transplantation is the only curative therapy available for PSC. Survival rates at 5 years are excellent at approximately 85%.[81,82] The decision and timing for liver transplantation referral in PSC patients is in general similar to that of patients with other causes of advanced liver disease, predominantly centered on the model for end-stage liver disease score.[43] However, special prioritization may be granted through an appeal process to the United Network for Organ Sharing review board for PSC patients with unique indications including limited stage CCA,[74] intractable pruritus, and recurrent bacterial cholangitis.[43] Unfortunately, PSC can recur in the transplanted allograft in 20% of patients,[81,83] and it may be associated with diminished graft survival.[83]

After transplantation, patients with PSC are at higher risk of bone loss[84]; therefore, bone mineral density monitoring should continue in these patients in the posttransplant setting. Also, after transplantation, patients may develop de novo IBD, and those with concurrent IBD appear to be at increased risk of disease exacerbation.[85]

FEATURES OF IBD IN PATIENTS WITH PSC

As mentioned earlier, approximately 70% to 85% of patients with PSC have concurrent IBD,[27,28,30] most commonly UC. However, a smaller proportion of PSC patients (~7%) have Crohn disease, typically with extensive colonic involvement. The frequency of PSC among patients with IBD is of approximately 5%.[86]

Although in most cases IBD is diagnosed before the PSC diagnosis, IBD can first present years after the diagnosis of PSC. Several traits of IBD are significantly more common among patients with IBD in the setting of PSC compared with those with IBD without concurrent PSC.[87] These features include pancolitis with predominant right-sided disease, rectal sparing, mild clinical symptoms or a quiescent course, increased risk of pouchitis after ileal pouch-anal anastomosis, a unique risk of peristomal varices after ileostomy, and an increased risk of colorectal neoplasia as mentioned earlier.[87] The increased risk of CRC in patients with IBD and concomitant PSC and CRC surveillance recommendations were discussed earlier.

SUMMARY

PSC is an uncommon but challenging liver disease that affects patient survival. Mortality in patients with PSC is not only attributable to progression to end-stage liver disease but also to development of malignancies, mainly biliary and CRCs. Although some advances in better understanding the pathogenesis and natural history of PSC have been made, to date, no effective therapeutic agent has been identified. Liver transplantation remains the only potentially curative option. Priority should be given to research efforts that will lead to the development or identification of effective medical therapies that would delay or halt disease progression, as well as toward determining an effective strategy to detect biliary malignancy much earlier in these patients.

REFERENCES

1. Quigley EM, LaRusso NF, Ludwig J, et al. Familial occurrence of primary sclerosing cholangitis and ulcerative colitis. Gastroenterology 1983;85:1160–5.
2. Bergquist A, Montgomery SM, Bahmanyar S, et al. Increased risk of primary sclerosing cholangitis and ulcerative colitis in first-degree relatives of patients with primary sclerosing cholangitis. Clin Gastroenterol Hepatol 2008;6:939–43.
3. Karlsen TH, Kaser A. Deciphering the genetic predisposition to primary sclerosing cholangitis. Semin Liver Dis 2011;31:188–207.
4. Melum E, Franke A, Schramm C, et al. Genome-wide association analysis in primary sclerosing cholangitis identifies two non-HLA susceptibility loci. Nat Genet 2011;43:17–9.
5. Karlsen TH, Franke A, Melum E, et al. Genome-wide association analysis in primary sclerosing cholangitis. Gastroenterology 2010;138:1102–11.
6. Folseraas T, Melum E, Rausch P, et al. Extended analysis of a genome-wide association study in primary sclerosing cholangitis detects multiple novel risk loci. J Hepatol 2012;57:366–75.

7. Spurkland A, Saarinen S, Boberg KM, et al. HLA class II haplotypes in primary sclerosing cholangitis patients from five European populations. Tissue Antigens 1999;53:459 69.

8. Wiencke K, Karlsen TH, Boberg KM, et al. Primary sclerosing cholangitis is associated with extended HLA-DR3 and HLA-DR6 haplotypes. Tissue Antigens 2007; 69:161–9.

9. Naess S, Shiryaev A, Hov JR, et al. Genetics in primary sclerosing cholangitis. Clin Res Hepatol Gastroenterol 2012;36(4):325–33.

10. Hashimoto E, Lindor KD, Homburger HA, et al. Immunohistochemical characterization of hepatic lymphocytes in primary biliary cirrhosis in comparison with primary sclerosing cholangitis and autoimmune chronic active hepatitis. Mayo Clin Proc 1993;68:1049–55.

11. Snook JA, Chapman RW, Sachdev GK, et al. Peripheral blood and portal tract lymphocyte populations in primary sclerosing cholangitis. J Hepatol 1989;9(1): 36–41.

12. Leon MP, Bassendine MF, Wilson JL, et al. Immunogenicity of biliary epithelium: investigation of antigen presentation to CD4+ cells. Hepatology 1996;24:561–7.

13. Angulo P, Peter JB, Gershwin ME, et al. Serum autoantibodies in patients with primary sclerosing cholangitis. J Hepatol 2000;32:182–7.

14. Terjung B, Sohne J, Lechtenberg B, et al. p-ANCAs in autoimmune liver disorders recognise human beta-tubulin isotype 5 and cross-react with microbial protein FtsA. Gut 2010;59:808–16.

15. Saarinen S, Olerup O, Broome U. Increased frequency of autoimmune diseases in patients with primary sclerosing cholangitis. Am J Gastroenterol 2000;95: 3195–9.

16. Bodenheimer HC Jr, LaRusso NF, Thayer WR Jr, et al. Elevated circulating immune complexes in primary sclerosing cholangitis. Hepatology 1983;3:150–4.

17. Senaldi G, Donaldson PT, Magrin S, et al. Activation of the complement system in primary sclerosing cholangitis. Gastroenterology 1989;97:1430–4.

18. Worthington J, Cullen S, Chapman R. Immunopathogenesis of primary sclerosing cholangitis. Clin Rev Allergy Immunol 2005;28:93–103.

19. Sasatomi K, Noguchi K, Sakisaka S, et al. Abnormal accumulation of endotoxin in biliary epithelial cells in primary biliary cirrhosis and primary sclerosing cholangitis. J Hepatol 1998;29:409–16.

20. Escorsell A, Pares A, Rodes J, et al. Epidemiology of primary sclerosing cholangitis in Spain. Spanish Association for the Study of the Liver. J Hepatol 1994;21: 787–91.

21. Levy C, Lindor KD. Primary sclerosing cholangitis: epidemiology, natural history, and prognosis. Semin Liver Dis 2006;26:22–30.

22. Bowlus CL, Li CS, Karlsen TH, et al. Primary sclerosing cholangitis in genetically diverse populations listed for liver transplantation: unique clinical and human leukocyte antigen associations. Liver Transpl 2010;16:1324–30.

23. Mitchell SA, Thuecon M, Orchard TR, et al. Cigarette smoking, appendectomy, and tonsillectomy as risk factors for the development of primary sclerosing cholangitis: a case control study. Gut 2002;51:567–73.

24. Loftus EV, Sandborn WJ, Tremaine WJ, et al. Primary sclerosing cholangitis is associated with nonsmoking: a case-control study. Gastroenterology 1996;110: 1496–502.

25. Van Erpecum KJ, Smits SJ, van de Meeberg PC, et al. Risk of primary sclerosing cholangitis is associated with nonsmoking behavior. Gastroenterology 1996;110: 1503–6.

26. Boonstra K, Beuers U, Ponsioen CY. Epidemiology of primary sclerosing cholangitis and primary biliary cirrhosis: a systematic review. J Hepatol 2012;56:1181–8.

27. Bambha K, Kim WR, Talwalkar J, et al. Incidence, clinical spectrum, and outcomes of primary sclerosing cholangitis in a United States community. Gastroenterology 2003;125:1364–9.

28. Boberg KM, Aadland E, Jahnsen J, et al. Incidence and prevalence of primary biliary cirrhosis, primary sclerosing cholangitis, and autoimmune hepatitis in a Norwegian population. Scand J Gastroenterol 1998;33:99–103.

29. Hurlburt KJ, McMahon BJ, Deubner H, et al. Prevalence of autoimmune liver disease in Alaska natives. Am J Gastroenterol 2002;97:2402–7.

30. Kaplan GG, Laupland KB, Butzner D, et al. The burden of large and small duct primary sclerosing cholangitis in adults and children: a population based analysis. Am J Gastroenterol 2007;102:1042–9.

31. Lindkvist B, Benito V, Gullberg B, et al. Incidence and prevalence of primary sclerosing cholangitis in a defined adult population in Sweden. Hepatology 2010;52: 571–7.

32. Kingham JG, Kochar N, Gravenor MB. Incidence, clinical patterns, and outcomes of primary sclerosing cholangitis in South Wales, United Kingdom. Gastroenterology 2004;126:1929–30.

33. Ponsioen CY, Vrouenraets SM, Prawirodirdjo W, et al. Natural history of primary sclerosing cholangitis and prognostic value of cholangiography in a Dutch population. Gut 2002;51:562–6.

34. Broome U, Olsson R, Loof L, et al. Natural history and prognostic factors in 305 Swedish patients with primary sclerosing cholangitis. Gut 1996;38:610–5.

35. Lee YM, Kaplan MM. Primary sclerosing cholangitis. N Engl J Med 1995;332: 924–33.

36. Tischendorf JJ, Hecker H, Kruger M, et al. Characterization, outcome and prognosis in 273 patients with primary sclerosing cholangitis: a single center study. Am J Gastroenterol 2007;102:107–14.

37. Boberg KM, Fausa O, Haaland T, et al. Features of autoimmune hepatitis in primary sclerosing cholangitis: an evaluation of 114 primary sclerosing cholangitis patients according to a scoring system for the diagnosis of autoimmune hepatitis. Hepatology 1996;23:1369–76.

38. Hov JR, Boberg KM, Karlsen TH. Autoantibodies in primary sclerosing cholangitis. World J Gastroenterol 2008;14:3781–91.

39. Van de Meeberg PC, Portincasa P, Wolfhagen FH, et al. Increased gall bladder volume in primary sclerosing cholangitis. Gut 1996;39:594–9.

40. Said K, Glaumann H, Bergquist A. Gallbladder disease in patients with primary sclerosing cholangitis. J Hepatol 2008;48:598–605.

41. Johnson KJ, Olliff JF, Olliff JP. The presence and significance of lymphadenopathy detected by CT in primary sclerosing cholangitis. Br J Radiol 1998;71:1279–82.

42. MacCarty RL, LaRusso NF, Wiesner RH, et al. Primary sclerosing cholangitis: findings on cholangiography and pancreatography. Radiology 1983;149:39–44.

43. Chapman R, Fevery J, Kalloo A, et al. Diagnosis and management of primary sclerosing cholangitis. AASLD practice guidelines. Hepatology 2010;51:660–78.

44. Angulo P, Pearce DH, Johnson CD, et al. Magnetic resonance imaging in patients with biliary disease: its role in primary sclerosing cholangitis. J Hepatol 2000;33: 520–7.

45. Berstad AE, Abakken L, Smith HJ, et al. Diagnostic accuracy of magnetic resonance and endoscopic retrograde cholangiography in primary sclerosing cholangitis. Clin Gastroenterol Hepatol 2006;4:514–20.

46. Fulcher AS, Turner MA, Franklin KJ, et al. Primary sclerosing cholangitis: evaluation with MR cholangiography - a case-control study. Radiology 2000;215:71–80.
47. Burak KW, Angulo P, Lindor KD. Is there a role for liver biopsy in primary sclerosing cholangitis? Am J Gastroenterol 2003;98:1155–8.
48. Bjornsson E, Olsson R, Bergquist A, et al. The natural history of small duct primary sclerosing cholangitis. Gastroenterology 2008;134:975–80.
49. Angulo P, Maor-Kendler Y, Lindor KD. Small-duct primary sclerosing cholangitis: a long term follow up study. Hepatology 2002;35:1494–500.
50. Lindor KD. Ursodiol for primary sclerosing cholangitis. N Engl J Med 1997;336: 691–5.
51. Olsson R, Boberg KM, de Muckadell OS, et al. High-dose ursodeoxycholic acid in primary sclerosing cholangitis: a 5-year multicenter, randomized, controlled study. Gastroenterology 2005;129:1464–72.
52. Lindor KD, Kowdley KV, Luketic VA, et al. High-dose ursodeoxycholic acid for the treatment of primary sclerosing cholangitis. Hepatology 2009;50:808–14.
53. European Association for the Study of the Liver. EASL Clinical Practice Guidelines: management of cholestatic liver diseases. J Hepatol 2009;51:237–67.
54. Okolicsanyi L, Fabris L, Viaggi S, et al. Primary sclerosing cholangitis: clinical presentations, natural history and prognostic variables: an Italian multicenter study. Eur J Gastroenterol Hepatol 1996;8:685–91.
55. Bjornsson E, Lindqvist-Ottosson J, Asztely M, et al. Dominant strictures in patients with primary sclerosing cholangitis. Am J Gastroenterol 2004;99:502–8.
56. Gotthardt D, Stiehl A. Endoscopic retrograde cholangiopancreatography in diagnosis and treatment of primary sclerosing cholangitis. Clin Liver Dis 2010;14: 349–58.
57. Kaya M, Petersen BT, Angulo P, et al. Balloon dilation compared to stenting of dominant strictures in primary sclerosing cholangitis. Am J Gastroenterol 2001; 96:1059–66.
58. Stiehl A, Rudolph G, Sauer P, et al. Development of dominant bile duct stenoses in patients with primary sclerosing cholangitis treated with ursodeoxycholic acid: outcome after endoscopic treatment. J Hepatol 2002;36:151–6.
59. Gluck M, Cantone NR, Brandabur JJ, et al. A twenty-year experience with endoscopic therapy for symptomatic primary sclerosing cholangitis. J Clin Gastroenterol 2008;42:1032–9.
60. Baluyut AR, Sherman S, Lehman GA, et al. Impact of endoscopic therapy on the survival of patients with primary sclerosing cholangitis. Gastrointest Endosc 2001;53:308–12.
61. Cameron JL, Pitt HA, Zinner MJ, et al. Resection of hepatic duct bifurcation and transhepatic stenting for sclerosing cholangitis. Ann Surg 1988;207:614–22.
62. Myburgh JA. Surgical biliary drainage in primary sclerosing cholangitis. The role of the Hepp-Couinaud approach. Arch Surg 1994;129:1057–62.
63. Angulo P, Therneau TM, Jorgesen A, et al. Bone disease in patients with primary sclerosing cholangitis. prevalence, severity and prediction of progression. J Hepatol 1998;29:729–35.
64. Zein CO, Jorgensen RA, Clarke B, et al. Alendronate improves bone mineral density in primary biliary cirrhosis: a randomized placebo-controlled trial. Hepatology 2005;42:762–71.
65. Jorgensen RA, Lindor KD, Sartin JS, et al. Serum lipid and fat-soluble vitamin levels in primary sclerosing cholangitis. J Clin Gastroenterol 1995;20:215–9.
66. Zein CO, Lindor KD, Angulo P. Prevalence and predictors of esophageal varices in patients with primary sclerosing cholangitis. Hepatology 2004;39:204–10.

67. Abraham SC, Kamath PS, Eghtesad B, et al. Liver transplantation in precirrhotic biliary tract disease: portal hypertension is frequently associated with nodular regenerative hyperplasia and obliterative portal venopathy. Am J Surg Pathol 2006;30:1454–61.

68. Boberg KM, Lind GE. Primary sclerosing cholangitis and malignancy. Best Pract Res Clin Gastroenterol 2011;25:753–64.

69. Bergquist A, Ekbom A, Olsson R, et al. Hepatic and extrahepatic malignancies in primary sclerosing cholangitis. J Hepatol 2002;36:321–7.

70. Burak K, Angulo P, Pasha TM, et al. Incidence and risk factors for cholangiocarcinoma in primary sclerosing cholangitis. Am J Gastroenterol 2004;99:523–6.

71. Claessen MM, Vleggaar FP, Tytgat KM, et al. High lifetime risk of cancer in primary sclerosing cholangitis. J Hepatol 2009;50:158–64.

72. Levy C, Lymp J, Angulo P, et al. The value of serum CA 19-9 in predicting cholangiocarcinoma in patients with primary sclerosing cholangitis. Dig Dis Sci 2005; 50:1734–40.

73. Kaya M, deGroen PC, Angulo P, et al. Treatment of cholangiocarcinoma complicating primary sclerosing cholangitis: the Mayo Clinic experience. Am J Gastroenterol 2001;96:1164–9.

74. Gores GJ, Nagorney DM, Rosen CB. Cholangiocarcinoma: is transplantation an option? for whom? J Hepatol 2007;47:455–9.

75. Buckles DC, Lindor KD, LaRusso NF. In primary sclerosing cholangitis gallbladder polyps are frequently malignant. Am J Gastroenterol 2002;97: 1138–42.

76. Harnois DM, Gores GJ, Ludwig J, et al. Are patients with cirrhotic stage primary sclerosing cholangitis at risk for the development of hepatocellular cancer? J Hepatol 1997;27:512–6.

77. Broome U, Lofberg R, Veress B, et al. Primary sclerosing cholangitis and ulcerative colitis: evidence for increased neoplastic potential. Hepatology 1995;22: 1404–8.

78. Soetikno RM, Lin OS, Heidenreich PA, et al. Increased risk of colorectal neoplasia in patients with primary sclerosing cholangitis and ulcerative colitis: a meta-analysis. Gastrointest Endosc 2002;56:48–54.

79. Brackmann S, Andersen SN, Aamodt G, et al. Relationship between clinical parameters and the colitis-colorectal cancer interval in a cohort of patients with colorectal cancer in inflammatory bowel disease. Scand J Gastroenterol 2009; 44(1):46–55.

80. Lindstrom L, Lapidus A, Ost A, et al. Increased risk of colorectal cancer and dysplasia in patients with Chrohn's colitis and primary sclerosing cholangitis. Dis Colon Rectum 2011;54:1392–7.

81. Graziadei IW, Wiesner RH, Marotta PJ, et al. Long term results of patients undergoing liver transplantation for primary sclerosing cholangitis. Hepatology 1999; 30:1121–7.

82. Wiesner RH. Liver transplantation for primary sclerosing cholangitis: timing, outcome, impact of inflammatory bowel disease and recurrence of disease. Best Pract Res Clin Gastroenterol 2001;15:667–80.

83. Campsen J, Zimmerman MA, Trotte JF, et al. Clinically recurrent primary sclerosing cholangitis following liver transplantation: a time course. Liver Transpl 2008;14:181–5.

84. Guichelaar MM, Kendall R, Malinchoc M, et al. Bone mineral density before and after OLT: long term follow up and predictive factors. Liver Transpl 2006;12: 1390–402.

85. Dvorchik I, Subotin M, Demetris AJ, et al. Effect of liver transplantation on inflammatory bowel disease in patients with primary sclerosing cholangitis. Hepatology 2002;35:380–4.
86. Mendes FD, Levy C, Enders FB, et al. Abnormal hepatic biochemistries in patients with inflammatory bowel disease. Am J Gastroenterol 2007;102:344–50.
87. Loftus EV, Harewood GC, Loftus CG, et al. PSC-IBD: a unique form of inflammatory bowel disease associated with primary sclerosing cholangitis. Gut 2005;54: 91–6.

Primary Biliary Cirrhosis
Therapeutic Advances

Frank Czul, MD[a], Adam Peyton, DO[b], Cynthia Levy, MD[b],*

KEYWORDS

- Primary biliary cirrhosis • Therapeutics • Ursodeoxycholic acid • Fibrates
- 6α-Ethyl-chenodeoxycholic acid

KEY POINTS

- Ursodeoxycholic acid is the only US Food and Drug Administration–approved medical treatment for PBC, and it is associated with significant biochemical, histologic, and survival benefits.
- The only definitive treatment for end-stage primary biliary cirrhosis (PBC) is liver transplantation.
- Approximately 40% of patients with PBC respond incompletely to treatment with ursodeoxycholic acid.
- Several agents show promise in the treatment of "poorly responsive" PBC, including obeticholic acid, fibrates, tetrathiomolybdate, and rituximab.

INTRODUCTION

Primary biliary cirrhosis (PBC) is an autoimmune liver disease characterized by progressive destruction of intrahepatic bile ducts associated with cholestasis, portal inflammation, and fibrosis, which may lead to biliary cirrhosis, portal hypertension, and eventually to liver transplantation or death.[1] Histologically, focal bile duct lymphocytic infiltration and destruction with granuloma formation, termed the florid duct lesion, are considered essentially pathognomonic for PBC. Although the exact pathogenetic mechanism of PBC remains incompletely understood, PBC is thought to result from a combination of genetic predisposition and environmental triggers.[2]

The disease predominantly affects women, who are usually diagnosed in their 50s while in an asymptomatic state. Epidemiologic studies indicate annual incidence rates for PBC between 0.7 and 49 cases/1 million population and prevalence rates between

Disclosures: No competing interests to disclose.
a Department of Medicine, University of Miami Miller School of Medicine, Room 600D, Central Building, 1611 NW 12th Avenue, Miami, FL 33101, USA; b Division of Hepatology, University of Miami Miller School of Medicine, Miami, FL, USA
* Corresponding author. Division of Hepatology, Schiff Center for Liver Diseases, University of Miami Miller School of Medicine, 1500 Northwest 12th Avenue, Suite 1101, Miami, FL 33136.
E-mail address: clevy@med.miami.edu

Clin Liver Dis 17 (2013) 229–242
http://dx.doi.org/10.1016/j.cld.2012.12.003
1089-3261/13/$ – see front matter © 2013 Elsevier Inc. All rights reserved.

liver.theclinics.com

6.7 and 402 cases/1 million population.[3] In the United States, national estimates for incidence and prevalence of PBC are ≈3500 new cases each year with 47,000 prevalent cases among the white population.[4]

Individuals with asymptomatic disease consist of 20% to 60% of all first-time diagnoses, based largely on increased use of screening liver biochemistry studies.[5] It has been suggested that symptoms develop within 5 years in most asymptomatic patients, although one third of patients may remain symptom free for many years. However, at 20 years after diagnosis, less than 5% remain asymptomatic.[6] Pruritus and fatigue are early symptoms and occur in 20% to 50% of patients.[7] Although it seems that symptomatic individuals may have poorer outcomes compared with asymptomatic patients, it is the cumulative development of complications of end-stage liver disease and portal hypertension that has been consistently associated with decreased survival.[6] PBC can be divided into 3 distinct phases (**Fig. 1**) and, as each phase advances, survival or time to transplantation diminishes.[8] Liver failure (ascites, variceal bleeding, hepatic encephalopathy, or hyperbilirubinemia >6 mg/dL) has been estimated to occur in 15% at 5 years according to a large community-based study of 770 patients in northeast England.[6]

The diagnosis of PBC is suspected based on cholestatic serum liver tests and largely confirmed by the presence of antimitochondrial antibodies (AMA), which are directed against the E2 subunit of the pyruvate dehydrogenase complex found in the inner mitochondrial membrane. Considered the serologic hallmark of PBC, AMA positivity is detected in 90% to 95% of patients with PBC and less than 1% of normal control subjects.[9,10] Several AMA subtypes have been described, with the M2 subtype being the most specific for PBC.[11,12]

In the small subset of AMA-negative patients with PBC, up to 85% will test positive for antinuclear antibodies that are frequently PBC specific, such as the anti-gp210 (rimlike pattern) and anti-sp100 (multiple nuclear dot pattern).[13–15] However, in general, patients who are AMA negative have similar clinical, biochemical, and histologic features compared with AMA-positive patients, and they have similar response rates to ursodeoxycholic acid (UDCA) therapy.[16,17] In unclear cases when both AMA and antinuclear antibodies may be negative, a liver biopsy can be used to substantiate and to assist in the diagnosis, while also providing important prognostic information.

PBC has 4 histologic stages (**Table 1**), but the liver is not affected uniformly and a single biopsy sample may demonstrate the presence of different stages of the

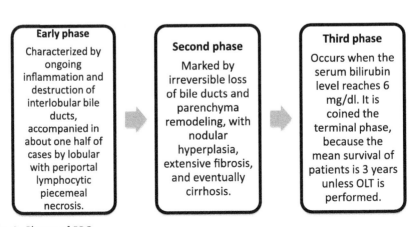

Fig. 1. Phases of PBC.

Table 1
Histologic characteristics and staging of PBC
Stage 1	Inflammation localized to portal triads; florid duct lesion may be seen
Stage 2	Extension of inflammation beyond the portal triads into the lobular parenchyma and reduction in number of normal bile ducts
Stage 3	Fibrous septa linking adjacent portal tracts
Stage 4	Biliary cirrhosis

disease. If this is the case, the most advanced stage of those present is assigned, according to convention.[18]

MANAGEMENT

The management of PBC encompasses disease-specific therapy, symptomatic treatment, and the management of end-stage liver disease complications. This article will focus on disease-specific treatment strategies. All patients with PBC and abnormal liver biochemistry should be considered for specific therapy.

Medical Therapy

UDCA

UDCA is the only drug approved for primary biliary cirrhosis by the US Food and Drug Administration.[19] UDCA, the 7-β epimer of chenodeoxycholic, is a hydrophilic naturally occurring bile acid that seems to have fewer hepatotoxic properties than endogenous bile acids.[20]

Mechanism of action Bile duct destruction leads to the retention of hydrophobic bile acids within the hepatocyte, most likely contributing to the gradual deterioration in liver function observed in patients with PBC. After oral administration, UDCA may reduce the ileal absorption of these endogenous bile acids by competitive inhibition at the level of the terminal ileum.[21] Eventually, UDCA and its conjugates become the predominant bile acids in bile, accounting for up to 60% of the total biliary bile acids.[22] In humans, the half-life of UDCA is 3.5 to 5.8 days, and the predominant route of elimination from the body is via feces.[23]

Multiple mechanisms of action have been proposed in experimental models (**Fig. 2**). In rat livers, UDCA has been shown to promote choleresis by (1) down-regulating bile acids uptake through basolateral membrane, (2) up-regulating synthesis and insertion of basolateral and canalicular export pumps, and (3) down-regulating bile acid synthesis.[24] In addition, UDCA modulates the expression of enzymes involved in bile acid metabolism. Thus, UDCA may exert beneficial effects in cholestatic liver disease by stimulating the elimination of toxic compounds from the hepatocytes and reducing cytotoxicity of bile acids. Of interest, such transcriptional regulatory effect by UDCA is mediated at least in part through nuclear receptors Pregnane X receptor (PXR) and farnesoid X receptor (FXR), as reviewed in an article by Emina Halilbasic and colleagues elsewhere in this issue.

Furthermore, UDCA has antiapoptotic properties, which are of great interest given the role of apoptotic bodies in perpetuating autoantigen production in PBC,[24,25] and exerts immunomodulatory effects by reversing aberrant expression of human leukocyte antigen class I molecules on hepatocytes and class II on cholangiocytes.[24,26]

Dosage The approved dosage in the United States is 13 to 15 mg/kg/d. Some studies initially used a regimen of administration 3 or 4 times a day, but it has been shown

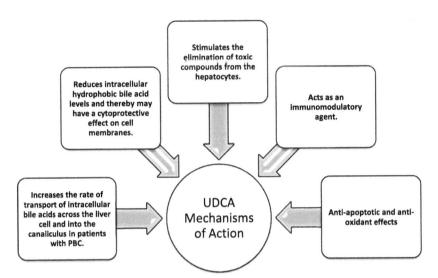

Fig. 2. Overview of the mechanisms of action of UDCA. The effects of UDCA in liver are multifaceted and correlated. Certainly, each of these proposed mechanisms might have varying contributions in different hepatobiliary disorders.

that a regimen of once or twice a day provides equivalent results. Anecdotal experience at the Mayo Clinic suggests that initiation of the drug at the full dose may precipitate pruritus and loose stool, but a gradual initiation of the drug during a period of 1 to 2 weeks eliminates these problems. Thus, for example, therapy might be started at a dosage of 250 mg/d with an increase in the dose every 3 to 4 days until the target dosage of 13 to 15 mg/kg/d is reached.[20]

Efficacy Without UDCA, the median survival free of liver transplantation is 10 to 15 years, which is poorer than that of an age- and sex-matched control population.[4,6,27]

Several randomized trials, combined analyses, and long-term observational studies have shown that UDCA not only improves biochemical liver indices[28,29] but also delays histologic progression, delays development of esophageal varices, and prolongs survival without liver transplantation.[30,31] Most studies indicate that patients treated with the recommended dosage of UDCA for a sufficient period have longer survival free of transplantation and overall survival, particularly the group of patients who have biochemical response to UDCA.[8]

Further corroborating the beneficial effect of UDCA on the survival of patients with PBC, the proportion of liver transplantations performed for PBC and the proportion of patients with PBC currently on a wait list for a transplant have been decreasing in the recent decades in both the United States and Europe.[32,33] Likewise, the percentage of transplantations for PBC decreased from 11.5% to 4.5% in the Netherlands, which may be at least in part because of an effect of UDCA on survival.[34]

Suboptimal response to UDCA Results of therapy can be monitored through the analysis of serum liver biochemistries. An initial response is typically followed by slow, continued improvement. Among responders to UDCA, an initial improvement will usually be seen within 1 month to 6 weeks. Most of the expected improvement will occur within 3 months of therapy initiation. However, normalization of biochemical values will occur within 2 years in only 20% of patients; such normalization will occur in an additional 15% of patients after 5 years.[35]

Observational studies have shown that the biochemical response to UDCA correlates with the long-term outcome. Biochemical response has been defined in varying ways (**Table 2**), but this is an evolving field and a uniform set of criteria to define response to UDCA is yet to be determined.[28,36–40] Regardless of how biochemical response is defined, ≈40% of patients with PBC respond incompletely to treatment with UDCA.[41] Nonresponders can be identified by their persistently abnormal liver biochemical tests and/or worsening liver histology despite treatment with UDCA for at least 12 months.

Numerous combination regimens have been studied to manage incomplete responders. Importantly, an increment in the dose of UDCA in patients who had incomplete response to UDCA was not found to be of any benefit in this subpopulation of patients.[42]

Methotrexate

Methotrexate (MTX) is an antimetabolite, immunosuppressive agent with anti-inflammatory effects. MTX has been extensively evaluated in patients with PBC, and data are conflicting.

In a double-blind randomized placebo-controlled study by Combes and colleagues[43] in 2005, MTX therapy was added to UDCA without evidence of a clinically important benefit of MTX therapy on transplant-free survival, time to clinical deterioration, or time to subclinical progression. Furthermore, there was no discernible benefit of MTX on prevalence of varices or histologic liver stage. On the other hand, there was also no evidence of substantial toxic effects of MTX therapy, beyond a slight increase in low-grade bone marrow suppression.

A recent Cochrane database meta-analysis including 370 patients shows that MTX compared with placebo has no significant effect on mortality or liver transplantation in patients with PBC. Moreover, despite an apparent improvement in pruritus scores, the drug failed to show a positive effect on biochemical markers.[44] Thus, given the potential for substantial adverse effects and the paucity of data supporting the use of MTX, this drug cannot be routinely recommended at this time.

Colchicine

Colchicine is a plant alkaloid shown to inhibit migration of granulocytes into inflamed areas and decrease metabolic and phagocytic activity of granulocytes. In addition, colchicine is an antimitotic and antifibrotic agent that retards the microtubule-mediated transport of procollagen and enhances collagenase activity.

Table 2	
Definition of biochemical response to UDCA in patients with PBC	
Criteria	**Definition**
Paris I	ALP <3 times ULN, aspartate aminotransferase <2 times ULN and bilirubin ≤1 mg/dL after 1 y of UDCA
Barcelona	ALP decline of >40% toward baseline value or a normal level after 1 y of UDCA treatment
Rotterdam	Normalization of bilirubin and albumin concentrations after treatment with UDCA when one or both parameters were abnormal before treatment, or normal bilirubin or albumin concentrations after treatment when both were abnormal at entry
Paris II	ALP and aspartate aminotransferase ≤1.5 times ULN and normal total bilirubin after 1 y of UDCA therapy
Toronto	ALP <1.67 times ULN at 2 y of UDCA therapy

Despite early excitement, a Cochrane meta-analysis from 2004 performed a combined analysis of 8 trials comparing colchicine versus placebo and demonstrated no significant difference in the rates of death or liver transplantation. On this meta-analysis, the same outcome was evaluated comparing colchicine plus UDCA versus placebo plus UDCA, again demonstrating no benefit of adding colchicine.[45] However, in a recent follow-up study, Leung and colleagues[46] showed, albeit in a small subset (N = 18), that treatment with the combination of UDCA and colchicine led to sustained clinical remission in 60% of the patients, perhaps indicating that this combination may be beneficial in a highly selected subgroup of patients.

Azathioprine

Azathioprine is an immunosuppressant, suppressing delayed hypersensitivity and cellular cytotoxicity more than antibody responses. The immunosuppressive action of azathioprine depends on its conversion to active 6-mercaptopurine by thiopurine S-methyl-transferase.

Azathioprine has been used for patients with PBC, but the therapeutic responses in randomized clinical trials have been conflicting. In light of insufficient evidence to support use of azathioprine for patients with PBC, this drug is currently only considered for patients with overlap syndrome with autoimmune hepatitis. Because patients with a thiopurine methyl-transferase deficiency could potentially have life-threatening hematopoietic toxicity, prescription of azathioprine should be monitored by laboratory tests, including full blood count and liver function.[47]

Budesonide

Budesonide is a nonhalogenated glucocorticoid absorbed in the small intestine. Of an oral dose, 90% is metabolized during the first liver pass in healthy individuals. After hepatic uptake, budesonide is metabolized to 2 major metabolites: 16-hydroxy-prednisolone and 6-hydroxy-budesonide. Glucocorticoid activity of these metabolites is only 1% to 10%. Compared with prednisolone, glucocorticoid receptor binding activity of budesonide is 15 to 20 times higher, so its effect on liver inflammation may be greater. In patients with inflammatory bowel disease, oral budesonide has been shown to exert fewer systemic side effects than do conventional corticosteroids.[48]

A multicenter randomized open study of 3 years' duration showed budesonide (6 mg/d) combined with UDCA to be more effective in improving and stabilizing the stage of liver histology than did UDCA alone in patients with stage I to III PBC. Fibrosis, assessed by both liver histology and serum amino-terminal propeptide of type III procollagen, decreased significantly in the combination group.[49] Leuschner and colleagues[50] had previously shown the same positive effect of combination therapy on liver histology (stage, fibrosis, and inflammation) and laboratory values but with a higher dose of budesonide (9 mg/d) during 2 years of therapy.

Combination therapy may be beneficial for all patients with PBC with precirrhotic liver disease, but for asymptomatic patients with stable early PBC who are receiving UDCA therapy, the potential systemic glucocorticoid effects would carry an unnecessary risk for diabetes and osteoporosis during long-term use. Patients with stage IV PBC are no longer subjects for combination therapy because significant increases in budesonide plasma levels were observed in late-stage PBC and were associated with serious side effects. Moreover, with the use of budesonide in cirrhotic patients, a concern exists for increasing the risk of portal vein thrombosis.[51]

Mycophenolate mofetil

Mycophenolate mofetil (MMF) is an ester prodrug of mycophenolic acid that inhibits inosine monophosphate dehydrogenase and guanylate synthetase. Disruption of the de novo purine synthetic pathway results in T- and B-lymphocyte fixation in the S phase of the cell cycle, resulting in failure to proliferate.[52] A pilot investigation performed by Talwarkar and colleagues[53] in 2006 demonstrated that adjuvant therapy with oral MMF at a dosage up to 3 g/d is not associated with significant clinical benefit in patients with incomplete response to UDCA monotherapy. Despite statistically significant differences between end-of-treatment and baseline values of serum alkaline phosphatase (ALP), only 37% of patients experienced at least a 30% reduction in serum levels. Most patients tolerated MMF with no serious adverse effects.

Tetrathiomolybdate

Tetrathiomolybdate (TM), which is an anticopper drug, was developed originally for treating the neurologic presentation of Wilson disease. TM has antiangiogenic, antifibrotic, anti-inflammatory, and immunomodulatory effects.[54]

In a double-blind, placebo-controlled trial involving 28 patients with PBC and incomplete response to UDCA, TM met the predefined primary outcome measures for efficacy. TM therapy significantly reduced alanine aminotransferase and aspartate aminotransferase levels compared with the placebo group but did not cause reduction in serum ALP.[54] Instead, it led to a significant drop in serum levels of tumor necrosis factor-α. During therapy averaging a little longer than 1 year in 13 patients taking TM, 7 cases of bone marrow suppression were reported. These events were expected given the degree of copper depletion that investigators attempted to achieve. Copper depletion, if excessive, lowers bone marrow hematopoiesis. Nevertheless, these episodes were easily overcome by drug holiday and dose reduction.[54] TM needs to be further evaluated in larger clinical trials to determine whether it improves survival and time to transplantation.

Orthotopic Liver Transplantation

PBC is a common, albeit decreasing, indication for liver transplantation. Untreated asymptomatic patients can expect median survival of 10 to 16 years, whereas in symptomatic patients this drops to 7 years.[55] Several prognostic models have been developed to predict survival in the absence of transplantation, but these models are rarely applied to individual patients.

The liver transplantation burden of PBC in the United States decreased between 1995 and 2006. This is despite an increase in total liver transplantations. The absolute number of liver transplantations in the United States increased an average of 249 transplants per year. However, the absolute number of transplants performed for PBC decreased an average of 5.4 cases per year. The trends for the absolute number of individuals added to the transplant wait list showed a similar pattern: (1) an increase in total listings for transplants of all diagnoses ($\beta = 265$; $P = .001$) and (2) a decrease in PBC ($\beta = -12.1$; $P<.001$).[32]

The prevalence of recurrent PBC post transplant ranges between 9% and 35% with a mean time that ranges between 1.6 and 6.5 years.[56] Factors proposed to affect the rate of recurrence include increased donor and recipient age, increased warm ischemia time, male recipient gender, use of tacrolimus as the mainstay for immunosuppression, and specific human leukocyte antigen alleles in donor and recipient.[32,57] Alternatively, use of azathioprine may be associated with protection against recurrence.[57] In the most recent era, higher rates of recurrence have been described compared with the prior decade: 10-year cumulative recurrence rate 55% to 70% versus 13% to 20%, respectively. This effect is likely a result of increased awareness of recurrent PBC as a clinical entity and widespread use of tacrolimus as preferential immunosuppression since 1999.[56] Despite the possibility of recurrence, OLT has greatly improved survival in patients with PBC with a reported survival rate of 92% and 85% at 1 and 5 years, respectively.[10,58–60]

New Approaches

Fibrates

Fibrates (fenofibrate, bezafibrate) are traditionally used for the treatment of hyperlipidemia. The mechanism of action of fibric acid derivatives in PBC is thought to be related to anti-inflammatory effects via peroxisome proliferator-activated receptor-α, a member of the nuclear hormone receptor superfamily, and possibly through increase in the expression of multiple drug resistance gene-3, both of which ameliorate hepatobiliary inflammation in PBC.[61] Furthermore, bezafibrate increases biliary phospholipid secretion into the bile by up-regulating the expression of phosphatidylcholine flippase on the canalicular membrane and restoring the ratio of phospholipid and bile salts to a harmless level.[62] Although bezafibrate is not available in the United States, fenofibrate is currently Food and Drug Administration approved for the management of hyperlipidemia.

Two prospective, multicenter randomized open studies in noncirrhotic patients with PBC were performed in Japan in 2008 to evaluate the efficacy of bezafibrate. The first compared UDCA and bezafibrate monotherapy (45 patients), and the other evaluated the addition of bezafibrate to patients who were refractory to UDCA (21 patients). Results after 52 weeks suggested that bezafibrate monotherapy (400 mg/d PO) was as effective as UDCA (600 mg/d PO). Moreover, bezafibrate combined with UDCA was effective in improving and maintaining liver enzyme levels among patients with inadequate response to long-term treatment with UDCA.[63]

In 2009, Walker and colleagues[64] reported the first European experience with a fibric acid derivative in PBC. The investigators reviewed the effect of fenofibrate 200 mg/d given to 16 patients who previously failed to respond to UDCA 13 to 15 mg/kg/d. These patients received combination therapy for a mean of 22.8 months. Both ALP and IgM levels dropped significantly, with 89% of patients normalizing serum ALP levels.

Recently, efficacy and safety of fenofibrate in patients with PBC and incomplete response to UDCA were evaluated in a pilot study involving 2 large US centers. Twenty patients with PBC and ALP >2 times the upper limit of normal (ULN) despite ongoing UDCA therapy for >1 year were treated with fenofibrate (160 mg/d) in addition to UDCA (13–15 mg/kg/d). At the end of 48 weeks, combination therapy induced significant biochemical improvement; median serum ALP decreased significantly from 351 (214–779) U/L at baseline to 177 (60–384) U/L at the end of the study ($P<.05$). Aspartate aminotransferase and IgM also decreased significantly, whereas bilirubin and albumin remained unchanged.[65] The decrease in serum IgM supports the hypothesis that fenofibrate altered the biology of PBC, because production of IgM in PBC is thought to be disease specific.

Recent work from Tokyo elegantly demonstrated that fibrates not only improve serum liver biochemistry studies and IgM in patients with PBC and incomplete response to UDCA but also do so through down-regulation of sinusoidal bile acid transporters, inhibition of bile acid synthesis, and up-regulation of canalicular transporters, thus acting as an agonist for both peroxisome proliferator-activated receptor-α and PXR pathways and inducing choleresis.[66]

Given these promising results, larger randomized, placebo-controlled studies of fibrates in PBC should be pursued to clarify its role in the overall management of the disease.

6α-Ethyl-chenodeoxycolic acid

6α-Ethyl-chenodeoxycolic acid (obeticholic acid) is a novel derivate of the primary human ethyl-chenodeoxycolic bile acid that has been chemically modified to make it more active. It is expected to work mainly by activating the farnesoid X receptor (FXR), which controls the production of bile. By activating FXR, obeticholic acid is expected to reduce the production of bile in the liver, preventing it from building up and damaging the liver tissue.

An international, double-blind, placebo-controlled, parallel-group, dose-response study was conducted to evaluate the effects of obeticholic acid on ALP and other liver enzymes and its safety in patients with PBC with persistently high ALP levels (>1.5 times ULN) while receiving a stable UDCA dose. In this study, 165 patients were randomized to placebo, obeticholic acid 10 mg, 25 mg or 50 mg once daily for 12 weeks, given in addition to their prior UDCA therapy.[67] Study subjects in all obeticholic acid dose groups showed statistically significant improvement in mean serum ALP levels compared with baseline values, and dose-related worsening of pruritus was the most important adverse event. A phase 3 trial is now ongoing.

Antiretrovirals

Several bacteria, viruses, and xenobiotics have been implicated in the pathogenesis of PBC. As such, a human β-retrovirus closely related to the mouse mammary tumor virus was directly cloned from biliary epithelium of patients with PBC.

In previous uncontrolled pilot studies, lamivudine monotherapy was of little use in treating PBC, whereas significant but not substantial improvements were observed using twice-daily combination therapy consisting of zidovudine 300 mg and lamivudine 150 mg. This regimen was associated with normalization of hepatic biochemistry studies in a proportion of patients with near normal liver tests and a reduction in mean necroinflammatory scores, bile duct damage, and ductopenia.[68]

In a subsequent study, Mason and colleagues[69] randomized 59 patients with an ALP level >1.5 times ULN despite being receiving UDCA therapy to either zidovudine 300 mg plus lamivudine 150 mg twice daily or placebo for 6 months. None of the patients had normalized ALP, and no significant differences were observed in rates of normalization of serum aminotransferase levels. Additional studies using a triple regimen of antiretrovirals are awaited.

Rituximab

Rituximab is a genetically engineered chimeric murine/human monoclonal antibody against protein CD20 that is primarily found on the surface of B cells. Rituximab is used in the treatment of many lymphomas, leukemia, transplant rejection, and some autoimmune disorders.

In a previous study, 14 patients with PBC refractory to UDCA (13–15 mg/kg/d for 6 months) received 2 rituximab infusions (1 g at days 1 and 15) and were followed for up to 12 months. The primary outcome of this study was the proportion of patients with normalization and/or ≥25% improvement in ALP at 6 months. Twelve and 8 patients completed 6 and 12 months of follow-up, respectively. Although rituximab was well tolerated, 1 patient withdrew because of asthma exacerbation during the first infusion. Effective B-cell depletion was observed in all patients. ALP normalization and/or ≥25% improvement was observed in 25% of patients at 6 and 12 months. Pruritus and fatigue also improved.[70]

Recently, Tsuda and colleagues[71] studied the safety and potential efficacy of rituximab on 6 patients with incomplete response to UDCA followed for 52 weeks. The investigators demonstrated a decrease in serum ALP lasting up to 36 weeks after rituximab treatment, perhaps suggesting a longstanding effect on bile duct injury. Their results indicate that rituximab is safe, transiently reverses several of the immunologic abnormalities that are characteristic of PBC, and may have a potential therapeutic effect in this difficult-to-treat PBC population.

In summary, selective B-cell depletion with rituximab shows promise as a therapy for PBC, but larger controlled studies are necessary to confirm its long-term efficacy and safety.

Vitamin D

Previous studies have shown that macrophage phagocytosis of apoptotic cells is impaired even in early-stage PBC, and vitamin D3 supplementation has been shown to enhance macrophage function.[72,73] A study was conducted to determine whether treatment with high-dose vitamin D3 improves macrophage phagocytosis of apoptotic cells in PBC. Twelve subjects with noncirrhotic PBC were randomized to receive placebo or vitamin D3 1000 IU/d for 3 months. The initial mean serum vitamin D3 levels were slightly lower in the treatment group (30.8 vs 38.0 ng/mL, $P = .029$), but at the end of study, the mean serum 25-hydroxyvitamin D3 levels were significantly higher in the treatment group (44.8 vs 26.2 ng/mL, $P<.010$, respectively). At baseline, mean macrophage phagocytosis of apoptotic cells (percent phagocytosis) was equivalent for treatment and placebo groups. At the end of the study, the percent phagocytosis was significantly higher in the vitamin D3 treatment group. This study showed that high-dose vitamin D3 supplementation might improve both PBC macrophage function and cholestasis.[74] Although larger studies have not been conducted to date, recent work from France indicates that correction of low vitamin D levels in those patients with PBC with vitamin D deficiency does not seem to improve their response to UDCA.[75]

SUMMARY

Tremendous progress has been made in recent years outlining the natural history and epidemiology of PBC. Furthermore, we have refined our diagnostic accuracy and treatment of this chronic progressive illness. Although most cases respond well to standard treatment with UDCA, a large portion of patients remain clinically challenging. Through the steadfast efforts of our colleagues, we are on the cusp of breakthroughs for newer treatments and a better understanding of the pathogenesis of this condition. Consequently, we have begun to alter the natural history and outcomes for our patients with PBC. With that being said, currently liver transplantation remains the only potentially curative option and thus we still have much work to do for our patients.

REFERENCES

1. Crosignani A, Battezzati PM, Invernizzi P, et al. Clinical features and management of primary biliary cirrhosis. World J Gastroenterol 2008;14(21):3313–27.
2. Selmi C, Mayo MJ, Bach N, et al. Primary biliary cirrhosis in monozygotic and dizygotic twins: genetics, epigenetics, and environment. Gastroenterology 2004;127(2):485–92.
3. Lazaridis KN, Talwalkar JA. Clinical epidemiology of primary biliary cirrhosis: incidence, prevalence, and impact of therapy. J Clin Gastroenterol 2007;41(5):494–500.
4. Kim WR, Lindor KD, Locke GR 3rd, et al. Epidemiology and natural history of primary biliary cirrhosis in a US community. Gastroenterology 2000;119(6):1631–6.

5. Inoue K, Hirohara J, Nakano T, et al. Prediction of prognosis of primary biliary cirrhosis in Japan. Liver 1995;15(2):70–7.
6. Prince M, Chetwynd A, Newman W, et al. Survival and symptom progression in a geographically based cohort of patients with primary biliary cirrhosis: follow-up for up to 28 years. Gastroenterology 2002;123(4):1044–51.
7. Talwalkar JA, Souto E, Jorgensen RA, et al. Natural history of pruritus in primary biliary cirrhosis. Clin Gastroenterol Hepatol 2003;1(4):297–302.
8. Corpechot C, Carrat F, Bahr A, et al. The effect of ursodeoxycholic acid therapy on the natural course of primary biliary cirrhosis. Gastroenterology 2005;128(2):297–303.
9. Mattalia A, Quaranta S, Leung PS, et al. Characterization of antimitochondrial antibodies in health adults. Hepatology 1998;27(3):656–61.
10. Lindor KD, Gershwin ME, Poupon R, et al. Primary biliary cirrhosis. Hepatology 2009;50(1):291–308.
11. Berg PA, Klein R. Heterogeneity of antimitochondrial antibodies. Semin Liver Dis 1989;9(2):103–16.
12. Berg PA, Klein R. Mitochondrial antigen/antibody systems in primary biliary cirrhosis: revisited. Liver 1995;15(6):281–92.
13. Invernizzi P, Podda M, Battezzati PM, et al. Autoantibodies against nuclear pore complexes are associated with more active and severe liver disease in primary biliary cirrhosis. J Hepatol 2001;34(3):366–72.
14. Muratori L, Granito A, Muratori P, et al. Antimitochondrial antibodies and other antibodies in primary biliary cirrhosis: diagnostic and prognostic value. Clin Liver Dis 2008;12(2):261–76, vii.
15. Nakamura M, Kondo H, Mori T, et al. Anti-gp210 and anti-centromere antibodies are different risk factors for the progression of primary biliary cirrhosis. Hepatology 2007;45(1):118–27.
16. Invernizzi P, Crosignani A, Battezzati PM, et al. Comparison of the clinical features and clinical course of antimitochondrial antibody-positive and -negative primary biliary cirrhosis. Hepatology 1997;25(5):1090–5.
17. Kim WR, Poterucha JJ, Jorgensen RA, et al. Does antimitochondrial antibody status affect response to treatment in patients with primary biliary cirrhosis? Outcomes of ursodeoxycholic acid therapy and liver transplantation. Hepatology 1997;26(1):22–6.
18. Scheuer PJ. Primary biliary cirrhosis: diagnosis, pathology and pathogenesis. Postgrad Med J 1983;59(Suppl 4).106–15.
19. Heathcote EJ. Management of primary biliary cirrhosis. The American Association for the Study of Liver Diseases practice guidelines. Hepatology 2000;31(4):1005–13.
20. Lindor K. Ursodeoxycholic acid for the treatment of primary biliary cirrhosis. N Engl J Med 2007;357(15):1524–9.
21. Poupon R. Primary biliary cirrhosis: a 2010 update. J Hepatol 2010;52(5):745–50.
22. Paumgartner G, Beuers U. Ursodeoxycholic acid in cholestatic liver disease: mechanisms of action and therapeutic use revisited. Hepatology 2002;36(3):525–31.
23. Lazaridis KN, Gores GJ, Lindor KD. Ursodeoxycholic acid 'mechanisms of action and clinical use in hepatobiliary disorders. J Hepatol 2001;35(1):134–46.
24. Roma MG, Toledo FD, Boaglio AC, et al. Ursodeoxycholic acid in cholestasis: linking action mechanisms to therapeutic applications. Clin Sci (Lond) 2011;121(12):523–44.

25. Rodrigues CM, Ma X, Linehan-Stieers C, et al. Ursodeoxycholic acid prevents cytochrome c release in apoptosis by inhibiting mitochondrial membrane depolarization and channel formation. Cell Death Differ 1999;6(9):842–54.

26. Bergamini A, Dini L, Baiocchi L, et al. Bile acids with differing hydrophilic-hydrophobic properties do not influence cytokine production by human monocytes and murine Kupffer cells. Hepatology 1997;25(4):927–33.

27. Balasubramaniam K, Grambsch PM, Wiesner RH, et al. Diminished survival in asymptomatic primary biliary cirrhosis. A prospective study. Gastroenterology 1990;98(6):1567–71.

28. Corpechot C, Abenavoli L, Rabahi N, et al. Biochemical response to ursodeoxycholic acid and long-term prognosis in primary biliary cirrhosis. Hepatology 2008; 48(3):871–7.

29. Gong Y, Huang ZB, Christensen E, et al. Ursodeoxycholic acid for primary biliary cirrhosis. Cochrane Database Syst Rev 2008;(3):CD000551.

30. Poupon RE, Lindor KD, Cauch-Dudek K, et al. Combined analysis of randomized controlled trials of ursodeoxycholic acid in primary biliary cirrhosis. Gastroenterology 1997;113(3):884–90.

31. Lindor KD, Jorgensen RA, Therneau TM, et al. Ursodeoxycholic acid delays the onset of esophageal varices in primary biliary cirrhosis. Mayo Clin Proc 1997; 72(12):1137–40.

32. Lee J, Belanger A, Doucette JT, et al. Transplantation trends in primary biliary cirrhosis. Clin Gastroenterol Hepatol 2007;5(11):1313–5.

33. Liermann Garcia RF, Evangelista Garcia C, McMaster P, et al. Transplantation for primary biliary cirrhosis: retrospective analysis of 400 patients in a single center. Hepatology 2001;33(1):22–7.

34. Kuiper EM, Hansen BE, Metselaar HJ, et al. Trends in liver transplantation for primary biliary cirrhosis in the Netherlands 1988-2008. BMC Gastroenterol 2010;10:144.

35. Jorgensen RA, Dickson ER, Hofmann AF, et al. Characterisation of patients with a complete biochemical response to ursodeoxycholic acid. Gut 1995;36(6): 935–8.

36. Corpechot C, Chazouilleres O, Poupon R. Early primary biliary cirrhosis: biochemical response to treatment and prediction of long-term outcome. J Hepatol 2011;55(6):1361–7.

37. Pares A, Caballeria L, Rodes J. Excellent long-term survival in patients with primary biliary cirrhosis and biochemical response to ursodeoxycholic acid. Gastroenterology 2006;130(3):715–20.

38. Kumagi T, Guindi M, Fischer SE, et al. Baseline ductopenia and treatment response predict long-term histological progression in primary biliary cirrhosis. Am J Gastroenterol 2010;105(10):2186–94.

39. Kuiper EM, Hansen BE, de Vries RA, et al. Improved prognosis of patients with primary biliary cirrhosis that have a biochemical response to ursodeoxycholic acid. Gastroenterology 2009;136(4):1281–7.

40. Azemoto N, Kumagi T, Abe M, et al. Biochemical response to ursodeoxycholic acid predicts long-term outcome in Japanese patients with primary biliary cirrhosis. Hepatol Res 2011;41(4):310–7.

41. Kaplan MM, Poupon R. Treatment with immunosuppressives in patients with primary biliary cirrhosis who fail to respond to ursodiol. Hepatology 2009;50(2):652.

42. Angulo P, Jorgensen RA, Lindor KD. Incomplete response to ursodeoxycholic acid in primary biliary cirrhosis: is a double dosage worthwhile? Am J Gastroenterol 2001;96(11):3152–7.

43. Combes B, Emerson SS, Flye NL, et al. Methotrexate (MTX) plus ursodeoxycholic acid (UDCA) in the treatment of primary biliary cirrhosis. Hepatology 2005;42(5): 1184–93.

44. Giljaca V, Poropat G, Stimac D, et al. Methotrexate for primary biliary cirrhosis. Cochrane Database Syst Rev 2010;(5):CD004385.

45. Gong Y, Gluud C. Colchicine for primary biliary cirrhosis. Cochrane Database Syst Rev 2004;(2):CD004481.

46. Leung J, Bonis PA, Kaplan MM. Colchicine or methotrexate, with ursodiol, are effective after 20 years in a subset of patients with primary biliary cirrhosis. Clin Gastroenterol Hepatol 2011;9(9):776–80.

47. Gong Y, Christensen E, Gluud C. Azathioprine for primary biliary cirrhosis. Cochrane Database Syst Rev 2007;(3):CD006000.

48. Greenberg GR, Feagan BG, Martin F, et al. Oral budesonide for active Crohn's disease. Canadian Inflammatory Bowel Disease Study Group. N Engl J Med 1994;331(13):836–41.

49. Rautiainen H, Karkkainen P, Karvonen AL, et al. Budesonide combined with UDCA to improve liver histology in primary biliary cirrhosis: a three-year randomized trial. Hepatology 2005;41(4):747–52.

50. Leuschner M, Maier KP, Schlichting J, et al. Oral budesonide and ursodeoxycholic acid for treatment of primary biliary cirrhosis: results of a prospective double-blind trial. Gastroenterology 1999;117(4):918–25.

51. Hempfling W, Grunhage F, Dilger K, et al. Pharmacokinetics and pharmacodynamic action of budesonide in early- and late-stage primary biliary cirrhosis. Hepatology 2003;38(1):196–202.

52. Sievers TM, Rossi SJ, Ghobrial RM, et al. Mycophenolate mofetil. Pharmacotherapy 1997;17(6):1178–97.

53. Talwalkar JA, Angulo P, Keach JC, et al. Mycophenolate mofetil for the treatment of primary biliary cirrhosis in patients with an incomplete response to ursodeoxycholic acid. J Clin Gastroenterol 2005;39(2):168–71.

54. Askari F, Innis D, Dick RB, et al. Treatment of primary biliary cirrhosis with tetrathiomolybdate: results of a double-blind trial. Transl Res 2010;155(3): 123–30.

55. Devlin J, O'Grady J. Indications for referral and assessment in adult liver transplantation: a clinical guideline. British Society of Gastroenterology. Gut 1999; 45(Suppl 6):VI1–22.

56. Mendes F, Couto CA, Levy C. Recurrent and de novo autoimmune liver diseases. Clin Liver Dis 2011;15(4):859–78.

57. Jacob DA, Neumann UP, Bahra M, et al. Long-term follow-up after recurrence of primary biliary cirrhosis after liver transplantation in 100 patients. Clin Transplant 2006;20(2):211–20.

58. Jacob DA, Bahra M, Schmidt SC, et al. Mayo risk score for primary biliary cirrhosis: a useful tool for the prediction of course after liver transplantation? Ann Transplant 2000;13(3):35–42.

59. MacQuillan GC, Neuberger J. Liver transplantation for primary biliary cirrhosis. Clin Liver Dis 2003;7(4):941–56, ix.

60. Neuberger J. Liver transplantation for primary biliary cirrhosis. Autoimmun Rev 2003;2(1):1–7.

61. Dohmen K, Mizuta T, Nakamuta M, et al. Fenofibrate for patients with asymptomatic primary biliary cirrhosis. World J Gastroenterol 2004;10(6):894–8.

62. Iwasaki S, Akisawa N, Saibara T, et al. Fibrate for treatment of primary biliary cirrhosis. Hepatol Res 2007;37(Suppl 3):S515–7.

63. Iwasaki S, Ohira H, Nishiguchi S, et al. The efficacy of ursodeoxycholic acid and bezafibrate combination therapy for primary biliary cirrhosis: a prospective, multicenter study. Hepatol Res 2008;38(6):557–64.

64. Walker LJ, Newton J, Jones DE, et al. Comment on biochemical response to ursodeoxycholic acid and long-term prognosis in primary biliary cirrhosis. Hepatology 2009;49(1):337–8 [author reply: 338].

65. Levy C, Peter JA, Nelson DR, et al. Pilot study: fenofibrate for patients with primary biliary cirrhosis and an incomplete response to ursodeoxycholic acid. Aliment Pharmacol Ther 2011;33(2):235–42.

66. Honda A, Ikegami T, Nakamuta M, et al. Anticholestatic effects of bezafibrate in patients with primary biliary cirrhosis treated with ursodeoxycholic acid. Hepatology 2012. [Epub ahead of print].

67. Mason A, Luketic V, Lindor K, et al. 2 Farnesoid-X receptor agonists: a new class of drugs for the treatment of PBC? an international study evaluating the addition of INT-747 to ursodeoxycholic acid. J Hepatol 2010;52:S1–2.

68. Mason AL, Farr GH, Xu L, et al. Pilot studies of single and combination antiretroviral therapy in patients with primary biliary cirrhosis. Am J Gastroenterol 2004;99(12):2348–55.

69. Mason AL, Lindor KD, Bacon BR, et al. Clinical trial: randomized controlled trial of zidovudine and lamivudine for patients with primary biliary cirrhosis stabilized on ursodiol. Aliment Pharmacol Ther 2008;28(7):886–94.

70. Myers R, Shaheen AA, Swain MG, et al. Rituximab for primary biliary cirrhosis (PBC) refractory to ursodeoxycholic acid (UDCA). Hepatology 2007;46(S1):532A–631A.

71. Tsuda M, Moritoki Y, Lian ZX, et al. Biochemical and immunologic effects of rituximab in patients with primary biliary cirrhosis and an incomplete response to ursodeoxycholic acid. Hepatology 2012;55(2):512–21.

72. Allina J, Hu B, Sullivan DM, et al. Anti-CD16 autoantibodies and delayed phagocytosis of apoptotic cells in primary biliary cirrhosis. J Autoimmun 2008;30(4):238–45.

73. Allina J, Stanca CM, Garber J, et al. T cell targeting and phagocytosis of apoptotic biliary epithelial cells in primary biliary cirrhosis. J Autoimmun 2006;27(4):232–41.

74. Allina J, Stanca CM, Delisser M, et al. High dose vitamin D3 treatment enhances macrophage phagocytosis of apoptotic cells and lowers bilirubin levels in PBC. Hepatology 2008;48(S1):706A.

75. Corpechot C, Gaouar F, Chazoilleres O, et al. Is biochemical response to ursodeoxycholic acid therapy impacted by vitamin D plasma level in patients with primary biliary cirrhosis? Hepatology 2012;56(S1):1137A.

Cholestatic Liver Disease Overlap Syndromes

Marlyn J. Mayo, MD

KEYWORDS

- Overlap • Variant • Biliary cirrhosis • Sclerosing cholangitis • Autoimmune hepatitis

KEY POINTS

- Primary biliary cirrhosis (PBC) and primary sclerosing cholangitis (PSC) may share some clinical features with autoimmune hepatitis (AIH), but when substantial features of AIH are present, prognosis can be affected and immunosuppressive treatment with corticosteroids may be warranted.
- Standard diagnostic criteria for overlap syndrome are lacking. Proposed criteria for overlapping AIH include the presence of (1) alanine aminotransferase (ALT) > 5 × upper limit of normal (ULN), (2) IgG > 2 × ULN and/or positive anti–smooth muscle antibody, (3) liver biopsy with moderate or severe periportal or periseptal inflammation and International Autoimmune Hepatitis Group (IAIHG) simplified criteria for the diagnosis of AIH.
- AIH and PSC commonly overlap in children and this combination should be actively excluded in the pediatric population.
- The presence of severe interface hepatitis in PBC portends a worse prognosis and should prompt evaluation for possible AIH overlap and consideration of treatment with immunosuppression.
- Drug-induced liver injury and IgG4 disease may masquerade as AIH or PSC and are important to consider in the differential diagnosis of the overlap or variant syndromes.

Overlap syndrome refers to the simultaneous presence in a single patient of what is considered 2 distinct diseases. Both diseases may be present at the initial diagnosis, or they may become clinically apparent in sequential fashion. Most cases of overlap in adults are between PBC and AIH, whereas in children most are between PSC and AIH. PBC and PSC are virtually never seen together in the same patient. The term, *overlap syndrome*, is sometimes used synonymously with the term, *variant syndrome*, but overlap syndrome is more than making an observation that one disease has some features of another. The implication is that true overlap requires treatment of both diseases.

Dr Mayo has no financial relationships with any commercial company that has a direct financial interest in the subject matter or materials discussed in this article.
Department of Internal Medicine, Division of Digestive and Liver Diseases, UT Southwestern, 5323 Harry Hines Boulevard, Dallas, TX 75390-9151, USA
E-mail address: marlyn.mayo@utsouthwestern.edu

Clin Liver Dis 17 (2013) 243–253
http://dx.doi.org/10.1016/j.cld.2012.12.006
1089-3261/13/$ – see front matter © 2013 Elsevier Inc. All rights reserved.

liver.theclinics.com

Each of the major autoimmune hepatobiliary diseases (PBC, AIH, and PSC) has its characteristic clinical, biochemical, serologic, and histologic profiles (**Table 1**), although none of these individual features is exclusive. The clinician's responsibility lies in assimilating as much data as needed to determine where on the spectrum of autoimmune hepatobiliary diseases an individual patient is positioned and weighing that information against an individual's comorbidities and personal situation to determine the most appropriate therapy. Overlap syndromes are rare and not clearly defined, so there is a stark paucity of data to guide management. As such, overlap syndromes is a field of hepatology where the art of clinical judgment frequently presides over the science of medicine.

A firm grasp of the range of clinical presentation for each of the autoimmune hepatobiliary diseases is needed to be able to differentiate what is within the reported spectrum of each disease versus which features indicate the presence of 2 distinct diseases. The clinical spectrum of each of these diseases is described, with attention to which features are or highly specific for each condition versus which features are not discriminating. The descriptions are not meant to provide a complete clinical review of each disease (more comprehensive descriptions of these entities can be found in the articles by Czul and colleagues and Zein elsewhere in this issue) but are meant to highlight or devalue the clinical criteria often considered in the diagnosis of overlap syndromes.

CLINICAL SPECTRUM OF PBC
Epidemiology

PBC is defined as a chronic cholestatic liver disease in which the small-sized to medium-sized bile ducts are the target of inflammatory destruction. The large, extrahepatic ducts should never be affected in PBC. The median age of presentation in the United States for PBC is 52 and the disease has never been reported in a prepubertal child. More than 90% of the patients are women. Approximately 15% to 20% of patients with PBC also have limited scleroderma (Calcinosis, Raynaud's phenomenon, Esophageal dysmotility, and Telangiectasias [CREST syndrome]), a syndrome that is not associated with AIH or PSC.

Laboratory

Because the disease is cholestatic, the degree of ALP elevation should be higher than the degree of transaminase elevation. One exception is that in early PBC, the alkaline phosphatase (ALP) may be normal and only mild elevation (<2 × ULN) of transaminases seen. Once the disease is well established, the ALP rises and the transaminases may also rise to 1 to 4 times the ULN. Elevation of transaminases above 500 IU/mL is

Table 1
Classical clinical features of the autoimmune hepatobiliary diseases

	PBC	PSC	Type I AIH
Symptoms	Itch, fatigue, asymptomatic	Itch, fatigue, jaundice, recurrent cholangitis	Episodic abdominal pain, nausea, arthralgias
Serology	AMA	pANCA/pANNA	ANA
Liver enzymes	Elevated ALP	Elevated ALP	Elevated AST and ALT
Histology	Nonsuppurative granulomatous cholangitis	Fibrosing obliteration of bile ducts	Lymphoplasmactyic interface hepatitis
Therapy	Ursodeoxycholic acid	None	Corticosteroids

generally not seen in PBC and should prompt consideration of overlap of another liver condition, such as AIH or drug-induced liver injury. Bilirubin becomes elevated as a patient advances to cirrhosis and steadily climbs. It is thus an excellent prognostic marker. Antimitochondrial antibodies (AMAs) detected by immunofluorescence are present in 95% of persons (**Table 2**). Antipyruvate dehydrogenase (PDC-E2) is slightly less sensitive (90%) but more specific (99%) in patients with chronic liver disease. When anti-M2 ELISAs are applied to the general population, however, the positive predictive value drops. In one series of AIH patients, 5 of 166 tested positive for AMAs without any bile duct changes on liver biopsy.[1] Although long-term follow-up is lacking from this particular series, there are other cases that describe AMA positivity in otherwise classical AIH patients who never develop overt PBC after long-term follow-up.[2] Most PBC patients have elevated IgM and many have a more modest elevation of IgG.

Histology

Liver biopsy is not necessary to make the diagnosis in PBC if patients are middle-aged women with positive AMAs and chronic cholestasis and no suspicion for a different liver disease. The American Association for the Study of Liver Diseases (AASLD) diagnostic criteria include chronically cholestatic liver tests with either positive AMAs or compatible liver biopsy.[3] The European Association for the Study of the Liver (EASL) diagnostic criteria require the presence of at least 2 out of 3 of the following: (1) ALP at least 2 × ULN or γ-glutamyltransferase (GGT) at least 5 × ULN, (2) positive AMAs, and (3) a liver biopsy with a florid duct lesion. If a liver biopsy is performed, non-suppurative destructive cholangitis is the classical finding. Due to the patchy nature of histologic involvement of the disease, however, these lesions may be missed, particularly if fewer than 10 portal tracts are present on the biopsy specimen. With worsening ductopenia, the chance of finding an inflamed duct on biopsy also diminishes. Granulomas, particularly in the portal tract areas, are highly suggestive of PBC but often not present. Granulomas are not usually found in AIH. Although elevated IgG, interface hepatitis, and plasma cell infiltrates are characteristic features of AIH, they are also found in many patients with classical PBC. A pathologist may suggest consideration of overlap based on the presence of exuberant interface hepatitis and/or

Table 2			
Autoantibodies in the autoimmune hepatobiliary diseases			
	PBC	PSC	AIH[a]
ANA (>1:40)	20%–50%	8%–77%	70%–80%
AMA (>1:40 or anti–PDC-E2)	90%–95%[b]	0%–9%	Few
pANCA/pANNA	0%–10%	25%–95%	50%–96%
ASMA	0%–10%	0%–83%	—
LKM	—	—	3%–4%
Anti–LC-1	—	—	4%
Anti–SLA/LP	Few	Few	10%–30%

Abbreviations: ASMA, anti smooth muscle antibody; Anti-LC-1, anti liver-cytosol antibodies; LKM, liver kidney microsomal antibodies; Anti-SLA/LP, anti soluble liver antigen/liver pancreas.
  [a] Approximately 10% do not have any autoantibodies.
  [b] Whereas 5% may be AMA negative, these same persons are usually ANA positive.
  Data from Hov JR, Boberg KM, Karlsen TH. Autoantibodies in primary sclerosing cholangitis. World J Gastroenterol 2008;14(24):3781–91.

presence of plasma cells, but this is not sufficient evidence alone because up to 30% of patients with PBC have severe interface hepatitis.[4–6] Additional clinical evidence is needed to support the diagnosis. Alternatively, overlap between AIH and PBC should have interface hepatitis, and EASL has proposed that this is mandatory for the diagnosis of AIH + PBC overlap.[7]

CLINICAL SPECTRUM OF AIH
Epidemiology

AIH is most clearly defined by the revised IAIHG scoring system, which incorporates age, female gender, interface hepatitis, and response to steroids. The diagnosis requires liver biopsy. The majority of patients (60%–75%) are women but it can present at any age, including young children.

Laboratory

Transaminases are elevated predominantly. AIH is one of the few diseases that can cause ALT to rise over 1000 IU/mL, whereas uncomplicated PBC or PSC should not result in transaminases over 500 IU/mL. IgG is often elevated in AIH, and the degree of elevation is more pronounced than is typical for PBC or PSC. Elevation of serum IgG correlates with plasma cell infiltration on biopsy and may not be present at all.

Histology

Whereas the small bile ducts may have some intraepithelial lymphocytes in AIH, florid cholangitis or granulomatous destruction of the small bile ducts is only seen in PBC. The large ducts are also not affected by the AIH process. An irregular lumen of the extrahepatic ducts found by cholangiogram in patients with AIH should prompt consideration of overlap with PSC, pruning of the ducts from cirrhosis, or IgG4 disease. Children seem to be at particular risk for overlap of AIH and PSC. Approximately 30% of children with AIH have acute or chronic cholangitis on liver biopsy.

CLINICAL SPECTRUM OF PSC
Epidemiology

PSC typically affects persons in the 4th decade of life but may also affect children and older individuals. Approximately 60% to 70% of patients are male. Inflammatory bowel disease is present in 75%, whereas fewer than 10% of patients with PBC or AIH have IBD.

Laboratory

A cholestatic pattern of elevated ALP and GGT is typical. Bilirubin may fluctuate over the course of the disease, and acute elevations suggest a dominant stricture may have developed. Transaminases are modestly elevated but also rise in the setting of acute cholangitis. The autoantibody, perinuclear antineutrophil cytoplasmic antibodies/perinuclear antineutrophil nuclear antibody (pANCA/pANNA), helps differentiate PSC from PBC but is often found in AIH and thus is not a good discriminating factor between AIH and PSC. Approximately half of patients with PSC have elevated IgG and/or IgM. Because IgG4 cholangiopathy may masquerade as PSC and is treated in a completely different manner (immunosuppression), an elevated serum total IgG in any patient with apparent PSC should be subtyped.

Histology

Liver biopsy findings in PSC are usually nonspecific, although fibrosing obliteration (onion skinning) of medium-large sized ducts may be seen. Lymphocytic infiltration of the portal tracts and bile ducts is also seen but does not help differentiate the disease from PBC or AIH or even viral hepatitis. The diagnosis of PSC is made by detecting multiple areas of stricturing with or without dilation on cholangiogram. Magnetic resonance cholangiopancreatography (MRCP) is preferred as the initial diagnostic test in persons whom therapeutic intervention is not anticipated because of its lower risk compared with ERCP or PTC. Liver biopsy is not necessary once the diagnosis is confirmed with cholangiography unless there is a clinical suspicion of overlap with AIH.

DEFINITION AND PREVALENCE OF OVERLAP SYNDROMES

Published reports of overlap syndromes suffer from lack of uniform diagnostic criteria and are descriptive and retrospective. Most case series apply IAIHG revised criteria[8] published in 1999 to patients with PSC or PBC to define who has overlap with AIH. The IAIHG criteria were not created with that intended application, however, leading the IAIHG to publish a position paper stating, "The IAIHG suggests that patients with autoimmune liver disease should be categorized according to the predominating feature(s) as AIH, PBC, and PSC/small duct PSC respectively, and that those with overlapping features are not considered as being distinct diagnostic entities. The IAIHG scoring system should not be used to establish subgroups of patients."[9] The original AIH criteria were revised with the intent of being able to better distinguish PBC from AIH, although many of the criteria (eg, female gender or lack of other liver diseases) do not discriminate between AIH or PBC. In 2008, the IAIHG published simplified criteria for the diagnosis of AIH, including just the variables of autoantibodies, immunoglobulins, absence of viral hepatitis, and histology (**Table 3**).[10] These criteria were

Table 3	
Proposed criteria for the diagnosis of AIH overlap with PBC or PSC	
French Criteria[11]	**IAIHG Simplified Criteria[10]**
ALT > 5 × ULN	ANA or ASMA ≥1:40 → 1 Point ≥1:80 → 2 Points LKM ≥1:40 → 2 Points SLA Positive → 2 points
IgG > 2 × ULN and/or positive anti–smooth muscle antibody	IgG >ULN → 1 point >1.1 × ULN → 2 points Absence of viral hepatitis → 2 points
Liver biopsy with moderate or severe periportal or periseptal inflammation	Compatible histology: interface hepatitis (lymphocytic/lymphoplasmocytic infiltrates in portal tracts extending into the lobule) → 1 point Typical histology: interface hepatitis, emperipolesis and rosettes → 2 points
Scoring At least 2 out of 3 criteria must be present for a diagnosis of overlapping AIH features and the presence of interface hepatitis is required.	Scoring The sum of all the points from autoantibodies is limited to 2 points. Total score ≥6: Probable AIH (88% sensitivity, 97% specificity) ≥7: Definite AIH (81% sensitivity, 99% specificity)

Abbreviations: SLA, soluble liver antigen; ASMA, anti smooth muscle antibody.

intended for clinical diagnosis at the bedside rather than defining subjects for clinical trials. The criteria were established on a training set of 250 AIH patients and 193 controls from 11 centers and validated using data of an additional 109 AIH patients and 284 controls and predicted AIH with 88% sensitivity and 97% specificity at cutoff value of greater than or equal to 6. There were patients included in their study cohort who were believed to have some kind of overlap syndrome.

An alternative set of criteria has been used to establish the diagnosis of AIH overlap in some studies. This score requires 2 of the following: (1) ALT > 5 × ULN, (2) IgG > 2 × ULN and/or positive anti–smooth muscle antibody, (3) liver biopsy with moderate or severe periportal or periseptal inflammation (see **Table 3**).[11]

PBC + AIH Overlap

When the revised IAIHG criteria are applied to PBC, approximately 2% to 19% of patients meet criteria for AIH. A large Italian study applied the revised criteria to 142 PBC patients and found that 3 (2%) scored as probable or definite AIH.[12] In a similar study of 137 PBC patients performed at Mayo Clinic, 19% had probable AIH, although none had definite AIH.[6] When the simplified AIH score[10] was applied to 77 patients with autoimmune cholestatic disease, the sensitivity of the simplified IAIHG score was found similar to the revised IAIHG score (53.8% vs 61.5%) to detect overlap with AIH.[13]

PSC + AIH Overlap

When the original IAIHG criteria were applied to 114 Norwegian PSC patients, 33 had probable AIH and 2% had definite AIH.[14] These findings were reproduced in a Mayo Clinic study of 211 PSC patients, where 19% had probable AIH and 2% had definite AIH, although the percent of probable AIH dropped to 6% when the revised criteria were used.[15] Similar findings were obtained in Holland, where 14% of Dutch PSC patients met the revised criteria for AIH.[16] AIH overlap may be more common in small duct PSC than in large duct PSC. In one Scandinavian study, 7 of 26 (27%) of PSC-AIH overlap cases were small duct PSC.[17]

The reverse approach to diagnosing PSC + AIH overlap is to perform cholangiography in patients with established AIH. Prevalence of PSC overlap in adult AIH patients using this strategy varies from rare to 10%.[18,19] In the Canadian study where 10% were found to have abnormalities, ductular irregularities were associated with advanced fibrosis on biopsy, hinting to some investigators that perhaps pruning of ducts may have played a role. Routine screening of adult AIH patients for PSC overlap with MRCP is controversial and insufficient data are present to recommend it for all AIH patients at this time. The presence of cholestatic enzymes in a patient with AIH, however, should prompt consideration of MRCP to exclude PSC overlap. Children, in contrast, seem to have a higher likelihood of PSC + AIH overlap, with prevalence rates reported up to 50%. The combination of PSC + AIH in children is referred to as autoimmune sclerosing cholangitis. In a 16-year prospective study,[20] 27 of 55 children presenting with presumed AIH in the United Kingdom were reclassified as PSC + AIH after investigation with cholangiography. Thus, routine performance of cholangiography in children presenting with AIH is justified.

DIFFERENTIAL DIAGNOSIS: IGG4 DISEASE

IgG4 disease is a systemic disorder of unknown cause that may cause both sclerosing cholangitis and hepatitis. Thus, it may be mistaken for PSC + AIH overlap syndrome and is important to consider in the differential diagnosis of both disorders. The disease is characterized by IgG4-positive lymphoplasmacytic infiltration with fibrosis of multiple organs, including the biliary and pancreatic ducts, liver, lymph nodes (abdominal, thoracic, and head and neck), kidneys, and lung. In one of the largest series of IgG4 disease, 27 of 114 (23.7%) patients presented with predominant hepatobiliary/pancreatic disease.[21] When it involves the biliary tree, IgG4 disease has a predilection for the distal common bile duct. The small bile ducts may be involved, particularly in those who have intrahepatic strictures on cholangiography, but, in contrast to PBC, the biliary epithelium is usually intact.[22] The biliary disease has been reported to be more likely in older men compared with PSC, although head and neck IgG4 disease has been reported more common in women.[21] The AASLD recommends that a serum IgG4 should be checked for any patient with suspected PSC. An elevated serum polyclonal IgG4 is found in most, but not all, persons with IgG4 disease. Identification of the IgG4+ plasma cells in the diseased tissue establishes a definitive diagnosis. In a Canadian series of 168 patients with sclerosing cholangitis, 22% had elevated serum IgG4 and this was associated with higher ALP, a prior history of pancreatitis, and prior history of biliary intervention.[23] In a Japanese series of type 1 AIH patients, 2 of 60 (3.3%) had elevated IgG4 and one of these went on to develop sclerosing cholangitis 5 years later.[24] IgG4 disease responds well to corticosteroid therapy. One small series (N = 4) reported excellent response to rituximab in those who do not respond to corticosteroids.[25]

DIFFERENTIAL DIAGNOSIS: DRUG-INDUCED LIVER DISEASE

Drug-induced liver injury may present with several autoimmune features, such as antinuclear antibody (ANA) positivity, cholangitis, female predominance, interface hepatitis, and elevated globulins. Thus, the possibility of drug-induced liver disease should be entertained when faced with what seems to be an overlap with AIH. Several medications are well known to lead to a chronic hepatitis that mimics AIH, including α-methyldopa, nitrofurantoin, oxyphenisatin, and hydralazine and minocycline. Several reports of infliximab eliciting an AIH syndrome have emerged.[26–29] Infliximab is often used to treat inflammatory bowel disease and thus may be given to patients with associated PSC.

TREATMENT OF OVERLAP SYNDROMES
PBC + AIH Overlap

As stated previously, the designation of overlap implies that both disorders are present in sufficient quantity to justify treatment. There are no large randomized controlled trials to guide treatment, however. Given the rarity of overlap syndromes, even small randomized trials likely require international collaboration. One North American study demonstrated that patients with PBC + AIH overlap may be managed with ursodeoxycholic acid (UDCA) alone[30] AIH overlap in that study was defined by the presence of 2 or more of the following: (1) ALT > 5 × ULN; (2) IgG > 2 × ULN or positive anti–smooth muscle antibody; and (3) moderate to severe lobular inflammation on pretreatment liver biopsy. Of the 16 patients who had PBC with features of AIH, changes in serum biochemistry and immunoglobulin levels were similar to 315 patients with classical PBC and there was little change in histology over 2-year follow-up. One caveat is that 2-year follow-up may be too short an interval to detect progression in a group of 16 patients.

In other larger studies with longer follow-up, the presence of interface hepatitis in PBC has been associated with faster progression to cirrhosis. In one study of 44 subjects treated with UDCA for 4 years, severe interface hepatitis and lobular inflammation were associated with progression of fibrosis over a 4-year period. Whereas florid duct lesions, granulomas, and lobular inflammation improved over time, the interface hepatitis did not respond to UDCA treatment.[5] In another study, 26 patients with AIH + PBC followed for a mean of 6 years had worse clinical outcomes than 109 patients with classical PBC.[31] Complications of portal hypertension, death or need for transplantation were more common in the patients with PBC and probable or definite AIH. This study suggests that even without meeting other criteria for overlap syndrome, the presence of severe interface hepatitis alone may indicate a need for additional therapy besides UDCA. Studies are lacking to identify exactly what that therapy should be. Several small uncontrolled studies have demonstrated, however, that patients who have PBC + AIH overlap respond biochemically and histologically to steroids and that this may decrease progression to cirrhosis.[11,32–35] In one study of 12 patients with PBC + AIH overlap, 9 of 12 achieved biochemical remission with steroid therapy and their progression to cirrhosis was slower than expected compared with classical AIH.[32] Sequential therapy, where either UDCA or prednisone is tried first and then the other added if there is lack of adequate response, has minimalist appeal. In one study, 9 patients who failed to respond to initial monotherapy (3 UDCA alone and 6 prednisone alone) were treated with combination UDCA plus prednisone for 18 months and experienced reduction in biochemistries.[34] Recent EASL guidelines recommend adding steroids to UDCA if a biochemical response has not been evident after 3 months of UDCA.[7]

Budesonide (6 mg/d) plus mycophenolate mofetil (1.5 g/d) was used to treat a cohort of 15 French patients with PBC with suboptimal response to UDCA who also had significant interface hepatitis without cirrhosis.[36] Biochemistries normalized in 41% and improved (ALT <70 IU/L) in 47%. Histologic inflammation and fibrosis were also improved after 3 years of therapy. This regimen may offer improvement for PBC + AIH patients with reduced steroid side effects but remains to be tested in larger trials. Adding mycophenolate mofetil (1–3 g/d) to UDCA was not beneficial to PBC non-UDCA responders in the absence of significant interface hepatitis; it only resulted in insignificant improvements in ALP and AST.[37]

PSC + AIH Overlap

Both AASLD and EASL guidelines recommend the use of steroids in patients with AIH/PSC overlap, although the quality of evidence supporting those recommendations is primarily expert opinion. Children with AIH/PSC, called *autoimmune sclerosing cholangitis*, seem to benefit the most from steroid therapy. In the aforementioned 16-year prospective British study, 23 of 27 children with PSC + AIH demonstrated a good biochemical response to steroids.[20] All of the 17 children who had follow-up liver biopsies demonstrated improved inflammation without progression to cirrhosis. Response of the PSC component of the overlap syndrome was not evident: 9 follow-up cholangiograms were unchanged and 8 showed progressive cholangiopathy. In adults, the overlap of PSC + AIH seems to carry an intermediate prognosis: better than classical PSC alone, but worse than classical AIH, even if a biochemical response to steroids is seen. In one study of 7 PSC + AIH overlap patients treated with UDCA plus steroids/azathioprine, liver enzymes improved and survival was better compared with a group of 34 PSC patients treated with UDCA alone.[38] Another study, however, found that PSC + AIH patients were at increased risk of death (hazard ratio 2.14) compared with classical AIH (hazard ratio 2.08) despite a good biochemical response to steroids.[39] A study including 16 adult PSC + AIH overlap patients confirmed that the biliary disease continues to progress despite biochemical response to steroids.[40]

SUMMARY

Because knowledge of the pathogenesis of all 3 autoimmune hepatobiliary disorders—PBC, AIH, and PSC—is limited, their definitions are limited to clinical criteria that are imperfect and lack absolute specificity. Without precisely clear boundaries, they must be considered on a continuum of disease, and the possibility of overlap should be considered when several features of another disease are present. Severe interface hepatitis in PBC portends a worse prognosis and should prompt evaluation for possible AIH overlap syndrome and consideration of treatment with immunosuppression. AIH and PSC commonly overlap in children and a high index of suspicion should be maintained for this combination in the pediatric population.

REFERENCES

1. Czaja AJ, Muratori P, Muratori L, et al. Diagnostic and therapeutic implications of bile duct injury in autoimmune hepatitis. Liver Int 2004;24(4):322–9.
2. O'Brien C, Joshi S, Feld JJ, et al. Long-term follow-up of antimitochondrial antibody-positive autoimmune hepatitis. Hepatology 2008;48(2):550–6.
3. Lindor KD, Gershwin ME, Poupon R, et al. Primary biliary cirrhosis. Hepatology 2009;50(1):291–308.
4. Poupon R. Autoimmune overlapping syndromes. Clin Liver Dis 2003;7(4):865–78.
5. Degott C, Zafrani ES, Callard P, et al. Histopathological study of primary biliary cirrhosis and the effect of ursodeoxycholic acid treatment on histology progression. Hepatology 1999;29(4):1007–12.
6. Talwalkar JA, Keach JC, Angulo P, et al. Overlap of autoimmune hepatitis and primary biliary cirrhosis: an evaluation of a modified scoring system. Am J Gastroenterol 2002;97(5):1191–7.
7. EASL Clinical Practice Guidelines: management of cholestatic liver diseases. J Hepatol 2009;51(2):237–67.
8. Alvarez F, Berg PA, Bianchi FB, et al. International Autoimmune Hepatitis Group Report: review of criteria for diagnosis of autoimmune hepatitis. J Hepatol 1999;31(5):929–38.
9. Boberg KM, Chapman RW, Hirschfield GM, et al. Overlap syndromes: the International Autoimmune Hepatitis Group (IAIHG) position statement on a controversial issue. J Hepatol 2011;54(2):374–85.
10. Hennes EM, Zeniya M, Czaja AJ, et al. Simplified criteria for the diagnosis of autoimmune hepatitis. Hepatology 2008;48(1):169–76.
11. Chazouilleres O, Wendum D, Serfaty L, et al. Primary biliary cirrhosis-autoimmune hepatitis overlap syndrome: clinical features and response to therapy. J Hepatology 1998;28(2):296–301.
12. Muratori L, Cassani F, Pappas G, et al. The hepatitic/cholestatic "overlap" syndrome: an Italian experience. Autoimmunity 2002;35(8):565–8.
13. Gatselis NK, Zachou K, Papamichalis P, et al. Comparison of simplified score with the revised original score for the diagnosis of autoimmune hepatitis: a new or a complementary diagnostic score? Dig Liver Dis 2010;42(11):807–12.
14. Boberg KM, Fausa O, Haaland T, et al. Features of autoimmune hepatitis in primary sclerosing cholangitis: an evaluation of 114 primary sclerosing cholangitis patients according to a scoring system for the diagnosis of autoimmune hepatitis. Hepatology 1996;23(6):1369–76.
15. Kaya M, Angulo P, Lindor KD. Overlap of autoimmune hepatitis and primary sclerosing cholangitis: an evaluation of a modified scoring system. J Hepatol 2000;33(4):537–42.
16. van Buuren HR, van Hoogstraten HJE, Terkivatan T, et al. High prevalence of autoimmune hepatitis among patients with primary sclerosing cholangitis. J Hepatol 2000;33(4):543–8.

17. Olsson R, Glaumann H, Almer S, et al. High prevalence of small duct primary sclerosing cholangitis among patients with overlapping autoimmune hepatitis and primary sclerosing cholangitis. Eur J Intern Med 2009;20(2):190–6.

18. Lewin M, Vilgrain V, Ozenne V, et al. Prevalence of sclerosing cholangitis in adults with autoimmune hepatitis: a prospective magnetic resonance imaging and histological study. Hepatology 2009;50(2):528–37.

19. Abdalian R, Dhar P, Jhaveri K, et al. Prevalence of sclerosing cholangitis in adults with autoimmune hepatitis: evaluating the role of routine magnetic resonance imaging. Hepatology 2008;47(3):949–57.

20. Gregorio GV, Portmann B, Karani J, et al. Autoimmune hepatitis/sclerosing cholangitis overlap syndrome in childhood: a 16-year prospective study. Hepatology 2001;33(3):544–53.

21. Zen Y, Nakanuma Y. IgG4-related disease: a cross-sectional study of 114 cases. Am J Surg Pathol 2010;34(12):1812–9.

22. Naitoh I, Zen Y, Nakazawa T, et al. Small bile duct involvement in IgG4-related sclerosing cholangitis: liver biopsy and cholangiography correlation. J Gastroenterol 2011;46(2):269–76.

23. Alswat K, Al-Harthy N, Mazrani W, et al. The spectrum of sclerosing cholangitis and the relevance of IgG4 elevations in routine practice. Am J Gastroenterol 2012;107(1):56–63.

24. Umemura T, Zen Y, Hamano H, et al. Clinical significance of immunoglobulin G4-associated autoimmune hepatitis. J Gastroenterol 2011;46(Suppl 1):48–55.

25. Khosroshahi A, Bloch DB, Deshpande V, et al. Rituximab therapy leads to rapid decline of serum IgG4 levels and prompt clinical improvement in IgG4-related systemic disease. Arthritis Rheum 2010;62(6):1755–62.

26. van Casteren-Messidoro C, Prins G, van Tilburg A, et al. Autoimmune hepatitis following treatment with infliximab for inflammatory bowel disease. J Crohns Colitis 2012;6(5):630–1.

27. Subramaniam K, Chitturi S, Brown M, et al. Infliximab-induced autoimmune hepatitis in Crohn's disease treated with budesonide and mycophenolate. Inflamm Bowel Dis 2011;17(11):E149–50.

28. Goldfeld DA, Verna EC, Lefkowitch J, et al. Infliximab-induced autoimmune hepatitis with successful switch to adalimumab in a patient with Crohn's disease: the index case. Dig Dis Sci 2011;56(11):3386–8.

29. Ozorio G, McGarity B, Bak H, et al. Autoimmune hepatitis following infliximab therapy for ankylosing spondylitis. Med J Aust 2007;187(9):524–6.

30. Joshi S, Cauch-Dudek K, Wanless IR, et al. Primary biliary cirrhosis with additional features of autoimmune hepatitis: response to therapy with ursodeoxycholic acid. Hepatology 2002;35(2):409–13.

31. Silveira MG, Talwalkar JA, Angulo P, et al. Overlap of autoimmune hepatitis and primary biliary cirrhosis: long-term outcomes. Am J Gastroenterol 2007;102(6):1244–50.

32. Czaja AJ. Frequency and nature of the variant syndromes of autoimmune liver disease. Hepatology 1998;28(2):360–5.

33. Lohse AW, zum Buschenfelde KH, Franz B, et al. Characterization of the overlap syndrome of primary biliary cirrhosis (PBC) and autoimmune hepatitis: evidence for it being a hepatitic form of PBC in genetically susceptible individuals. Hepatology 1999;29(4):1078–84.

34. Chazouilleres O, Wendum D, Serfaty L, et al. Long term outcome and response to therapy of primary biliary cirrhosis-autoimmune hepatitis overlap syndrome. J Hepatol 2006;44(2):400–6.

35. Wu CH, Wang QH, Tian GS, et al. Clinical features of the overlap syndrome of autoimmune hepatitis and primary biliary cirrhosis: retrospective study. Chin Med J (Engl) 2006;119(3):238–41.
36. Rabahi N, Chretien Y, Gaouar F, et al. Triple therapy with ursodeoxycholic acid, budesonide and mycophenolate mofetil in patients with features of severe primary biliary cirrhosis not responding to ursodeoxycholic acid alone. Gastroenterol Clin Biol 2010;34(4–5):283–7.
37. Talwalkar JA, Angulo P, Keach JC, et al. Mycophenolate mofetil for the treatment of primary biliary cirrhosis in patients with an incomplete response to ursodeoxy-cholic acid. J Clin Gastroenterol 2005;39(2):168–71.
38. Boberg KM, Egeland T, Schrumpf E. Long-term effect of corticosteroid treatment in primary sclerosing cholangitis patients. Scand J Gastroenterol 2003;38(9): 991–5.
39. Al-Chalabi T, Portmann BC, Bernal W, et al. Autoimmune hepatitis overlap syndromes: an evaluation of treatment response, long-term outcome and survival. Aliment Pharmacol Ther 2008;28(2):209–20.
40. Luth S, Kanzler S, Frenzel C, et al. Characteristics and long-term prognosis of the autoimmune hepatitis/primary sclerosing cholangitis overlap syndrome. J Clin Gastroenterol 2009;43(1):75–80.

IgG4-Associated Cholangitis

Marina G. Silveira, MD

KEYWORDS

- Sclerosing cholangitis • Autoimmune pancreatitis • Chronic liver disease
- Autoimmune disease • Corticosteroids

KEY POINTS

- IgG4-associated cholangitis (IAC) is the hepatobiliary manifestation of IgG4-associated systemic disease, characterized by IgG4-positive lymphoplasmacytic infiltration of the biliary tract.
- Multiorgan disease may be evident at diagnosis but can also evolve over months to years.
- Differential diagnoses of IAC, which may present with hilar strictures/hepatic masses or pancreatic mass, include cholangiocarcinoma and pancreatic cancer, respectively.
- The diagnosis is established based on a combination of clinical, serologic, radiological, and histologic findings.
- Steroid treatment is the mainstay of management, but because of frequent disease relapse after completion of therapy or as steroids are tapered, the use of steroid-sparing immunosuppressive agents may be necessary.

INTRODUCTION

IgG4-associated systemic disease (ISD) is a systemic disorder involving multiple organs associated with increased IgG4 serum levels or IgG4-positive plasma cell infiltrates. The seminal description of this relatively new clinical entity by Hamano and colleagues[1] in 2001 included patients with pancreatic involvement, but over the course of the last decade, reports have emerged describing involvement in several organs, including the biliary tree, gallbladder, liver, retroperitoneum, mediastinum, the salivary, parotid, and lacrimal glands, kidneys, lungs, lymphatic system, breast, prostate, stomach, small bowel, nervous system and meninges, thyroid gland, pituitary gland, periorbital tissues, skin, pericardium, and vascular system.[2–4] Typically, lesions in any of these organs are characterized by infiltrating T cells and IgG4-bearing plasma cells.[5] The histologic findings include lymphoplasmacytic infiltrates organized in a storiform pattern, on occasion resulting in tumefactive lesions

Financial disclosures: None.
No conflict of interest to disclose.
Division of Gastroenterology and Hepatology, Louis Stokes Cleveland VAMC, Case Medical Center, 10701 East Boulevard, 111E (W), Cleveland, OH 44106, USA
E-mail address: marina.silveira@va.gov

Clin Liver Dis 17 (2013) 255–268
http://dx.doi.org/10.1016/j.cld.2012.11.007
1089-3261/13/$ – see front matter Published by Elsevier Inc.

liver.theclinics.com

that can mimic malignancy, infiltration of IgG4-positive plasmacytes, obliterative phlebitis, and, as the disease progresses, fibrotic changes. Corticosteroids are effective in the initial inflammatory phase of the disease,[1] although a significant proportion of treated patients may relapse after steroid treatment or during the initial steroid taper. Although ISD is rare, disease presentation may include inflammatory masses mimicking malignancies, occasionally resulting in unnecessary surgical interventions,[6] which can be avoided by accurate diagnosis and prompt initiation of treatment.

IGG4-ASSOCIATED CHOLANGITIS

Autoimmune pancreatitis (AIP) and IgG4-associated cholangitis (IAC) are the most common manifestations of ISD. IAC is the biliary manifestation of ISD, and is often associated with AIP. Pancreaticobiliary manifestations of ISD may mimic pancreatic cancer, sclerosing cholangitis, or cholangiocarcinoma. Although rare, identification of this patient group is of crucial importance, especially to distinguish them from those with malignant pancreaticobiliary disease. This review focuses on IAC.

PATHOPHYSIOLOGY

The pathophysiology of ISD is not well known. Because it is associated with hypergammaglobulinemia, increased serum levels of IgG, increased levels of IgG4 or presence of autoantibodies (including antinuclear antibodies, and rheumatoid factor, although those are not disease-specific, as well as anticarbonic anhydrase II antibodies and antilactoferrin antibodies), and effective response to steroid therapy, it has been postulated that its pathogenesis may involve autoimmune mechanisms.[7]

Potential initiating mechanisms may include genetic risk factors, bacterial infection and molecular mimicry, and autoimmunity. Studies have shown that HLA serotypes DRB1*0405 and DQB1*0401 increase the susceptibility to IgG4-related disease in Japanese populations,[8] whereas substitution of aspartic acid at DQβ1-57 is associated with disease relapse in Korean populations.[9] One study showed that many patients with AIP (94%) have antibodies against the plasminogen-binding protein of *Helicobacter pylori*,[10] which could theoretically behave as autoantibodies by means of molecular mimicry in genetically predisposed persons.[2]

Autoimmunity is widely regarded as the initial immunologic stimulus for the type 2 helper (Th2) T-cell immune response that is associated with IgG4-related disease. In healthy individuals, IgG1 usually accounts for most of the total IgG, and IgG4 accounts for less than 5% of the total IgG.[11] IgG4 production is controlled primarily by Th2 T cells.[12] Physiologic IgG4 responses can be induced by prolonged or repeat antigen exposures.[13] The role of IgG4-type autoantibodies in the pathogenesis of IgG4-related diseases is not entirely clear. IgG4-related diseases may reflect an excessive production of antiinflammatory cytokines such as interleukin 10 (IL-10), triggering an overwhelming expansion of IgG4-producing plasma cells.[14] In AIP, increased peripheral inducible-memory T regulatory cells (Tregs) are positively correlated with serum levels of IgG4[15] and prominent infiltration of Tregs with upregulation of IL-10 can be seen in the livers of patients with IAC.[16]

CLINICAL FEATURES
Demographics

Studies pertaining to the epidemiology of ISD are limited and focus mainly on AIP. AIP is typically found in patients older than 60 years (range 40–80 years), and most of the patients are men. A large, national Japanese study reported a male/female ratio of

2.8:1.[17] Limited epidemiologic data exist on IAC. As in AIP, studies report IAC in mostly men older than 50 years,[18] but population-based studies have not been conducted. A few studies have reported the prevalence of IAC among patients presenting with primary sclerosing cholangitis (PSC), suggesting that approximately 7% to 9% of patients presenting as PSC have features of IAC.[19–21]

Clinical Manifestations

The clinical presentation of patients with IAC is highly variable. Because IAC is often seen in association with AIP, clinical manifestations of the disease may also include manifestations of pancreatic disease. Obstructive jaundice is a common clinical presentation in IAC, present in up to 75% of patients.[22] Patients can present with abdominal pain, weight loss, jaundice, pruritus, and biochemical signs of pancreatitis and cholestasis.[18] The cholestatic and some gastrointestinal symptoms of IgG4-associated disease of the pancreas and biliary tree are the result of stenoses of the pancreatic duct or biliary tree. Anorexia, steatorrhea, and new-onset diabetes are also reported in many cases.[21] Several reports have described patients whose presentation included pancreatic mass or hilar strictures/hepatic masses, highly concerning for pancreatic cancer and cholangiocarcinoma, respectively.

Laboratory Features

As seen in other chronic cholestatic diseases, the most common laboratory finding described is increased alkaline phosphatase, seen in as much as 90% of patients with IAC.[3] Increases in γ-glutamyltransferase level are also observed. Serum bilirubin levels are typically higher compared with patients with classic PSC.[23] Most patients have increased serum IgG4 levels (up to 80% of patients). Modest increases of IgG4 levels (>140 mg/dL) show a moderate sensitivity of 70% to 80% for diagnosing AIP and have been described in patients with PSC,[21] cholangiocarcinoma,[24] and pancreatic cancer.[25] A recent study from the Mayo Clinic investigated the ability of IgG4 to reliably distinguish IAC from cholangiocarcinoma.[24] Serum IgG4 levels more than twice the upper limits of normal provided a specificity of 97% and sensitivity of 50% in distinguishing IAC from cholangiocarcinoma. Serum IgG4 levels more than 4 times the upper limits of normal yielded a specificity of 100%, albeit at a decreased sensitivity of 26%.[24] It has been shown that some patients with IAC did not have increased levels of IgG4 initially but developed subsequently high levels during follow-up.[26] In a recent study to assess serial changes of serum IgG4 levels in ISD, fluctuations of serum IgG4 levels of more than 30 mg/dL were detected in half of the cases during follow-up.[27] Serum IgG4 levels decrease after steroid therapy in patients with ISD,[1] although normalization of the IgG4 levels may occur in only about half of the patients after 24 months of therapy.[27]

Recently, the diagnostic value of biliary IgG4 levels was evaluated in a study including 67 patients, 5 of whom were diagnosed with IAC.[28] In this small study, IgG4 was markedly increased in bile of patients with IAC compared with patients with other biliary disorders, including PSC. Further studies are needed to confirm the value of biliary IgG4 measurements as a diagnostic tool for IAC.

Radiographic Features

In patients with AIP, which is commonly associated with IAC, computed tomography or magnetic resonance imaging may reveal enlargement of the pancreas or may mimic a malignant pancreatic lesion.[29] Changes consistent with acute pancreatitis, atrophic pancreas, and diffuse pancreatic enhancement have been described less commonly.[18] Hilar involvement of the biliary ducts in IAC can mimic hilar cholangiocarcinoma. Hepatic masslike lesions have been reported in patients with hepatic involvement. Magnetic resonance cholangiopancreaticography (MRCP) can be used to diagnose many pancreaticobiliary diseases, but may have limited capacity to delineate the exact disease in the main pancreatic duct of patients with AIP. In 1 small study including 20 patients who underwent both MRCP and endoscopic retrograde cholangiopancreaticography (ERCP), MRCP findings were comparable with ERCP for showing pancreatic ductal abnormalities in only approximately half of patients with diffuse-type AIP.[30] The diagnostic performance of MRCP and ERCP was similar for focal-type AIP, when localized stenosis with upstream dilation was identified.[30] These investigators report that MRCP was useful for detection of pancreatic gland abnormalities as well as for follow-up of patients with AIP.

Endoscopic evaluation of the biliary tree and pancreatic duct by ERCP may disclose irregularities of the pancreatic duct and stenoses of the distal or proximal common bile duct and intrahepatic bile ducts (as shown in **Figs. 1** and **2**). One study has described bile duct strictures in 88% of patients with AIP, most commonly seen in the lower common bile duct.[23] Nonetheless, sclerosing changes can be observed both in the intrahepatic and extrahepatic bile ducts.[23,26,31] Segmental strictures, long strictures with prestenotic dilatation, and strictures of the distal common bile duct are commonly observed on cholangiography in patients with IAC. Multifocal intrahepatic biliary strictures may occur, but are less common than in typical PSC. A few studies have shown that the use of cholangiography alone to diagnose IAC and differentiate it from other important alternative diagnosis is suboptimal, but cholangiographic evaluation can provide important features that might support the diagnosis when diagnostic criteria are used.[32,33]

The value of biliary biopsies is still under debate, because a histologic diagnosis may not be made on many of these biopsy specimens. Nonetheless, strong IgG4-positive infiltrates in intraductal biopsies of the bile duct have been shown in cases of IAC.[18,34]

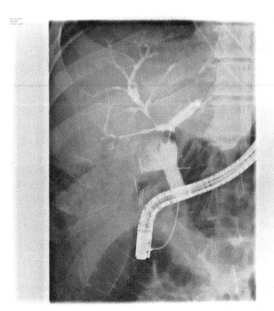

Fig. 1. Endoscopic retrograde cholangiogram showing segmental intrahepatic bile duct stricture. (*Courtesy of* Dr Todd H. Baron.)

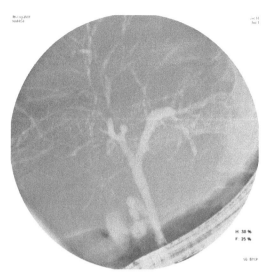

Fig. 2. Endoscopic retrograde cholangiogram showing multifocal intrahepatic biliary strictures. (*Courtesy of* Dr Todd H. Baron.)

Histologic Features

Although no single histologic feature is specific, a mix of lymphoplasmacytic inflammation, storiform fibrosis, and obliterative phlebitis is characteristic (**Fig. 3**).[35] Central to the diagnoses of ISD in pancreatic, biliary, or liver tissue is the immunohistochemical staining of more than 10 IgG4-positive cells per high-power field.[22] Because IAC can mimic presentation of cholangiocarcinoma, there are occasional surgical resections for this condition. In resected extrahepatic bile ducts, the wall is diffusely thickened (see **Fig. 3**). Peribiliary glands are encased in the fibroinflammatory process (**Fig. 4**). Phlebitis is present in adventitial veins (**Fig. 5**). The duct epithelium is preserved and neutrophils are unusual, unless biliary stents have altered the mucosal morphology.[35] Immunohistochemical staining reveals IgG4-positive cells (**Fig. 6**). Although it may be challenging to make a histologic diagnosis on small biliary biopsies,

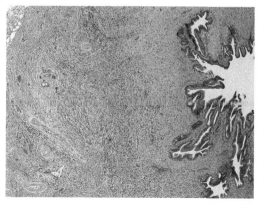

Fig. 3. Intact bile duct epithelium with wall thickened by storiform fibrosis and inflammation, low power. (*Courtesy of* Dr Thomas C. Smyrk.)

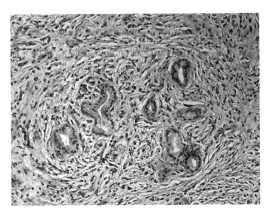

Fig. 4. Biliary glands encased in fibroinflammatory process. (*Courtesy of* Dr Thomas C. Smyrk.)

the histologic pattern is usually sufficient to suggest the correct diagnosis even in endoscopic biliary biopsy specimens (**Fig. 7**).[35]

Liver biopsy may reveal inflammatory infiltrates in the portal tracts, including lymphocytes, plasma cells, and eosinophils. As in the biliary ducts, immunohistochemical staining reveals IgG4-positive plasma cells. Most reports have shown that the number of IgG4-positive plasma cells in extrahepatic bile ducts affected by IAC usually exceeds 30 per high-power field.[22] As for the peripheral bile ducts of small portal tracts, marked heterogeneity in the degree of IgG4-positive plasma cells is described, and several portal tracts may lack the IgG4 cells entirely.[36] Obliterative phlebitis and cholangitis with periductal fibrosis have been found to be common features.

DIAGNOSIS

Although the diagnosis of IAC is often established based on a combination of clinical, serologic, radiological, and histologic findings, strict criteria for IAC are lacking.[22] Multiple diagnostic criteria have been proposed, following the initial Japanese consensus criteria[37] for the diagnosis of AIP (summarized in **Table 1**). The HISORt (histology, imaging, serology, other organ involvement, and response to

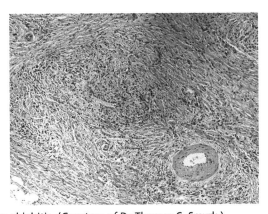

Fig. 5. Obliterative phlebitis. (*Courtesy of* Dr Thomas C. Smyrk.)

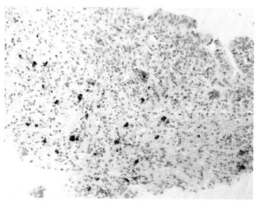

Fig. 6. Bile duct biopsy with immunohistochemical staining showing more than 10 IgG4-positive cells per high-power field. (*Courtesy of* Dr Thomas C. Smyrk.)

corticosteroid) criteria[29] for AIP (summarized in **Table 2**) and its variant criteria for IAC[18] (summarized in **Table 3**), as well as the Asian consensus criteria[38] (summarized in **Table 4**) have been the most commonly applied criteria for diagnosing AIP and IAC. Recently, experts in IAC in Japan have established separate criteria for the diagnosis of IAC[39] (summarized in **Table 5**).

The HISORt criteria for IAC[18] seem to be most helpful in clinical practice. The use of these criteria (summarized in **Table 3**) allows for a practical approach to the diagnosis and management of IAC. A definitive diagnosis can be established if there is (1) typical histology from a previous pancreaticobiliary resection or from core biopsy of the pancreas or if (2) classic imaging findings of AIP/IAC are observed in conjunction with increased serum IgG4 levels. In patients who do not meet either criteria for definitive IAC but in whom there is a high index of suspicion, after every effort has been made to exclude malignancy, a response of the biliary stricture to steroid therapy after 4 weeks confirms the diagnosis.[18]

At present, the criteria are valuable tools in clinical practice but cannot exclude entirely other disorders. The most relevant differential diagnoses of pancreaticobiliary ISD are pancreatic cancer and, less commonly, cholangiocarcinoma, which should be

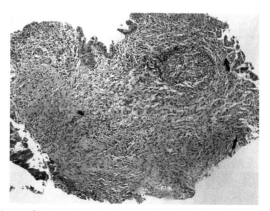

Fig. 7. Bile duct biopsy showing lymphoplasmacytic infiltration. (*Courtesy of* Dr Thomas C. Smyrk.)

Table 1
Japanese Pancreas Society criteria

Mandatory criteria	Typical imaging: diffuse enlargement of pancreas along with diffuse (>33%) main pancreatic duct narrowing with irregular wall
Supportive criteria (at least 1)	1. Serology: autoantibodies, increased γ-globulins or IgG 2. Histopathology: lymphoplasmacytic infiltrate and pancreatic fibrosis

From Members of the Criteria Committee for Autoimmune Pancreatitis of the Japan Pancreas Society. Diagnostic criteria for autoimmune pancreatitis by the Japan Pancreas Society. J Jpn Pancreas Soc 2002;17:585–7 [in Japanese]; with permission.

excluded before a diagnosis of IAC can be established. PSC must also be excluded, as well as secondary sclerosing cholangitis.

NATURAL HISTORY

Limited data exist on the prognosis and natural history of IAC, because most case series do not report long-term follow-up. Without treatment, IAC may be self-limited or it may progress to biliary cirrhosis.[18] Compared with patients with PSC, it seems that the prognosis of patients with IAC is more favorable,[20] potentially because of the responsiveness of the biliary strictures to steroids. Only 1 case of liver transplantation for established IAC has been reported,[40] although an older report describes a patient presenting with a distal stricture of the common bile duct with associated pancreatic pseudotumors (and therefore presumed IAC) eventually requiring liver transplantation.[41] One study has described that patients with a diagnosis of PSC with increased IgG4 levels manifested an increased severity of liver disease and shorter time to transplant.[21]

Table 2
The HISORt criteria

Histology	At least 1 of the following: 1. Periductal lymphoplasmacytic infiltrate with obliterative phlebitis and storiform fibrosis 2. Lymphoplasmacytic infiltrate with storiform fibrosis showing abundant ($\geq$10 cells/high-power field) IgG4-positive cells
Pancreatic imaging	Typical: diffusely enlarged gland with delayed (rim) enhancement; diffusely irregular, attenuated main pancreatic duct Others: focal pancreatic mass/enlargement; focal pancreatic duct stricture; pancreatic atrophy; pancreatic calcification; or pancreatitis
Serology	Increased serum IgG4 level (normal, 8–140 mg/dL)
Other organ involvement	Hilar/intrahepatic biliary strictures, persistent distal biliary stricture, parotid/lacrimal gland involvement; mediastinal lymphadenopathy; retroperitoneal fibrosis
Response to steroid therapy	Resolution/marked improvement of pancreatic/extrapancreatic manifestation with steroid therapy

From Chari ST, Smyrk TC, Levy MJ, et al. Diagnosis of autoimmune pancreatitis: the Mayo Clinic experience. Clin Gastroenterol Hepatol 2006;4:1011; [quiz: 934]; with permission.

Table 3
The HISORt criteria for IAC

Histology of bile duct	Lymphoplasmacytic sclerosing cholangitis on resection specimens (lymphoplasmacytic infiltrate with $\geq$10 IgG4-positive cells/HPF within and around bile ducts with associated obliterative phlebitis and storiform fibrosis). Bile duct biopsy specimens often do not provide sufficient tissue for a definitive diagnosis; however, presence of $\geq$10 IgG4-positive cells/HPF is suggestive of IAC
Imaging of bile duct	One or more strictures involving intrahepatic, proximal extrahepatic, or intrapancreatic bile ducts Fleeting/migrating biliary strictures
Serology	Increased serum IgG4 level (normal, 8–140 mg/dL)
Other organ involvement	Pancreas: classic features of AIP on imaging or histology; suggestive pancreatic imaging findings: focal pancreatic mass/enlargement without pancreatic duct dilation, multiple pancreatic masses, focal pancreatic duct stricture without upstream dilatation, pancreatic atrophy Retroperitoneal fibrosis Renal lesions: single or multiple parenchymal low-attenuation lesions (round, wedge-shaped, or diffuse patchy) Salivary/lacrimal gland enlargement
Response to steroid therapy	Normalization of liver enzyme increase or resolution of stricture (although complete resolution of stricture may not be seen early in the course of treatment or in patients with predominantly fibrotic strictures)

Abbreviation: HPF, high-power field.
From Ghazale A, Chari ST, Zhang L, et al. Immunoglobulin G4-associated cholangitis: clinical profile and response to therapy. Gastroenterology 2008;134:713; with permission.

TREATMENT

The goals of treatment in the initial inflammatory phase of IAC/AIP are symptom alleviation (eg, jaundice and abdominal discomfort), improvement of radiological and biochemical parameters and confirmation of diagnosis in select patients receiving

Table 4
Asian diagnostic criteria

Imaging (both required)	1. Pancreatic parenchyma: diffuse/segmental/focal enlargement of the gland, occasionally with a mass or hypoattenuating rim 2. Pancreaticobiliary ducts: diffuse/segmental/focal pancreatic ductal narrowing, often with stenosis of the bile duct
Serology (1 required)	1. High levels of serum IgG or IgG4 2. Detection of autoantibodies
Histopathology of pancreatic biopsy lesions	Lymphoplasmacytic infiltration with fibrosis, with abundant IgG4-positive cell infiltration
Optional	Response to steroid therapy
Diagnosis	When imaging criteria and either serology or histopathology criteria are satisfied

From Otsuki M, Chung JB, Okazaki K, et al. Asian diagnostic criteria for autoimmune pancreatitis: consensus of the Japan-Korea Symposium on Autoimmune Pancreatitis. J Gastroenterol 2008;43:404; with permission.

Table 5
Japanese IgG-4 sclerosing cholangitis diagnostic criteria

Diagnostic items	1.	Biliary tract imaging shows diffuse or segmental narrowing of the intrahepatic or extrahepatic bile duct associated with the thickening of bile duct wall
	2.	Increased serum IgG4 levels (>135 mg/dL)
	3.	Coexistence of AIP, IgG4-related dacryoadenitis/sialoadenitis, or IgG4-related retroperitoneal fibrosis
	4.	Histology shows:
		a. Marked lymphocytic and plasmacyte infiltration and fibrosis
		b. Infiltration of IgG4-positive cells (>10 cells/high-power field)
		c. Storiform fibrosis
		d. Obliterative phlebitis
		Option: effectiveness of steroid therapy (as determined at specialized facility)
Diagnosis (once PSC, malignant diseases, and secondary sclerosing cholangitis have been excluded)		Definite: combinations of (1) and (3); (1), (2) and (4) a/b; (4) a/b/c; (4) a/b/d
		Probable: combination of (1), (2), and option
		Possible: combination of (1) and (2)

From Ohara H, Okazaki K, Tsubouchi H, et al. Clinical diagnostic criteria of IgG4-related sclerosing cholangitis 2012. J Hepatobiliary Pancreat Sci 2012;19:538; with permission.

a diagnostic steroid trial.[42] Patients with IAC usually show a dramatic response to corticosteroid therapy. Although spontaneous resolution has also been described,[18] and it is possible that long-standing biliary strictures from IAC may not show steroid responsiveness, steroid therapy is the first-line and mainstay treatment of IAC. No randomized clinical studies are available. Recommendations for the steroid regimen and duration of treatment are highly variable.[42] Commonly used treatment recommendations include those described by Mayo Clinic investigators[43] and Kamisawa and colleagues,[44] which are summarized in **Table 6**. Although pretreatment (and often, prediagnosis) biliary stenting is performed in many patients with quick resolution of symptoms, steroid treatment generally improves jaundice without need for drainage in IAC/AIP. Rare nonresponders to therapy may require prolonged biliary stent placement.[18]

Disease recurrence is common during the tapering phase or after discontinuation of therapy. Relapse rates after a successful course of steroids vary greatly, from approximately 30% to more than 50%.[45] Relapse can also occur in patients experiencing

Table 6
Proposed treatment regimens

Ghazale & Chari,[43] 2007	Prednisone 40 mg/d for 4 wk, repeat laboratory tests and imaging in 4–6 wk after initiating treatment, and, if there is clinical and radiological response, taper by 5 mg every week to complete a treatment course of 11 wk
Kamisawa et al,[44] 2009	Prednisolone 0.6 mg/kg/d, tapering gradually to 5 mg/d over 3–6 mo, and then continuing maintenance steroids (2.5–10 mg/d) for at least 6 mo and possibly up to 3 y

spontaneous resolutions, and after surgical resection for suspicion of cancer. Most relapses occur within the first 3 years.[44,46] Early predictors of relapse seem to be increasing levels of alkaline phosphatase and IgG4.[27] Persistent increase in serum IgG4 levels may be a predictor for relapse.[27,44] Proximal bile duct involvement has also been described as a predictor of disease relapse.[18,44] Management of recurrent disease is controversial. On the suspicion of relapse, steroid therapy can be reinitiated or the original dose can be resumed. Steroid-sparing immunosuppression with azathioprine,[18,47,48] 6-mercaptopurine, or mycophenolate mofetil[18,48–50] is subsequently used for long-term immunosuppression. There is some experience with successful use of immunosuppressive drugs in refractory cases with frequent relapses, including budesonide and rituximab.[48,51,52] A treatment algorithm for management of disease relapse for patients with firmly established AIP or IAC has recently been proposed by researchers from the Mayo Clinic.[48] The proposed algorithm includes a repeat course of steroids for all patients and reassessment of disease activity at 6 to 8 weeks. The investigators suggest that patients who have evidence of rapid, near-complete resolution, should proceed with steroid taper with or without maintenance treatment, or initiate an immunomodulator and proceed with steroid taper (with an overlap period of ≥ 8 weeks). In patients with incomplete remission, or unable to wean prednisone (requiring prednisone doses of 20 mg/d or higher to maintain remission), treatment with rituximab is recommended. Rituximab is also recommended for patients with steroid intolerance at any time or immunomodulator intolerance (if unable to change to a different immunomodulator class).[48] Many questions about the management of IAC/AIP remain unanswered, particularly with regards to the optimal management of recurrent relapsers, the role of immunomodulators in the maintenance of remission, and disease management in patients who are intolerant of corticosteroids or whose disease is refractory to corticosteroids. Larger clinical studies are needed to help refine clinical indications and dosing protocols for the treatment of IAC/AIP.

SUMMARY

IAC is the hepatobiliary manifestation of a recently described inflammatory systemic disease, characterized by IgG4-positive lymphoplasmacytic infiltration of the biliary tract. The diagnosis is established based on a combination of clinical, serologic, radiological, and histologic findings. Often, patients present with obstructive jaundice, and imaging reveals stenoses of the distal or proximal common bile duct and intrahepatic bile ducts, often in association with parenchymal pancreatic findings and irregularities of the pancreatic duct. Serum levels of IgG4 are often greater than twice the upper limits of normal. Steroid treatment is the mainstay of management, but despite exquisite steroid sensitivity, relapse is common after discontinuation of therapy or during tapering of steroids.

REFERENCES

1. Hamano H, Kawa S, Horiuchi A, et al. High serum IgG4 concentrations in patients with sclerosing pancreatitis. N Engl J Med 2001;344:732–8.
2. Stone JH, Zen Y, Deshpande V. IgG4-related disease. N Engl J Med 2012;366:539–51.
3. Maillette de Buy Wenniger L, Rauws EA, Beuers U. What an endoscopist should know about immunoglobulin-G4-associated disease of the pancreas and biliary tree. Endoscopy 2012;44:66–73.

4. Kawa S, Okazaki K, Kamisawa T, et al. Japanese consensus guidelines for management of autoimmune pancreatitis: II. Extrapancreatic lesions, differential diagnosis. J Gastroenterol 2010;45:355–69.

5. Zhang L, Notohara K, Levy MJ, et al. IgG4-positive plasma cell infiltration in the diagnosis of autoimmune pancreatitis. Mod Pathol 2007;20:23–8.

6. Hardacre JM, Iacobuzio-Donahue CA, Sohn TA, et al. Results of pancreaticoduodenectomy for lymphoplasmacytic sclerosing pancreatitis. Ann Surg 2003;237: 853–8 [discussion: 8–9].

7. Okazaki K, Kawa S, Kamisawa T, et al. Japanese consensus guidelines for management of autoimmune pancreatitis: I. Concept and diagnosis of autoimmune pancreatitis. J Gastroenterol 2010;45:249–65.

8. Kawa S, Ota M, Yoshizawa K, et al. HLA DRB10405-DQB10401 haplotype is associated with autoimmune pancreatitis in the Japanese population. Gastroenterology 2002;122:1264–9.

9. Park do H, Kim MH, Oh HB, et al. Substitution of aspartic acid at position 57 of the DQbeta1 affects relapse of autoimmune pancreatitis. Gastroenterology 2008;134: 440–6.

10. Frulloni L, Lunardi C, Simone R, et al. Identification of a novel antibody associated with autoimmune pancreatitis. N Engl J Med 2009;361:2135–42.

11. Aalberse RC, Stapel SO, Schuurman J, et al. Immunoglobulin G4: an odd antibody. Clin Exp Allergy 2009;39:469–77.

12. Nirula A, Glaser SM, Kalled SL, et al. What is IgG4? A review of the biology of a unique immunoglobulin subtype. Curr Opin Rheumatol 2011;23:119–24.

13. Robinson DS, Larche M, Durham SR. Tregs and allergic disease. J Clin Invest 2004;114:1389–97.

14. Okazaki K, Uchida K, Koyabu M, et al. Recent advances in the concept and diagnosis of autoimmune pancreatitis and IgG4-related disease. J Gastroenterol 2011;46:277–88.

15. Miyoshi H, Uchida K, Taniguchi T, et al. Circulating naive and CD4+CD25high regulatory T cells in patients with autoimmune pancreatitis. Pancreas 2008;36: 133–40.

16. Zen Y, Fujii T, Harada K, et al. Th2 and regulatory immune reactions are increased in immunoglobin G4-related sclerosing pancreatitis and cholangitis. Hepatology 2007;45:1538–46.

17. Nishimori I, Tamakoshi A, Otsuki M, Research Committee on Intractable Diseases of the Pancreas Ministry of Health, Labour, and Welfare of Japan. Prevalence of autoimmune pancreatitis in Japan from a nationwide survey in 2002. J Gastroenterol 2007;42(Suppl 18):6–8.

18. Ghazale A, Chari ST, Zhang L, et al. Immunoglobulin G4-associated cholangitis: clinical profile and response to therapy. Gastroenterology 2008;134:706–15.

19. Toosi MN, Heathcote J. Pancreatic pseudotumor with sclerosing pancreatocholangitis: is this a systemic disease? Am J Gastroenterol 2004;99:377–82.

20. Takikawa H, Takamori Y, Tanaka A, et al. Analysis of 388 cases of primary sclerosing cholangitis in Japan: presence of a subgroup without pancreatic involvement in older patients. Hepatol Res 2004;29:153–9.

21. Mendes FD, Jorgensen R, Keach J, et al. Elevated serum IgG4 concentration in patients with primary sclerosing cholangitis. Am J Gastroenterol 2006;101: 2070–5.

22. Bjornsson E, Chari ST, Smyrk TC, et al. Immunoglobulin G4 associated cholangitis: description of an emerging clinical entity based on review of the literature. Hepatology 2007;45:1547–54.

23. Nakazawa T, Ohara H, Sano H, et al. Clinical differences between primary sclerosing cholangitis and sclerosing cholangitis with autoimmune pancreatitis. Pancreas 2005;30:20–5.
24. Oseini AM, Chaiteerakij R, Shire AM, et al. Utility of serum immunoglobulin G4 in distinguishing immunoglobulin G4-associated cholangitis from cholangiocarcinoma. Hepatology 2011;54:940–8.
25. Ghazale A, Chari ST, Smyrk TC, et al. Value of serum IgG4 in the diagnosis of autoimmune pancreatitis and in distinguishing it from pancreatic cancer. Am J Gastroenterol 2007;102:1646–53.
26. Hirano K, Shiratori Y, Komatsu Y, et al. Involvement of the biliary system in autoimmune pancreatitis: a follow-up study. Clin Gastroenterol Hepatol 2003;1:453–64.
27. Tabata T, Kamisawa T, Takuma K, et al. Serial changes of elevated serum IgG4 levels in IgG4-related systemic disease. Intern Med 2011;50:69–75.
28. Vosskuhl K, Negm AA, Framke T, et al. Measurement of IgG4 in bile: a new approach for the diagnosis of IgG4-associated cholangiopathy. Endoscopy 2012;44:48–52.
29. Chari ST, Smyrk TC, Levy MJ, et al. Diagnosis of autoimmune pancreatitis: the Mayo Clinic experience. Clin Gastroenterol Hepatol 2006;4:1010–6 [quiz: 934].
30. Kamisawa T, Tu Y, Egawa N, et al. Can MRCP replace ERCP for the diagnosis of autoimmune pancreatitis? Abdom Imaging 2009;34:381–4.
31. Nishino T, Toki F, Oyama H, et al. Biliary tract involvement in autoimmune pancreatitis. Pancreas 2005;30:76–82.
32. Nishino T, Oyama H, Hashimoto E, et al. Clinicopathological differentiation between sclerosing cholangitis with autoimmune pancreatitis and primary sclerosing cholangitis. J Gastroenterol 2007;42:550–9.
33. Kalaitzakis E, Levy M, Kamisawa T, et al. Endoscopic retrograde cholangiography does not reliably distinguish IgG4-associated cholangitis from primary sclerosing cholangitis or cholangiocarcinoma. Clin Gastroenterol Hepatol 2011;9:800–803.e2.
34. Alexander S, Bourke MJ, Williams SJ, et al. Diagnosis of autoimmune pancreatitis with intraductal biliary biopsy and treatment of stricture with serial placement of multiple biliary stents. Gastrointest Endosc 2008;68:396–9.
35. Smyrk TC. Pathological features of IgG4-related sclerosing disease. Curr Opin Rheumatol 2011;23:74–9.
36. Deshpande V, Sainani NI, Chung RT, et al. IgG4-associated cholangitis: a comparative histological and immunophenotypic study with primary sclerosing cholangitis on liver biopsy material. Mod Pathol 2009;22:1287–95.
37. Members of the Criteria Committee for Autoimmune Pancreatitis of the Japan Pancreas Society. Diagnostic criteria for autoimmune pancreatitis by the Japan Pancreas Society. J Jpn Pancreas Soc 2002;17:585–7 [in Japanese].
38. Otsuki M, Chung JB, Okazaki K, et al. Asian diagnostic criteria for autoimmune pancreatitis: consensus of the Japan-Korea Symposium on Autoimmune Pancreatitis. J Gastroenterol 2008;43:403–8.
39. Ohara H, Okazaki K, Tsubouchi H, et al. Clinical diagnostic criteria of IgG4-related sclerosing cholangitis 2012. J Hepatobiliary Pancreat Sci 2012;19:536–42.
40. Clendenon JN, Aranda-Michel J, Krishna M, et al. Recurrent liver failure caused by IgG4 associated cholangitis. Ann Hepatol 2011;10:562–4.
41. Stathopoulos G, Nourmand AD, Blackstone M, et al. Rapidly progressive sclerosing cholangitis following surgical treatment of pancreatic pseudotumor. J Clin Gastroenterol 1995;21:143–8.

42. Pannala R, Chari ST. Corticosteroid treatment for autoimmune pancreatitis. Gut 2009;50:1430–9.
43. Ghazale A, Chari ST. Optimising corticosteroid treatment for autoimmune pancreatitis. Gut 2007;56:1650–2.
44. Kamisawa T, Shimosegawa T, Okazaki K, et al. Standard steroid treatment for autoimmune pancreatitis. Gut 2009;58:1504–7.
45. Sah RP, Chari ST. Autoimmune pancreatitis: an update on classification, diagnosis, natural history and management. Curr Gastroenterol Rep 2012;14:95–105.
46. Sah RP, Chari ST, Pannala R, et al. Differences in clinical profile and relapse rate of type 1 versus type 2 autoimmune pancreatitis. Gastroenterology 2010;139: 140–8 [quiz: e12–3].
47. Church NI, Pereira SP, Deheragoda MG, et al. Autoimmune pancreatitis: clinical and radiological features and objective response to steroid therapy in a UK series. Am J Gastroenterol 2007;102:2417–25.
48. Hart PA, Topazian MD, Witzig TE, et al. Treatment of relapsing autoimmune pancreatitis with immunomodulators and rituximab: the Mayo Clinic experience. Gut 2012. [Epub ahead of print].
49. Mannion M, Cron RQ. Successful treatment of pediatric IgG4 related systemic disease with mycophenolate mofetil: case report and a review of the pediatric autoimmune pancreatitis literature. Pediatr Rheumatol Online J 2011;9:1.
50. Sodikoff JB, Keilin SA, Cai Q, et al. Mycophenolate mofetil for maintenance of remission in steroid-dependent autoimmune pancreatitis. World J Gastroenterol 2012;18:2287–90.
51. Topazian M, Witzig TE, Smyrk TC, et al. Rituximab therapy for refractory biliary strictures in immunoglobulin G4-associated cholangitis. Clin Gastroenterol Hepatol 2008;6:364–6.
52. Khosroshahi A, Carruthers MN, Deshpande V, et al. Rituximab for the treatment of IgG4-related disease: lessons from 10 consecutive patients. Medicine 2012;91: 57–66.

Secondary Sclerosing Cholangitis
Pathogenesis, Diagnosis, and Management

Mohamad H. Imam, MBBS[a], Jayant A. Talwalkar, MD, MPH[a],
Keith D. Lindor, MD[b],*

KEYWORDS

- Liver transplantation • Clinical management • Cholangiopathy • Complications
- Outcomes

KEY POINTS

- Secondary sclerosing cholangitis (SSC) is a rare disease entity with complex pathogenesis.
- Common causes for SSC include obstruction, infection, ischemia, and critical illness.
- Although initially asymptomatic, patients with SSC may present later with pruritus, abdominal pain, and jaundice.
- The cholangiographic finding of isolated peripheral ductal abnormalities suggests SSC over primary sclerosing cholangitis.
- Management should address the underlying cause of SSC, and liver transplantation is an option for advanced disease.

INTRODUCTION

Secondary sclerosing cholangitis (SSC) is a chronic disease with phenotypical, clinical, and cholangiographic resemblance to idiopathic primary sclerosing cholangitis (PSC). Conversely, a known pathologic process underlies SSC, leading to inflammation, obliterative fibrosis of the bile ducts, stricture formation, and progressive destruction of the biliary tree that ultimately leads to biliary cirrhosis. Without timely intervention, the natural history of SSC is less favorable than that of PSC.

The most common disease processes and causes underlying SSC include stones in the biliary ducts, surgery, chemotherapy, blunt trauma, and recurrent or autoimmune pancreatitis.[1] A new form of SSC, sclerosing cholangitis in critically ill patients (SC-CIP), is associated with rapid progression to liver cirrhosis. Patients with this form of sclerosing cholangitis generally do not have a history of preceding biliary or liver

[a] Cholestatic Liver Diseases Study Group, Division of Gastroenterology and Hepatology, Mayo Clinic, 200 First Street SW, Rochester, MN 55905, USA; [b] College of Health Solutions, Arizona State University, 500 North 3rd Street, Phoenix, AZ 85004-0698, USA
* Corresponding author.
E-mail address: Keith.Lindor@asu.edu

Clin Liver Dis 17 (2013) 269–277
http://dx.doi.org/10.1016/j.cld.2012.11.004
1089-3261/13/$ – see front matter Published by Elsevier Inc.

liver.theclinics.com

disease and do not show evidence of obstructive injury to the bile duct. Therapeutic options for SSC remain limited, and patients with SSC who do not receive liver transplantation have significantly reduced survival compared with those with PSC.

This article describes the epidemiology, pathogenesis, common causes, diagnostic modalities, management, and outcomes in patients with SSC.

Epidemiology

Because of a common perception that SSC is a rare disease, relevant epidemiologic data confirming the prevalence of SSC are lacking. From the authors' experience at the Mayo Clinic in Rochester, MN, USA, only 31 cases were described through a decade of diligent patient follow-up. In this population, the major causes of SCC were postcholecystectomy trauma, chronic pancreatitis, and intraductal stones. Patients with SSC who did not undergo transplantation had a shorter period of survival (72 months) than those with PSC (89 months).[2]

Pathogenesis

Primary hepatocellular bile has an intricately modulated content comprising a set alkalinity and fluidity that is adjusted by the intrahepatic bile duct epithelium, which in turn affects the reabsorption of bile acids, amino acids, and glucose and the secretion of electrolytes and water.

Orchestration of hepatocytes and cholangiocytes (epithelial cells of bile duct) is essential for bile formation. Bile is first secreted by hepatocytes as primary bile, which is modified later by cholangiocytes through secretion of electrolytes and fluids.[3,4] Anatomically, the liver consists of a convoluted network of intrahepatic ducts that are required for bile secretion. In these ducts an increase in alkalinity and fluidity occurs; this is in contrast to the acidification and concentration that occurs in the gallbladder. Specific sections of intrahepatic bile ducts are often targeted by biliary abnormalities, and hence different functional properties of these segments can be affected accordingly.[5,6]

The intrahepatic bile duct epithelium transport function is synchronized by several factors, including neurotransmitters, neuropeptides, and hormones. This intrahepatic biliary epithelium is the primary target of cholestatic insults, which may include autoimmune diseases, toxic agents, ischemia, infections, and even genetic diseases. Characteristic findings in cholangiopathy include cholangiocyte apoptosis, proliferation, inflammation, and fibrosis. The pathogenic cascade involving the development of SSC targets cholangiocytes. Through production of various proinflammatory mediators, cholangiocyte proliferation and death may contribute to the process of inflammation, resulting in chronic liver destruction. These afflictions of cholangiocytes are often produced by toxins, ischemia, trauma, or apoptosis. SSC is characterized by damage to the peribiliary circulation, proliferation of cholangiocytes, alterations in cholangiolar secretions and transport processes, and, finally, activation of fibrosis. Specific molecular pathways that lead to fibrosis are still under investigation.[7]

COMMON CAUSES

Unlike PSC, the origin of which is still under investigation, common causes for SSC are evident and can be treated accordingly. Common causes include obstruction, ischemic insult, infections, and immunologic disease. Imaging and diagnostic modalities can help differentiate secondary causes, and can hence aid in implementing the appropriate treatment in a timely and effective manner. **Table 1** provides a summary of common causes and their related pathogenesis.

Table 1
Causes and related pathogenesis of SSC

Causes	Related Pathogenesis
Cytomegalovirus/parasites (mainly in AIDS or organ transplant recipients)	Infection leading to chronic inflammation
Autoimmune pancreatitis, hypereosinophilic syndrome	Immunologic modulation
Cholecystitis, biliary stones, polyps, tumors, arterial aneurysms, pancreatic disease, and strictures	Obstruction leading to a cycle of biliary stasis and suppurative cholangitis
Echinococcosis	Hydatid cyst rupture leading to necrosis and fibrosis of biliary epithelium
Allograft rejection, vasculitis, thrombotic obstruction, advanced AIDS, liver transplantation, hypoxia, massive transfusions, hereditary telangiectasias, radiotherapy, and chemotherapy	Ischemia caused by direct effect of trauma or subsequent massive transfusions, medications, or hypotension
Critical illness (SC-CIP)	Interference with the biliary blood supply

Obstruction

Obstruction of the biliary tree has numerous causes, which may include cholecystitis, biliary stones, polyps, tumors, arterial aneurysms, pancreatic disease, and strictures inflicted through surgery or trauma. Obstructive cholangiopathy is characterized by bile stasis, which eventually leads to inflammation and fibrosis. The timing at which this sequence occurs often depends on the extent and duration of the obstruction. Along with stasis, the external pressure effect and the possibility of superimposed infection may also lead to aggravated injury. Eventually, the patient develops a vicious cycle of biliary stasis and suppurative cholangitis.

Gallbladder and bile duct abnormalities can be associated with portal hypertension in some patients, which leads to extrinsic obstruction of the common bile duct. Moreover, this may be the pathogenesis that underlies bile duct obstruction in cirrhosis and liver fibrosis.[8] Patients with this disease, termed *portal biliopathy*, are often symptomatic at diagnosis, and liver histology shows minimal or no abnormalities. Cholangiography is the preferred modality for diagnosing patients with portal biliopathy, in whom abnormalities in the common bile duct are often prominent.[9] Recommendations for treatment include biliary balloon dilatation, and possibly surgery if persistent obstruction is present.[10,11]

Infectious and Inflammatory

Recurrent pyogenic cholangitis is caused by the development of strictures or pigmented stones that lead to obstruction of the biliary tract and, subsequently, recurrent episodes of bacterial cholangitis. This disease entity is also referred to as *Oriental cholangiohepatitis*.[12] Ultrasonography may be used initially to diagnose ductal stones or dilatation; this can then be followed by a contrast computed tomography to identify central ductal dilation and peripheral ductal tapering.[13,14] Conversely, endoscopic retrograde cholangiopancreatography (ERCP) and magnetic retrograde cholangiopancreatography are not recommended because of the increased risk of sepsis. This can be managed through conservative measures and antibiotic therapy, with surgery indicated in patients experiencing persistent symptoms or decompensation or those developing peritonitis.[15]

In patients with immunodeficiency, susceptibility to parasitic infections may predispose to SSC. For example, patients with advanced AIDS often develop a cholangiopathy caused by biliary infection with *Cryptosporidium parvum* or Microsporidia, which presents with papillary stenosis and features of SSC.[16,17] Moreover, in patients undergoing organ transplantation, cryptosporidiosis has been described to cause SSC and viral infection, with cytomegalovirus as the second leading cause of SSC in AIDS cholangiopathy.[17–20]

Echinococcosis can be complicated by hydatid cyst rupture, which may lead to necrosis of biliary epithelia and fibrosis through toxin mediated mechanisms.[21] Hepatic stellate cells seem to have a role in interacting with parasitic antigens, leading to liver fibrosis.[22] Leakage of fluid from the hydatid cyst through a biliary fistula may also cause SSC.[23]

A histologic finding of a heterogeneous population of plasma cells, fibroblasts, macrophages, and eosinophils may denote the presence of a rare pathologic entity referred to as *hepatic inflammatory pseudotumor*. Despite associations with Crohn disease, its pathophysiology remains obscure.[24,25]

Ischemia

The biliary system is a highly vascular network, which necessitates the maintenance of an adequate blood supply to avoid injury. The right and left hepatic arteries form the major blood supply to the extrahepatic biliary system, except for the gallbladder, which receives its blood supply from the retroduodenal artery and is less vascular than the remaining biliary formation.

Ischemic cholangitis is an umbrella term that can comprise several causes with a common pathophysiology, including allograft rejection, vasculitis, thrombotic obstruction, advanced AIDS, liver transplantation, hypoxia, massive transfusions, hereditary telangiectasias, radiotherapy, and chemotherapy.[1,26] After trauma, a patient may develop ischemic cholangitis either from the direct effects of the trauma on the biliary tree or as a result of subsequent massive transfusions, medications, or hypotension. In patients undergoing liver transplantation, ischemic injury may result from destruction of small arteries and thrombosis of larger arteries; this may occur in up to 19% of patients undergoing transplant. The risk for biliary ischemia is even higher in liver transplantation from donation after cardiac death, in which donor age and cold ischemic time act as major risk factors for the development of ischemic cholangiopathy.[27] Chemotherapy can affect the bile ducts through ischemia and hence lead to secondary sclerosing cholangitis; common agents include floxuridine, paclitaxel, 5-fluorouracil, formaldehyde, and yttrium 90.[1,26,28]

Sclerosing Cholangitis in Critically Ill Patients

Patients with life-threatening illnesses are prone to developing secondary sclerosing cholangitis, a disease entity coined as *SC-CIP*. Surprisingly, this pathogenetic process persists even after recovery from the primary illness, and leads to rapid development of cholestasis despite the absence of baseline liver disease. Investigators have suggested that the underlying pathogenesis is centered on interference with the biliary blood supply.[29] Cholangiography may initially show simple filling defects, but later stages may be confused with PSC, an important differential to consider when assessing patients. Casts are the hallmark of sclerosing cholangitis in critically ill patients and may be useful in distinguishing it from different disease entities. Once this disease develops, the outcomes are truly detrimental, with rapid progression to cirrhosis and an urgent need for transplantation.[30]

Immunologic

Several autoimmune disorders may be involved in the pathogenesis of SSC. One disorder is autoimmune pancreatitis, a distinct primary pancreatic disease with no gold standard for diagnosis but features of autoimmunity, such as the presence of hypergammaglobulinemia, elevated serum immunoglobulin G 4 (IgG4) levels, and elevated liver enzymes.[31–33] IgG4 levels are the most important in distinguishing auto-immune pancreatitis from pancreatic cancer.[32] On histology, autoimmune hepatitis shows diffuse lymphoplasmacytic infiltration with acinar atrophy, obliterative phlebitis, and marked fibrosis.[34] A varying array of symptoms may occur in patients with auto-immune pancreatitis, often related to strictures or pancreatitis; obstructive jaundice may be present in a little fewer than half of the patients with autoimmune pancreatitis.

Patients with eosinophilic infiltration from hypereosinophilic syndrome commonly present with features of sclerosing cholangitis. Infiltration of the liver with eosinophils may occur in several liver diseases or as an immune response to other pathogenetic processes. The role of this infiltration in inducing biliary fibrosis remains uncertain. Patients with SSC from hypereosinophilic syndrome show good response to steroids, reflected by a decrease in sclerosing cholangitis and eosinophilic infiltration.[1,35]

Fibrotic tissue is mast cell–rich, reflecting the role of mast cells in the production of fibrogenic factors, such as heparin, tryptase, stem cell factor, and histamine.[36–39] In patients with systemic mastocytosis, this infiltration of mast cells could lead to sclerosing cholangitis.[35,40]

Children with a diagnosis of cystic fibrosis may present with changes concordant with PSC. This finding can be explained by the increased expression of cystic fibrosis transmembrane conductance regulator (CFTR) gene.[41] Although some older studies contradict this theory, showing a lack of association between CFTR mutations and PSC,[42] more recent reports convey a link between CFTR dysfunction in the pediatric population and the development of PSC.[43,44]

Langerhans cell histiocytosis (LCH), also known as *histiocytosis X*, has been linked in several reports to PSC.[45,46] Patients with LCH may develop end-stage liver disease and hence require liver transplantation. Outcomes of patients with LCH after liver transplantation for advanced liver disease show good outcomes, but further study is required in a larger cohort of patients.[47]

CLINICAL SYMPTOMS AND DIAGNOSIS

Most patients at the initial stages of the disease are asymptomatic, with elevated alka-line phosphatase and gamma glutamyltransferase levels. Several symptoms may occur as the disease progresses, which may include pruritus, abdominal pain, and jaundice. In patients with SSC, recurrent episodes of bacterial cholangitis from ascending infection are common.[48–50]

After the identification of abnormal liver test results, patients should undergo ultraso-nography to detect biliary abnormalities relating to obstruction. If the underlying cause is not obstruction and the ultrasound shows no findings, the use of ERCP is recommen-ded. Findings on ERCP are similar to those for PSC, with ductal dilatation and beading.

RADIOLOGIC DIFFERENTIATION

Cholangiographic findings may be helpful in distinguishing SSC from PSC. Diffuse ductal narrowing and multifocal strictures suggest PSC, whereas isolated peripheral ductal abnormalities suggest SSC. Recurrent pyogenic cholangitis may show sudden ductal cutoff, intrahepatic bile collections, and ductal stones. Autoimmune pancreatitis may show changes to the pancreatic duct, whereas AIDS cholangiopathy is characterized by papillary stenosis and accompanying intrahepatic disease.

MANAGEMENT, COMPLICATIONS, AND OUTCOMES

The management of SSC depends on the underlying cause. Patients with recurrent pyogenic cholangitis may benefit from prompt supportive care and institution of empiric antibiotics, followed by monitoring. If decompensation occurs or the disease is persistent, surgical intervention may be necessary. Surgery focuses on drainage and exploration of the bile ducts. Endoscopic intervention may also be used when needed, and long-term drainage may be the only option in a few patients with widespread disease.[15,51,52]

Conversely, therapeutic options in patients with AIDS cholangiopathy are limited, because none have been shown to be beneficial in improving survival. Patients usually have advanced immunosuppression from AIDS, which contributes greatly to the poor prognosis in this subset of patients. Average survival is estimated merely as 12 months and is not affected by endoscopic interventions.[18,53] AIDS cholangiopathy has not been shown to benefit from antimicrobial therapy, and hence prognosis depends on the status of the underlying immunosuppression, with decreased viral load and improved counts being favorable signs.[17]

In symptomatic patients with portal biliopathy who develop obstructive jaundice from stones or stricture endoscopic sphincterotomy, balloon dilatation of the stricture or portosystemic shunting may be instituted.[10,11,54–58]

Despite the common notion perceived through retrospective study of patients with SSC that these patients are at no increased risk of developing cholangiocarcinoma, several case reports have shown an increased occurrence in patients with subtypes of SSC.[2,59,60] The possibility exists that the detection rate of cholangiocarcinoma in this population remains minimal because of the poor outcomes caused by comorbidities. Advances in diagnostic modalities may lead to increased diagnosis of cholangiocarcinoma in patients with SSC.

Liver transplantation seems to be an appropriate method of management for patients with advanced SSC. A French study of 5 patients with SSC requiring liver transplantation after biliary surgery who were followed up for 39 months posttransplant showed excellent outcomes with no recurrence.[61]

SUMMARY

Because of the reversible nature of secondary sclerosing cholangitis, a high suspicion for the diagnosis should be maintained, especially in patients with PSC with unclear diagnostic features.

REFERENCES

1. Abdalian R, Heathcote EJ. Sclerosing cholangitis: a focus on secondary causes. Hepatology 2006;44:1063–74.
2. Gossard AA, Angulo P, Lindor KD. Secondary sclerosing cholangitis: a comparison to primary sclerosing cholangitis. Am J Gastroenterol 2005;100:1330–3.
3. Strazzabosco M. New insights into cholangiocyte physiology. J Hepatol 1997;27: 945–52.

4. Tavoloni N. The intrahepatic biliary epithelium: an area of growing interest in hepatology. Semin Liver Dis 1987;7:280–92.
5. Nathanson MH, Boyer JL. Mechanisms and regulation of bile secretion. Hepatology 1991;14:551–66.
6. Alpini G, Glaser S, Robertson W, et al. Bile acids stimulate proliferative and secretory events in large but not small cholangiocytes. Am J Physiol 1997;273: G518–29.
7. Strazzabosco M, Spirli C, Okolicsanyi L. Pathophysiology of the intrahepatic biliary epithelium. J Gastroenterol Hepatol 2000;15:244–53.
8. O'Brien PH, Meredith HC, Vujic I, et al. Obstructive jaundice caused by cavernous transformation of the portal vein post neonatal omphalitis. J S C Med Assoc 1979;75:209–10.
9. Khuroo MS, Yattoo GN, Zargar SA, et al. Biliary abnormalities associated with extrahepatic portal venous obstruction. Hepatology 1993;17:807–13.
10. Chandra R, Kapoor D, Tharakan A, et al. Portal biliopathy. J Gastroenterol Hepatol 2001;16:1086–92.
11. Chaudhary A, Dhar P, Sarin SK, et al. Bile duct obstruction due to portal biliopathy in extrahepatic portal hypertension: surgical management. Br J Surg 1998;85: 326–9.
12. Seel DJ, Park YK. Oriental infestational cholangitis. Am J Surg 1983;146:366–70.
13. Lim JH, Ko YT, Lee DH, et al. Oriental cholangiohepatitis: sonographic findings in 48 cases. AJR Am J Roentgenol 1990;155:511–4.
14. Chan FL, Man SW, Leong LL, et al. Evaluation of recurrent pyogenic cholangitis with CT: analysis of 50 patients. Radiology 1989;170:165–9.
15. Fan ST, Choi TK, Wong J. Recurrent pyogenic cholangitis: current management. World J Surg 1991;15:248–53.
16. Sheikh RA, Prindiville TP, Yenamandra S, et al. Microsporidial AIDS cholangiopathy due to Encephalitozoon intestinalis: case report and review. Am J Gastroenterol 2000;95:2364–71.
17. Yusuf TE, Baron TH. AIDS Cholangiopathy. Curr Treat Options Gastroenterol 2004;7:111–7.
18. Bouche H, Housset C, Dumont JL, et al. AIDS-related cholangitis: diagnostic features and course in 15 patients. J Hepatol 1993;17:34–9.
19. Abdo A, Klassen J, Urbanski S, et al. Reversible sclerosing cholangitis secondary to cryptosporidiosis in a renal transplant patient. J Hepatol 2003;38:688–91.
20. Campos M, Jouzdani E, Sempoux C, et al. Sclerosing cholangitis associated to cryptosporidiosis in liver-transplanted children. Eur J Pediatr 2000;159:113–5.
21. Sahin M, Eryilmaz R, Bulbuloglu E. The effect of scolicidal agents on liver and biliary tree (experimental study). J Invest Surg 2004;17:323–6.
22. Anthony B, Allen JT, Li YS, et al. Hepatic stellate cells and parasite-induced liver fibrosis. Parasit Vectors 2010;3:60.
23. Stamm B, Fejgl M, Hueber C. Satellite cysts and biliary fistulas in hydatid liver disease. A retrospective study of 17 liver resections. Hum Pathol 2008;39: 231–5.
24. Sasahira N, Kawabe T, Nakamura A, et al. Inflammatory pseudotumor of the liver and peripheral eosinophilia in autoimmune pancreatitis. World J Gastroenterol 2005;11:922–5.
25. Amankonah TD, Strom CB, Vierling JM, et al. Inflammatory pseudotumor of the liver as the first manifestation of Crohn's disease. Am J Gastroenterol 2001;96: 2520–2.
26. Deltenre P, Valla DC. Ischemic cholangiopathy. Semin Liver Dis 2008;28:235–46.

27. Foley DP, Fernandez LA, Leverson G, et al. Biliary complications after liver transplantation from donation after cardiac death donors: an analysis of risk factors and long-term outcomes from a single center. Ann Surg 2011;253:817–25.

28. Riaz A, Lewandowski RJ, Kulik LM, et al. Complications following radioembolization with yttrium-90 microspheres: a comprehensive literature review. J Vasc Interv Radiol 2009;20:1121–30 [quiz: 1131].

29. Engler S, Elsing C, Flechtenmacher C, et al. Progressive sclerosing cholangitis after septic shock: A new variant of vanishing bile duct disorders. Gut 2003; 52(5):688–93.

30. Ruemmele P, Hofstaedter F, Gelbmann CM. Secondary sclerosing cholangitis. Nat Rev Gastroenterol Hepatol 2009;6:287–95.

31. Hirano K, Komatsu Y, Yamamoto N, et al. Pancreatic mass lesions associated with raised concentration of IgG4. Am J Gastroenterol 2004;99:2038–40.

32. Hamano H, Kawa S, Horiuchi A, et al. High serum IgG4 concentrations in patients with sclerosing pancreatitis. N Engl J Med 2001;344:732–8.

33. Yoshida K, Toki F, Takeuchi T, et al. Chronic pancreatitis caused by an autoimmune abnormality. Proposal of the concept of autoimmune pancreatitis. Dig Dis Sci 1995;40:1561–8.

34. Kawaguchi K, Koike M, Tsuruta K, et al. Lymphoplasmacytic sclerosing pancreatitis with cholangitis: a variant of primary sclerosing cholangitis extensively involving pancreas. Hum Pathol 1991;22:387–95.

35. Marbello L, Anghilieri M, Nosari A, et al. Aggressive systemic mastocytosis mimicking sclerosing cholangitis. Haematologica 2004;89:ECR35.

36. Tsuneyama K, Kono N, Yamashiro M, et al. Aberrant expression of stem cell factor on biliary epithelial cells and peribiliary infiltration of c-kit-expressing mast cells in hepatolithiasis and primary sclerosing cholangitis: a possible contribution to bile duct fibrosis. J Pathol 1999;189:609–14.

37. Garbuzenko E, Berkman N, Puxeddu I, et al. Mast cells induce activation of human lung fibroblasts in vitro. Exp Lung Res 2004;30:705–21.

38. Garbuzenko E, Nagler A, Pickholtz D, et al. Human mast cells stimulate fibroblast proliferation, collagen synthesis and lattice contraction: a direct role for mast cells in skin fibrosis. Clin Exp Allergy 2002;32:237–46.

39. Gruber BL. Mast cells in the pathogenesis of fibrosis. Curr Rheumatol Rep 2003; 5:147–53.

40. Ishii M, Iwai M, Harada Y, et al. A role of mast cells for hepatic fibrosis in primary sclerosing cholangitis. Hepatol Res 2005;31:127–31.

41. O'Brien S, Keogan M, Casey M, et al. Biliary complications of cystic fibrosis. Gut 1992;33:387–91.

42. Gallegos-Orozco JF, E Yurk C, Wang N, et al. Lack of association of common cystic fibrosis transmembrane conductance regulator gene mutations with primary sclerosing cholangitis. Am J Gastroenterol 2005;100:874–8.

43. Henckaerts L, Jaspers M, Van Steenbergen W, et al. Cystic fibrosis transmembrane conductance regulator gene polymorphisms in patients with primary sclerosing cholangitis. J Hepatol 2009;50:150–7.

44. Pall H, Zielenski J, Jonas MM, et al. Primary sclerosing cholangitis in childhood is associated with abnormalities in cystic fibrosis-mediated chloride channel function. J Pediatr 2007;151:255–9.

45. Thompson HH, Pitt HA, Lewin KJ, et al. Sclerosing cholangitis and histiocytosis X. Gut 1984;25:526–30.

46. Ramos FJ, Perez-Arellano JL, Lopez-Borrasca A. Primary sclerosing cholangitis in histiocytosis X. Am J Med 1987;82:191.

47. Concepcion W, Esquivel CO, Terry A, et al. Liver transplantation in Langerhans' cell histiocytosis (histiocytosis X). Semin Oncol 1991;18:24–8.

48. Deltenre P, Valla DC. Ischemic cholangiopathy. J Hepatol 2006;44:806–17.

49. Sakrak O, Akpinar M, Bedirli A, et al. Short and long-term effects of bacterial translocation due to obstructive jaundice on liver damage. Hepatogastroenterology 2003;50:1542–6.

50. Sherlock S. Pathogenesis of sclerosing cholangitis: the role of nonimmune factors. Semin Liver Dis 1991;11:5–10.

51. Tanaka M, Ikeda S, Ogawa Y, et al. Divergent effects of endoscopic sphincterotomy on the long-term outcome of hepatolithiasis. Gastrointest Endosc 1996;43:33–7.

52. Gott PE, Tieva MH, Barcia PJ, et al. Biliary access procedure in the management of oriental cholangiohepatitis. Am Surg 1996;62:930–4.

53. Cello JP, Chan MF. Long-term follow-up of endoscopic retrograde cholangiopancreatography sphincterotomy for patients with acquired immune deficiency syndrome papillary stenosis. Am J Med 1995;99:600–3.

54. Thervet L, Faulques B, Pissas A, et al. Endoscopic management of obstructive jaundice due to portal cavernoma. Endoscopy 1993;25:423–5.

55. Perlemuter G, Bejanin H, Fritsch J, et al. Biliary obstruction caused by portal cavernoma: a study of 8 cases. J Hepatol 1996;25:58–63.

56. Hymes JL, Haicken BN, Schein CJ. Varices of the common bile duct as a surgical hazard. Am Surg 1977;43:686–8.

57. Mork H, Weber P, Schmidt H, et al. Cavernous transformation of the portal vein associated with common bile duct strictures: report of two cases. Gastrointest Endosc 1998;47:79–83.

58. Dhiman RK, Puri P, Chawla Y, et al. Biliary changes in extrahepatic portal venous obstruction: compression by collaterals or ischemic? Gastrointest Endosc 1999;50:646–52.

59. Chow LT, Ahuja AT, Kwong KH, et al. Mucinous cholangiocarcinoma: an unusual complication of hepatolithiasis and recurrent pyogenic cholangitis. Histopathology 1997;30:491–4.

60. Hocqueloux L, Gervais A. Cholangiocarcinoma and AIDS-related sclerosing cholangitis. Ann Intern Med 2000;132:1006–7.

61. Mohsine R, Blanchet MC, El Rassi Z, et al. Liver transplantation for secondary sclerosing cholangitis following biliary surgery. Gastroenterol Clin Biol 2004;28:181–4 [in French].

Alagille Syndrome and Other Hereditary Causes of Cholestasis

Jane L. Hartley, MBChB, MRCPCH, MMedSci, PhD[a], Paul Gissen, MD, PhD[b],
Deirdre A. Kelly, MD, FRCPI, FRRCP, FRCPCH[a],[*]

KEYWORDS

- Conjugated hyperbilirubinemia • Neonatal jaundice • Pruritus
- Hepatosplenomegaly • Fat-soluble vitamins

KEY POINTS

- Conjugated hyperbilirubinemia is always significant and must be investigated.
- Inherited disorders cause a significant proportion of cases presenting with pediatric liver disease.
- It is important to recognize the spectrum of severity in the inherited cholestatic disorders.
- Early and accurate diagnosis helps informed patient management and can prevent deterioration in some patients.
- Genetic diagnosis in all cases improves family counseling and management of future cases.

INTRODUCTION

Neonatal jaundice is common and is transient in most normal infants. Conjugated hyperbilirubinemia is always significant and caused by several diseases, of which extrahepatic biliary atresia (EHBA) is the single leading cause of morbidity and mortality in childhood liver disease.[1] However, recent advances in the understanding of the cause and pathogenesis of cholestasis highlighted the importance of genetic causes of cholestasis.

ALAGILLE SYNDROME

Alagille syndrome (AGS) (MIM118450) is a highly variable, autosomal dominant multisystem condition with an estimated frequency of 1 in 30,000.[2] It was initially described as a hepatic disease, but molecular testing has shown that the liver involvement is variable including no overt liver disease. Those who have significant liver disease present

[a] Liver Unit, Birmingham Children's Hospital, Steelhouse Lane, Birmingham B4 6NH, UK; [b] MRC Laboratory for Molecular Cell Biology, UCL Institute of Child Health, London, UK
[*] Corresponding author.
E-mail address: DEIRDRE.KELLY@bch.nhs.uk

Clin Liver Dis 17 (2013) 279–300
http://dx.doi.org/10.1016/j.cld.2012.12.004
1089-3261/13/$ – see front matter © 2013 Elsevier Inc. All rights reserved.

liver.theclinics.com

in the neonatal period with conjugated hyperbilirubinemia.[3] Overall, there is a 10% mortality rate from vascular accidents, cardiac disease, and liver disease.[4]

Approximately 95% of patients with AGS have mutations in *JAG1*, which encodes the NOTCH signaling pathway ligand Jagged-1.[5] Jagged/Notch interactions that occur at cell–cell contact points determine cell fate in early development. *NOTCH2* mutations were found to cause AGS in patients who did not have mutations in JAG1,[6] and renal disease is more common in patients with NOTCH2 than JAG1 defects.

There is a lack of genotype–phenotype correlation in AGS, and a range of phenotypes are found in affected members of the same family.[7] Thus, it is likely that additional genetic and/or environmental factors determine the final clinical phenotype. Before molecular testing, AGS was a clinical diagnosis consisting of intralobular bile duct paucity and at least 3 of 5 other major clinical features[8]: cholestasis, cardiac disease with peripheral pulmonary stenosis, skeletal anomalies with butterfly thoracic vertebrae, posterior embryotoxon seen on slit lamp examination of the eyes, and triangular facies.

Clinical Features

Hepatic features

Cholestasis in the neonatal period occurs in 95% of cases[3] but may be mild and not clinically apparent.[2,9] When the cholestasis is severe, it may be clinically difficult to distinguish from biliary atresia. It is essential to make the correct diagnosis, as a Kasai procedure performed in a child with AGS may cause deterioration of liver function.[10] The identification of other AGS clinical features may aid medical management in cases that are difficult to distinguish from biliary atresia.

The liver disease is often associated with severe pruritus, which significantly affects the child's quality of life,[11] and hypercholesterolemia with xanthoma on the extensor surfaces. Xanthoma and pruritus may improve with time.[11] Hepatocellular cancer may develop in those with cirrhosis, and patients should be screened for this condition with abdominal ultrasonography and alpha fetoprotein levels.[12]

Cardiac features

More than 90% of patients with AGS have cardiac anomalies, with the typical cardiac lesion being peripheral pulmonary stenosis (PPS), although most other congenital cardiac lesions have also been associated with AGS (eg, 16% of cases have tetralogy of Fallot).[13] Cardiac disease is an important determinant for early survival.[3]

Skeletal features

Classically, butterfly shape of the thoracic vertebrae is seen because of abnormal fusion of the spine leading to a sagittal cleft in 80% of cases.[14] Other vertebral anomalies may occur such as pointed anterior process of C1, spina bifida occulta, fusion of adjacent vertebrae, hemivertebrae, and absence of 12th ribs. There is no long-term clinical consequence of the vertebral changes. Craniosynostosis[15] and radioulnar synostosis[16] with shortening of the finger distal phalanges and a fusiform appearance may occur. Fractures have been reported in up to 28% of patients with AGS, with the majority affecting the lower limb bones.[17]

Ophthalmologic features

Posterior embryotoxon may be supportive of the diagnosis of AGS, occurring in 90% of cases,[18] but can also be found in up to 15% of the normal population and in other syndromes such as 22q11.2 deletion.[19] It has no long-term visual consequences. Other ocular findings may be iris hypoplasia, abnormalities of the optic discs, abnormal retinal vessels, and pigmentary retinopathy.

Facial features
Triangular face with deep-set eyes, pointed chin, hypertelorism, and prominent forehead are characteristic. The features may not be prominent in the first few years of life but evolve with age, and the protrusion of the mandible and chin becomes more prominent.[3]

Renal features
Intrinsic renal diseases with tubulointerstitial nephropathy and mesangiolipidosis may occur. Structural changes with cysts are common with simple benign cysts or multicystic dysplastic kidneys and renal failure.[20] Renal tubular acidosis may contribute to poor growth and chronic renal insufficiency. Renal vascular disease may require stenting.

Growth and nutrition
Poor growth, fat-soluble vitamin deficiency, and delayed puberty are common in children with AGS. Poor growth may be part of the genetic defect in AGS but is compounded by the high energy requirements needed to overcome the liver and cardiac diseases.[21,22] Cholestasis also results in poor absorption of long-chain fats. Children with AGS are susceptible to severe metabolic bone disease and require supplementation of vitamin D and other fat-soluble vitamins.

Vascular involvement
Intracranial vascular anomalies are seen in up to 15% of patients[3] and are detectable on magnetic resonance angiography (MRA). They are often asymptomatic but may lead to intracranial bleeding, accounting for 34% of mortality in patients with AGS.[4] Other vessels may also be involved with intra-abdominal aneurysms, narrowing of the carotid artery, and renal artery stenosis.

Learning difficulties
Gross motor delay occurs in 16% of children.[8] Mental retardation is prevalent, but when confounding factors (liver disease and nutrition) are eliminated, they may be no more common than in the general population.

Benign intracranial hypertension
The development of benign intracranial hypertension, which may lead to optic nerve atrophy and blindness, has been reported both pretransplant and posttransplant. Annual examination of the fundus is essential to detect early papilledema.[23]

Diagnosis

The diagnosis of AGS is made by identifying the constellation of clinical features, with the characteristic histology of paucity of the intralobular bile ducts and confirmed by molecular DNA analysis.

Liver
Biochemistry: Typically there is conjugated hyperbilirubinemia, which improves with time. The levels of hepatic transaminases may be up to 10 times the upper limit of normal. Levels of gamma glutamyl transferase (GGT) are extremely high, up to 20 times the upper limit of normal. Unless there is end-stage liver disease, synthetic function is maintained (prothrombin and albumin). The levels of cholesterol and triglycerides are often elevated.

Ultrasonography of the liver: This result is often normal, although occasionally a contracted gallbladder is seen.

Radioisotope excretion: In severe cholestasis, the pale stool and dark urine with a nonexcretory radioisotope scan may make the diagnosis difficult to distinguish from biliary atresia [1,3]

Histology: An adequate sample for assessment contains 6 to 20 portal tracts, and a diagnosis of paucity of intralobular bile ducts is when the ratio is less than 0.5 (normal ratio, 0.9–1.8). The paucity of bile ducts is progressive and hence in young infants may not be appreciated.[24] In young infants, ductular proliferation may also be seen, again making the differential diagnosis from biliary atresia difficult. Periportal and centrilobular fibrosis develop in 15% to 20% of patients, leading to biliary cirrhosis.

Cholangiogram (endoscopic retrograde cholangiopancreatography or surgically): This test demonstrates the patency of the extrahepatic biliary tree.

Identifying other clinical features also is highly supportive of AGS:

Cardiac features: Echocardiography identifies cardiac anomalies and PPS.

Ophthalmologic features: A slit lamp examination is required to identify the posterior embryotoxon.

Vertebral features: Thoracic spinal radiography identifies butterfly vertebrae.

Renal features: Ultrasound scan is used to identify structural lesions, biochemistry to identify renal function, and urinary analysis to identify renal tubular acidosis.

Cranial features: Magnetic resonance imaging (MRI) or MRA identifies intracranial vascular anomalies if there are intracranial concerns, although this is not a routine investigation.

Genetic diagnosis

Genetic diagnosis is performed through sequencing of *JAG1* and *NOTCH2* genes, with mutations found in 95% and 5% of patients with AGS, respectively. Although it is possible to perform antenatal genetic testing using DNA obtained from chorionic villous sampling or amniocentesis, it may be difficult to predict the severity of the disease in an affected fetus because of variable penetrance of the disease mutations.

Management

Cholestasis: Ursodeoxycholic acid may improve the biochemical cholestasis.[25]

Pruritus: typically this is more severe than in other causes of cholestasis and may be difficult to control. The skin should be kept moisturized; the child's skin should be covered and nails short to avoid excoriation. Rooms should be kept cool. The efficacy of antipruritic medication varies with each patient. Medications that have been shown to be effective are shown in **Table 1**. If there is no response to medication, then phototherapy may be useful in some cases, or partial external biliary diversion may be performed, although results are variable.

Table 1
Antipruritic therapy in children with cholestasis

Drug	Dose
Cholestyramine	1–4 g/d
Phenobarbitone	5–10 mg/kg/d
Rifampicin[26]	5–10 mg/kg/d
Ondansetron[27]	2–4 mg bid
Natrexone[28]	0.25–0.5 mg/kg/d
Antihistamines	These are ineffective but may cause sedation at night to provide symptomatic relief

Xanthomas: The number of xanthomas typically increases in the first few years, but they disappear when the cholestasis improves with a reduction in cholesterol levels. If the xanthomas are disfiguring or interfere with function (eg, inner canthus of the eye), lipid lowering medication may be beneficial. Partial external biliary diversion may lead to complete resolution in some patients without hepatic fibrosis.[29]

Nutrition: Growth failure is likely to be multifactorial. Cholestasis results in steatosis because of poor absorption of long-chain fats, and a high-energy feed containing mainly medium-chain triglycerides is required. Nutritional intake may be compromised in patients with AGS, and nasogastric or gastrostomic tube feeding may be required to achieve adequate caloric intake.[28]

Fat-soluble vitamins: Most children with AGS require supplementation of fat-soluble vitamins. Vitamin D deficiency is especially difficult to treat, and lower limb fractures are common. Vitamin E may be better absorbed in the water-soluble format (Vedrop). **Table 2** provides suggested vitamin doses.

Liver transplant: Liver transplant may be necessary if cirrhosis and chronic liver disease develop. Other indications include deterioration in quality of life, intense refractory pruritus, or malnutrition with recurrent bone fractures despite optimal nutrition.[11] Occasionally, early liver transplant is indicated before the development of severe pulmonary hypertension. Posttransplant survival rates are similar to other cholestatic indications, but few children achieve normal height posttransplant.[11]

Genetic counseling: Genetic counseling is necessary to identify other family members with AGS and to provide accurate information for further children, including prenatal diagnostic investigations.

Prognosis

Most estimates put overall mortality at 20% to 30%, due to cardiac disease, intercurrent infection, or progressive liver disease.[3,11] The largest outcomes study showed that in 163 children with AGS and liver involvement, 44 (33%) required liver transplant, with neonatal cholestasis at presentation more likely to result in a worse outcome.[11] Actuarial survival rates with native liver were 51% and 38% at 10 and 20 years, respectively, and overall survival rates were 68% and 62%, respectively.

The natural history of the cholestasis is that it typically worsens in the first few years and then starts to improve with relief of pruritus and xanthomas,[11] and hence liver transplant indicated for these reasons may not be required in later childhood.

PROGRESSIVE FAMILIAL INTRAHEPATIC CHOLESTASIS

This heterogeneous group of inherited cholestatic diseases is caused by mutations in the hepatocellular transport system genes involved in bile synthesis. They have characteristic clinical, biochemical, and histopathologic features. The genes for types 1, 2, and 3 have been characterized, leading to increased accuracy of diagnosis. Other genes involved in bile salt metabolism that are not directly associated with clinical

Table 2	
Fat-soluble vitamin supplementation for children with cholestasis	
Vitamin A	5000 units/d
Vitamin D/ergocalciferol	4000–8000 units/d
Vitamin E (polyethylene glycol)	25 IU/kg/d
Vitamin K	2.5 mg/d

disease could modify the phenotype of other forms of cholestasis. These modifier genes include the apical sodium-dependent bile acid transporter and the farsenoid X-receptor, a bile acid–activated transcription factor that mediates transcriptional repression of genes important in bile acid and cholesterol homeostasis.[30,31] Progressive familial intrahepatic cholestasis (PFIC) is a group of rare diseases thought to have an incidence of 1/50,000 to 1/100,000, with worldwide occurrence and equal sex distribution.

Nomenclature

PFIC1 (MIM211600) is also known as FIC1 deficiency or Byler disease and is caused by mutations in *ATP8B1*.[32] Benign recurrent intrahepatic cholestasis type I (MIM243300, BRIC1) is also caused by mutations in *ATP8B1* and is an allelic condition to PFIC1. ATP8B1 protein translocates phospholipids, such as phosphatidylserine, from the outer to the inner canalicular membrane leaflets.[33]

PFIC2 (MIM601847) is also known as bile salt export pump (BSEP) deficiency. It is caused by mutations in *ABCB11*.[34] Benign recurrent intrahepatic cholestasis type II (MIM605479, BRIC2) is also caused by mutations in *ABCB11* and is an allelic condition to PFIC2.[35] BSEP is the major canalicular bile salt export pump in man, which extracts bile salts from hepatocytes into canaliculi.

PFIC3 (MIM602347) is also known as MDR3 deficiency and is caused by mutations in *ABCB4*.[36] Unlike in PFIC1 and PFIC2, patients with PFIC3 have raised levels of GGT. ABCB4 encodes protein ABCB4, which translocates phosphatidyl choline and other membrane phospholipids from the inner to the outer canalicular membrane leaflet. Thus, phospholipids become available for extraction by bile salts.[37] Evidence shows that there exists a functional interdependence between ABCB4 and ATP8B1 whereby these 2 proteins together maintain hepatocyte canalicular membrane function.[38] Thus, a combined genotype of ATP8B1 and ABCB4 may determine the extent of clinical phenotype in PFIC.

Mutations in genes involved in PFIC and BRIC are found in a range of cholestatic conditions presenting in older age including intrahepatic cholestasis of pregnancy (ICP), drug-induced cholestasis, and gallstones.[39,40]

Clinical Features

PFIC1: Presentation is in the first months of life with recurrent episodes of jaundice, which becomes persistent. Pruritus may be severe with high serum bile acid levels. Due to the extrahepatic expression of *ATP8B1*, other clinical features include pancreatitis, diarrhea, sensorineural deafness, and short stature. The extrahepatic manifestations may become more evident or severe following liver transplant.[40]

PFIC2: Cholestasis is usually permanent from the time of presentation in infancy. It may present with coagulopathy secondary to fat-soluble vitamin K deficiency. Pruritus is a major clinical feature. Due to the expression of ABCB11 in the liver only, there are no extrahepatic manifestations.[41] Hepatocellular carcinoma has been reported in infancy and should be monitored with alpha fetoprotein levels and ultrasound scans.[42]

PFIC3: Cholestasis is variable, and only 30% of patients present with cholestasis in infancy. It may present at anytime during childhood or adult life with complications of chronic liver disease such as portal hypertension and liver failure. Pruritus is often mild.[43]

Diagnosis

Biochemistry: Both PFIC1 and PFIC2 have low-normal GGT levels despite marked cholestasis in contrast to the GGT levels in PFIC3, which may be up to 10 times normal.

The levels of hepatic transaminases in all 3 forms are raised (up to 10 times normal in PFIC1 and PFIC2 and up to 5 times normal for PFIC3). Cholesterol level tends to be low. Synthetic function is maintained until liver failure develops. Coagulopathy with abnormal prothrombin time is usually due to poor absorption of vitamin K.

Ultrasound scan of liver: There are no specific findings associated with PFIC, although cholelithiasis is the presenting feature of PFIC3 and may complicate PFIC2.

Histology

PFIC1: There is a bland canalicular cholestasis with no bile duct paucity or proliferation.[44] There is minimal inflammation. Biopsies taken later in childhood may show a more marked giant cell change with fibrosis. Electron microscopy shows paucity of canalicular microvilli and coarse granular bile (known as Bylers bile).

PFIC2: There is canalicular cholestasis with hepatocellular necrosis and giant cell transformation. There is portal fibrosis and inflammation from infancy. Bile duct loss can occur. On electron microscopy there is amorphous or filamentous bile. Immunohistochemical staining for BSEP is negative in patients with mutations causing abrogation of protein production.

PFIC3: There is portal fibrosis and ductular proliferation with a mixed inflammatory infiltrate. There may be bile plugs in the lobule, and some giant cell changes are seen. Later biopsies demonstrate biliary cirrhosis.

Genetic diagnosis

Identification of mutations in *ATP8B1* (PFIC1), *ABCB11* (PFIC2), or *ABCB4* (PFIC3) can aid clinical diagnosis in this group of conditions. Due to some clinical overlap, particularly between PFIC1 and PFIC2, some of the laboratories offer sequencing of all 3 genes simultaneously. Screening of large phenotype-specific gene panels is easier with new sequencing technologies.[45]

Management

Cholestasis: Ursodeoxycholic acid may be helpful in improving bile flow and reducing pruritus.

Pruritus: Antipruritic medication (see **Table 1**) is necessary for PFIC1 and PFIC2. For those with intractable pruritus and without fibrosis, nasobiliary drainage or biliary diversion is effective, although the extrahepatic manifestations of PFIC1 may be exacerbated. Bile adsorptive resins such as cholestyramine are the most effective in reducing pruritus but are unpalatable.

Nutrition: Cholestasis results in poor absorption of long-chain fats and a medium-chain triglyceride formula is necessary. Nasogastric feeding may be required if nutritional intake is suboptimal. It is essential to supplement with fat-soluble vitamins, as deficiency is common (see **Table 2**).

Liver transplant: Most patients require liver transplant in childhood. For those with PFIC2 and PFIC3 this is curative. For those with PFIC1 the extrahepatic manifestations may worsen, especially the diarrhea. Graft steatosis leading to cirrhosis and the need for retransplant occurs with PFIC1.[46] Recurrence of disease (jaundice and pruritus) has been recognized in children who underwent transplant for PFIC2 (BSEP; *ABCB11*). These patients developed anti-BSEP antibodies presumably because the acquired transporter acts as a neoantigen.[47]

BILE ACID SYNTHESIS DEFECTS

There are 16 enzymes involved in converting cholesterol to the primary bile acids, cholic and chenodeoxycholic acids,[48] and a defect in any could cause liver disease.

This review provides brief details on 2 bile synthesis defects; in-depth description of these rare but important disorders is given elsewhere.[49]

Clinical Features

3β-Hydroxy-Δ5-C27-steroid dehydrogenase deficiency (MIM607765)
This enzyme deficiency presents with severe neonatal hepatitis with cholestasis and acholic stool or mild cholestasis with fat-soluble vitamin deficiency at a later date.[50,51]

Δ4-3-Oxosteroid 5b-reductase deficiency (MIM235555)
This condition has a heterogeneous clinical presentation ranging from severe neonatal liver disease and coagulopathy[52] to chronic liver disease in later childhood.

Diagnosis

Diagnosis is made using fast atom bombardment mass spectroscopy (FAB-MS) of urine or plasma to identify the abnormal bile acid composition, noting the lack of primary bile acids with a high concentration of intermediary metabolites.

GGT level is typically low despite cholestasis. Histologically there are features of neonatal hepatitis and giant cell changes.[53] Δ4-3-Oxosteroid 3β-reductase deficiency has iron overload similar to neonatal hemochromatosis. Diagnosis is confirmed by gene sequencing, although this is not available routinely. It is likely that with the reduced cost of analysis and availability of whole-exome sequencing these methods will improve diagnosis.

Management

Replacement of the deficient primary bile acid reduces the formation of toxic intermediary compounds. Cholic acid and ursodeoxycholic acid are beneficial,[54] and in 24,25-dihydroxycholanoic cleavage enzyme deficiency the addition of chenodeoxycholic acid may also be beneficial, but there have been reports of hepatotoxicity.

Prognosis

There is progressive liver disease due to the formation of toxic metabolites leading to the requirement for liver transplant, which is avoided if treatment is started promptly.

NIEMANN-PICK TYPE C DISEASE

Niemann-Pick type C disease (NPC) (MIM257220) is an autosomal recessive lysosomal storage disorder caused by mutations in either the NPC1 or the NPC2 gene.[55] Abnormal trafficking and lysosomal accumulation of cholesterol and various sphingolipids was found in cells and tissues from patients with NPC.[56] It is a clinically heterogeneous neurovisceral condition with presentation from infancy with liver disease to adulthood when it tends to present with neurodegeneration. It has an estimated incidence of 1/120,000 live births.[57]

NPC1 is a membrane-bound glycoprotein that contains putative sterol-sensing domains and in brain is expressed in presynaptic astrocytic glial processes, where it localizes to lysosomes and late endosomes.[58] NPC2 is a soluble cholesterol-binding protein that is secreted, and therefore, it is thought that bone marrow transplant is able to modify NPC phenotype in patients with NPC2 mutations.[59,60] Together, NPC1 and NPC2 are required for the trafficking of lipids out of the lysosomes. Approximately 10% of patients have no mutations in either NPC1 or NPC2, and other genes may be involved in the NPC pathogenesis.

The underlying mechanism of liver or neurologic disease in NPC remains undetermined, although it has been suggested that a secondary sphingolipid accumulation may play a significant role in neurodegeneration.[61]

Clinical Features

Perinatal period: NPC may present prenatally with fetal hydrops and ascites.[62] Half the patients present with neonatal cholestasis in the first days or weeks of life.[63] In 10% of these patients, liver failure leads to death within the first 6 months. In others, the jaundice improves by 2 to 4 months, but there is progressive hepatosplenomegaly.

Early infancy (2 months – 2 years): NPC may present at this stage with isolated hepatosplenomegaly.[64] In some there is early-onset severe neurologic involvement with delay of developmental milestones and hypotonia, followed by loss of motor skills and mental regression. Some children have an intention tremor.

Late infancy (2–6 years): There may be isolated hepatomegaly or isolated splenomegaly. Language delay is frequent, and dysphagia, dysarthria, gait problems, clumsiness, and dementia develop. Cataplexy is common and may be the presenting feature at this age. Seizures are also common. Swallowing problems may be pronounced requiring the child to have a gastrostomy.

Juvenile period (6–15 years): This form of the disease is the most common. It may present with isolated splenomegaly, although in 10% of cases there is no organomegaly. The child has difficulty in writing, with reduced attention span, as well as dyspraxia, dysarthria, pyramidal signs, spasticity, and difficulty swallowing. Cataplexy, which is laughter-induced, and narcolepsy may occur.

Adult form: There are reports of isolated splenomegaly with no neurologic involvement presenting in adults, but these are rare cases. Many have neurologic symptoms similar to the juvenile-onset form, with at least a third having psychiatric presentation such as psychosis, delusions, and hallucinations. Seizures are rare at this age of presentation. The most common neurologic features are cerebellar ataxia and dysarthria.[65] Vertical supranuclear ophthalmoplegia is considered pathognomonic and may be found from an early age.

Diagnosis

Biochemistry: In the perinatal form there is variable conjugated hyperbilirubinemia, which improves with time. Levels of transaminases are usually raised up to 5 times normal, although they increase further with the development of liver failure. Prothrombin time and albumin levels are normal unless liver failure develops. Biochemical findings are normal in later presentations. There may be reduced cholesterol and raised chitotriosidase levels, although this is variable.[66]

Imaging: Imaging may show hepatosplenomegaly or features of chronic liver disease (heterogeneous liver and abdominal varices). MRI and computed tomographic scan results may be normal or may show cerebellar or cortical changes or white matter changes in the infantile form.

Histology: Foam cells are seen in the bone marrow and the liver but are difficult to detect in young infants.[62]

Filipin test: This test demonstrates the impaired cholesterol efflux and accumulation in late endosomes and lysosomes. Skin fibroblasts are cultured in low density lipoprotein–enriched medium and then stained with filipin (specifically forms complexes with unesterified cholesterol). In NPC there is positive fluorescence of cholesterol-filled perinuclear vesicles. There are proved cases in which the staining is abnormal but not as prominent (variant phenotype), and diagnosis is difficult based on filipin staining alone. Moreover, carriers with abnormal filipin staining have been described.[57,67]

Neurophysiologic tests: A full neurologic assessment is essential to identify muscle, motor, and reflex anomalies. Hearing and swallowing are abnormal. Ophthalmologic examination may diagnose the abnormal saccadic eye movement and vertical gaze.[68]

Genetics: Diagnosis is confirmed by identifying mutations in NPC1 (95% of cases) or NPC2 (5% of cases). Prenatal diagnosis and carrier testing is offered if the mutations are known.

Management

The treatment of NPC is supportive. Bone marrow or liver transplant does not influence the neurologic progress of the disease. A low-cholesterol diet and cholesterol-lowering medication reduce the cholesterol load in the liver but do not influence the neurologic progression.[68]

To reduce the glycolipid storage in NPC, an iminosugar inhibitor of glucosylceramide synthase (miglustat) has been developed, which reduces progression of the disease. It has no influence on systemic symptoms. The side effects include diarrhea, flatulence, weight loss, and tremor. It is recommended to commence miglustat at the onset of any neurologic symptoms.[68,69]

Prognosis

NPC is a severe disease leading to premature death, but the rate of progression is extremely variable. In the majority, jaundice is transient and resolves by 4 months. Splenomegaly persists but rarely results in hypersplenism. The age of onset of systemic symptoms has no relationship with the development of neurologic signs.[68] Within families there is variability in the onset of systemic symptoms, whereas the neurologic onset occurs at a similar age. Children with the filipin staining variant may have a milder phenotype.[62]

Children who present in the neonatal period with hydrops or acute liver failure die in infancy. Those presenting later in infancy often die in childhood, whereas those with the juvenile form may survive into adult life. The mean age of death in the adult-onset disease is 38 years.[57]

CITRIN DEFICIENCY (CITRULLINEMIA TYPE II)

Citrin deficiency (CD) or citrullinemia type II caused by mutations in SLC25A13 (MIM605814) is an autosomal recessive disorder that was described in Japan but is now recognized worldwide.[70] CD can present with neonatal cholestasis—neonatal intrahepatic cholestasis due to citrin deficiency (NICCD)—or with adult-onset disease, which is less common. Citrin is a mitochondrial aspartate glutamate carrier, which is expressed in the liver, heart, and kidneys. CD can lead to secondary dysfunction of argininosuccinate synthetase, a urea cycle enzyme; hyperammonemia; and coma.[71]

Clinical Features

Typically there is neonatal conjugated hyperbilirubinemia. This condition is associated with a diverse range of metabolic anomalies including gluconeogenesis, glycolysis, urea synthesis, and fatty acid synthesis, which may present with hypoglycemia, poor hepatic synthetic function, and failure to thrive.[70] Older children have food preferences with avoidance of sweets and rice and preference for peanuts and beans. Adults (citrullinemia type II) present with fatty liver, hepatitis, iron accumulation, and neurologic symptoms secondary to hyperammonemia.[71]

Diagnosis

Biochemistry: Plasma amino acids show elevated levels of galactose, citrulline, and methionine; however, these abnormalities often are not present after the newborn period.[72] There may be recurrent hypoglycemia and galactosuria.

Histology: There is neonatal hepatitis and steatosis.[73]

Ophthalmology: Some infants have cataracts.

Management

Treatment is based on dietary modifications with adequate calories to prevent hypoglycemia. When cholestatic, the infant should have fat-soluble vitamin supplementation and a medium-chain triglyceride feed. A lactose-free diet may be offered to patients with galactosuria. Thereafter, a high-protein, low-carbohydrate diet may be beneficial.[74] After the resolution of initial liver disease, patients may have recurrent nonspecific symptoms of nausea, vomiting, and abdominal pain, which are sometimes associated with hypoglycemic episodes. A high-protein diet may relieve these symptoms. There is no agreed management protocol, but it is important to ensure adequate calorie supply (with protein and fat) during episodes of illness.

Prognosis

Neonatal hepatitis resolves in most infants within the first year, although some require liver transplant.[75] In those whose symptoms resolve, there is a risk of developing the adult features of citrullinemia that may be provoked by alcohol ingestion.[76] Symptomatic adults have been treated successfully with liver transplant.[77]

ARTHROGRYPOSIS-RENAL DYSFUNCTION-CHOLESTASIS SYNDROME

Arthrogryposis-renal dysfunction-cholestasis (ARC) syndrome (MIM208085 and MIM613404) is an autosomal recessive multisystem disease caused by mutations in *VPS33B* and *VIPAS39* encoding VPS33B and VIPAR proteins that are involved in vesicular recycling of apical membrane proteins in polarized epithelial cells.[78–80]

Clinical Features

The classic features are arthrogryposis (skeletal contractures), Fanconi-like renal tubular dysfunction, and cholestasis.[81] Other clinical phenotypes include ichthyosis, failure to thrive (independent of liver or renal involvement), hypotonia, developmental delay, chronic diarrhea, and nephrogenic diabetes insipidus.[82]

Diagnosis

Biochemistry: There is conjugated hyperbilirubinemia at presentation, with a low level of GGT. Despite a normal platelet count, platelet function is abnormal and there is a high risk of bleeding in children who undergo liver biopsy.[83]

Histology: Molecular genetic investigations should replace liver biopsy in these children because of the risk of bleeding. Historical biopsies showed bile duct paucity with neonatal hepatitis.[81]

Genetics: Gene sequencing can confirm the diagnosis with mutations found in *VPS33B* and *VIPAS39* in approximately 70% and 30% percent of cases, respectively.

Management

Management is supportive with nutritional supplementation using a medium-chain triglyceride feed and fat-soluble vitamins. Renal support and correction of metabolic acidosis is necessary. The liver disease may progress to cirrhosis. There is no role in this multisystem disease for liver transplant.

Prognosis

Most infants die within the first year of life, although milder variants have been described.[80]

AAGENAES SYNDROME

This rare disease consists of lymphedema and severe neonatal cholestasis (MIM214900). It was first reported in the Norwegian population but is also found in other ethnic groups. The mode of inheritance is autosomal recessive, but the underlying molecular defect is still not known.[84]

Clinical Features

Conjugated hyperbilirubinemia is severe in the neonatal period and becomes episodic. Children may develop features of chronic liver disease with cirrhosis. Fat-soluble vitamin deficiency and pruritus are common. The lymphedema may manifest at birth or at anytime in childhood. It usually affects the lower limbs, hands, scrotum, and periorbital tissue. In older children it affects the small intestine and thorax.[85]

Diagnosis

Conjugated jaundice is associated with a raised GGT level and improves with time. In some, chronic liver disease may develop, but it is uncommon to need a liver transplant. Despite the lymphedema the albumin level is normal.

Prognosis

Life expectancy is reported as normal in the Norwegian cases; however, further delineation of an international cohort is required.[85]

NEONATAL ICHTHYOSIS-SCLEROSING CHOLANGITIS SYNDROME

Neonatal ichthyosis-sclerosing cholangitis (NISCH) (MIM607626) is an autosomal recessive multisystem disorder caused by mutations in *CLDN1* encoding the tight junction protein CLAUDIN1. It is thought that increased paracellular permeability leading to paracellular bile regurgitation leads to liver injury in NISCH.[86]

The liver disease in neonates with NISCH is variable and can comprise sclerosing cholangitis or neonatal hepatitis, as well as decreased scalp hair, scarring alopecia, sparse eyebrows and lashes, and ichthyosis. All patients present with neonatal cholestasis, which may mimic the signs of biliary atresia. Histologically, there is extensive fibrosis with ductular proliferation. The jaundice may clear by 3 to 6 months of age with intermittent jaundice returning 1 to 2 years later.[87]

Diagnosis

Biochemistry: Levels of serum alkaline phosphatase and GGT are elevated.

Imaging: Endoscopic or percutaneous cholangiography demonstrates medium to large beaded irregularity in intrahepatic bile ducts in all patients and in extrahepatic ducts in 80%.

Histology: Liver histology shows portal fibrosis with ductal proliferation and biliary cirrhosis.

Genetics: Diagnosis is confirmed by identification of mutations in *CLDN1*, which allows antenatal detection and carrier screening.

Management

Nutritional and supportive management is required. A Kasai portoenterostomy is not indicated. The disease is progressive and requires transplant in childhood. The skin is managed with topical applications to keep it moist, retinoids, and sunlight exposure.

Prognosis

The disease is progressive, requiring liver transplant at some stage. After transplant, the skin manifestations may improve.[88]

ALPHA1 ANTITRYPSIN DEFICIENCY

Alpha1 antitrypsin deficiency (A1ATD) (MIM613490) is a clinically heterogeneous condition manifesting as liver disease in infancy in 10% of cases or lung disease in adulthood. It is caused by mutations in SERPINA1.[89] It has an estimated incidence of 1 in 2500 and is the most common inherited metabolic disorder causing liver disease in infants in the Caucasian population.[90]

Clinical Features

Jaundice may present at any time in the first 4 months of life but usually in the neonatal period. The babies are small for gestational age, which helps distinguish them from babies with biliary atresia. The stools may be pale, but this is variable. There is hepatomegaly, but splenomegaly is unusual unless there is significant fibrosis. Up to 5% of those who present in infancy have late hemorrhagic disease of the newborn with intracranial bleeding. This condition can be avoided by the administration of intramuscular vitamin K.[91]

Diagnosis

Biochemistry: There is conjugated hyperbilirubinemia, which may improve with age. aspartate aminotransferase and alkaline phosphatase concentrations are elevated up to 10 times normal values. GGT levels may be elevated up to 5 times normal.

A1AT serum level: The serum level in patients with PiZZ phenotype is often reduced to less than 0.6 g/L (normal range, 0.8–1.8 g/L). However, as A1AT is an acute-phase reactant and therefore may be elevated in liver inflammation, these levels cannot be relied on and phenotype must be obtained in all patients with cholestasis.[92]

A1AT protease inhibitor (Pi) phenotype: This phenotype is assessed by isoelectric focusing on polyacrylamide gels. The normal phenotype is PiMM, and the most common homozygote form leading to A1AT is PiZZ. Other forms may also result in liver disease, including the PiSZ phenotype. It is essential that the test be performed in an experienced laboratory. Cytomegalovirus infection may cause a spurious Z band.

Genotype: This information is available in reference laboratories and is not a commonly used diagnostic tool, as it is not known what factors determine penetrance of the phenotype. There are polymerase chain reaction primers available for M, Z, and S alleles.

Liver biopsy: In early infancy, there is an acute hepatitis of varying severity, which may resemble idiopathic neonatal hepatitis, but giant cells are rarely prominent. Liver histology may mimic EHBA, with marked ductular reaction in the portal tracts. Fatty infiltration may be seen around portal tracts. There is hepatocellular necrosis and inflammatory cell infiltrate. Fibrosis may be present, with or without portal bridging. Periodic acid–Schiff-positive diastase-resistant granules are present in hepatocytes.

These granules are 2 to 20 nm in diameter and correspond to amorphous material within the endoplasmic reticulum, seen on electron microscopy. However, they may not be prominent in early biopsies and only become marked after 3 months of age.

With increasing age, the cholestasis, inflammation, and hepatocellular necrosis resolve. By age 1 to 2 years, inflammation becomes limited to expanded portal tracts and adjacent hepatocytes.

Management

Neonates presenting with A$_1$AT benefit from the general management of their cholestatic liver disease with nutritional support with medium-chain triglyceride feed and fat-soluble vitamin supplementation. Close follow-up throughout childhood at a specialist center is mandatory to detect signs of progressive liver disease and the possible need for transplant.

The family should be counseled as to the detrimental effects of cigarette smoking, with early development of emphysema, and alcohol consumption.

Prognosis

The prognosis is variable. With good nutrition and management of cholestasis, children may have resolution of their liver disease. However, if there is early fibrosis, then cirrhosis and portal hypertension may develop.[92]

NORTH AMERICAN INDIAN CHILDHOOD CIRRHOSIS

North American Indian childhood cirrhosis (NAIC) (MIM604901) is caused by mutations in *CIRH1A*, which encodes a protein with unknown function. All patients with NAIC have a homozygous mutation in CIRH1A that changes conserved Arg565 to Trp (R565W) in cirhin, which is a nucleolar protein of unknown function. It has been shown that cirhin may be a transcriptional regulatory factor of the nuclear factor (NF)-kappaB and could regulate multiple genes with NF-kappaB-responsive elements that are known to be important during development. In addition, cirhin was found to interact with a novel protein NOL11, which is required for ribosome biogenesis.[93,94]

Clinical Features

This cholestatic condition was first described in North American Indians in Quebec. Neonatal jaundice initially improves, but chronic liver disease develops with hepatosplenomegaly, pruritus, facial telangiectasia and portal hypertension.[95]

Diagnosis

Biochemistry: Levels of transaminases, alkaline phosphatase, and serum bile salts are elevated. GGT level is elevated. Serum cholesterol level is normal.

Histology: Electron microscopy shows widening of the pericanalicular microfilament cuff.[96]

Management

Supportive therapy should be provided during the cholestatic phase, with good nutrition and fat-soluble vitamin supplementation.

Prognosis

Biliary cirrhosis develops, but it is unusual to require liver transplant in childhood.

ZELLWEGER SYNDROME

Zellweger syndrome is a prototype for a large number of peroxisomal biosynthesis disorders that result in abnormal bile acid synthesis and accumulation of C_{27} bile acids that would normally undergo modification to chenodeoxycholic and cholic acids. Zellweger syndrome (MIM214100) is caused by recessive mutations in at least 20 different genes and has an incidence of approximately 1 in 100,000. It is found in all ethnicities and equally in men and women.[97]

Clinical Features

Zellweger syndrome is a multisystem disease including features of hypotonia, facial dysmorphism (high forehead and large fontanelles), developmental delay, seizures, and cystic malformation of the kidneys and brain. There is failure to thrive and feeding difficulties. The liver is not always involved initially, although a few infants have persistent conjugated jaundice.[97] Half the patients have hepatosplenomegaly with poor hepatic synthetic function.

Diagnosis

Biochemistry: Abnormal bile salt metabolites are identified on FAB-MS. Very-long-chain fatty acids are identified in the serum. GGT level is normal or low, and serum bile salt levels are also low.

Histology: The liver may be normal or have excess iron, hepatic fibrosis, or paucity of the bile ducts. Electron microscopy reveals the absence of peroxisomes, and the mitochondria are abnormal.

Management

Boluses of chenodeoxycholic and cholic acids may produce some improvement but does not prolong life.[98] Treatment is supportive, and liver transplant is contraindicated.

Prognosis

The severity of the phenotype can vary, and a milder presentation has been described.

CILIOPATHIES

Ciliopathies are a heterogeneous group of conditions in which the common pathologic condition is an abnormality in the primary cilium.[99] Autosomal dominant and recessive forms of polycystic kidney disease were the first described ciliopathies[99] and are also the most common, whereas others including Joubert, Meckel-Gruber, and Jeune syndromes are rare. Ciliopathies share common clinical features, which are variably expressed and hence have a diverse clinical phenotype. The hepatic features arise because of abnormalities in the formation of the ductal plate, which lead to the features of congenital hepatic fibrosis (CHF), Caroli disease or syndrome (when Caroli disease is associated with CHF), and polycystic liver disease.

Clinical Features

The clinical features that overlap in ciliopathies[99] are renal cystic disease, retinitis pigmentosa, polydactyly, situs inversus, developmental delay, Dandy-Walker malformation, posterior encephalocele, and hepatic disease.

The clinical presentation of ciliopathies is variable, usually with prolonged neonatal cholestasis. Progression of liver disease to portal hypertension presents with splenomegaly, signs of chronic liver disease, and variceal bleeding but may only be identified on screening for ciliopathy. The most common disorders include Meckel-Gruber syndrome, cerebellar vermis hypoplasia, oligophrenia, ataxia congenita, coloboma, hepatic fibrosis (COACH) syndrome, Jouberts syndrome, Jeune syndrome, oral–facial digital syndrome, and Bardet-Biedl syndrome, which occur with CHF. Others are well summarized in these reviews.[99]

Genetic diagnosis: Confirmation by conventional gene sequencing is difficult in this group of disorders because of a significant overlap in clinical features but may improve with novel methods of gene sequencing.[99]

SMITH-LEMLI-OPITZ SYNDROME

This defect in cholesterol biosynthesis (MIM270400) may present with multiple congenital anomalies or isolated neurodevelopmental abnormalities. Smith-Lemli-Opitz syndrome (SLOS) is caused by mutations in *DHCR7* encoding sterol delta-7-reductase. The incidence is estimated at 1/20,000 to 1/70,000 and is more common in Europeans. Liver involvement occurs in up to 16% of cases.[100]

Clinical Features

There are 2 distinct hepatic phenotypes, isolated hypertransaminasemia and progressive cholestasis, which is associated with early death.[100] Nonhepatic congenital phenotypes range from fetal lethality to minimal physical and mental impairment. The most common clinical features are failure to thrive, distinct facial features, postaxial polydactyly, photosensitivity of the skin, congenital heart defects, pyloric stenosis, renal malformation, ambiguous genitalia, holoprosencephaly, autistic features, and self-harming behavior.

Diagnosis

The diagnosis is suggested from the clinical features and facial dysmorphism.

Biochemistry: The level of 7-dehydrocholesterol (7DHC) in plasma is elevated as measured by gas chromatography–mass spectrometry. Other findings are a low/normal cholesterol level, isolated raised levels of transaminases, and a reduced level of GGT with cholestasis.

Imaging: Hepatomegaly with increased echogenicity is seen.

Histology: Findings range from hepatocyte degeneration in those with raised levels of transaminases to hepatocyte ballooning, macrovesicular fatty change, periportal fibrosis, and ductular proliferation in those with cholestasis.

Genetics: Confirmation of diagnosis by identification of mutations in *DHCR7* encoding sterol delta-7-reductase. The knowledge of mutations allows carrier testing and antenatal genetic diagnosis.

Management

Cholestasis requires nutritional support with medium-chain triglyceride feed and fat-soluble vitamin and cholesterol supplementation.[100] The excess production of 7DHC may be ameliorated by simvastatin use.

Prognosis

Those with progressive severe cholestasis are associated with a severe SLOS phenotype, whereas an isolated increase in the levels of transaminases is associated with a milder phenotype.

SUMMARY

Pediatric liver disease is rare but significant. The identification of causative genes has improved diagnosis; enabled the clinical phenotype to be extended, such as in AGS and ARC syndromes; and led to the understanding that the same gene may have multiple phenotypes such as in PFIC, BRIC, and ICP. These developments have increased the understanding of molecular pathways within the liver in the normal and disease states. One still needs to identify genotype–phenotype correlations and understand the role of genetic modifiers and the influence of environmental factors on disease severity, so as to aid clinical management and prognosis. The realization of the multiorgan involvement and complex genetics of the ciliopathies has expanded the understanding of gene interactions in the development of disease. In future, other pediatric liver diseases may be identified as having a genetic component as part of a multifactorial etiology. The challenge is to use the increased knowledge of molecular pathways to develop novel therapies for these devastating conditions.

REFERENCES

1. McKiernan PJ, Baker AJ, Kelly DA. The frequency and outcome of biliary atresia in the UK and Ireland. Lancet 2000;355(9197):25–9.
2. Kamath BM, Bason L, Piccoli DA, et al. Consequences of JAG1 mutations. J Med Genet 2003;40:891–5.
3. Emerick KM, Rand EB, Goldmuntz E, et al. Features of Alagille syndrome in 92 patients: frequency and relation to prognosis. Hepatology 1999;29:822–9.
4. Kamath BM, Spinner NB, Emerick KM, et al. Vascular anomalies in Alagille syndrome: a significant cause of morbidity and mortality. Circulation 2004; 109:1354–8.
5. Li L, Krantz ID, Deng Y, et al. Alagille syndrome is caused by mutations in human Jagged1, which encodes a ligand for Notch1. Nat Genet 1997;16(3): 243–51.
6. McDaniell R, Warthen DM, Sanchez-Lara PA, et al. NOTCH2 mutations cause Alagille syndrome, a heterogeneous disorder of the notch signaling pathway. Am J Hum Genet 2006;79(1):169–73.
7. Kamath BM, Krantz ID, Spinner NB, et al. Monozygotic twins with a severe form of Alagille syndrome and phenotypic discordance. Am J Med Genet 2002; 112(2):194–7.
8. Alagille D, Estrada A, Hadchouel M, et al. Syndromic paucity of intralobular bile ducts (Alagille syndrome or arteriohepatic dysplasia): review of 80 cases. J Pediatr 1987;110:195–200.
9. Krantz ID, Smith R, Collliton RP, et al. Jagged 1 mutations in patients ascertained with isolated congenital heart defects. Am J Med Genet 1999;84:56–60.
10. Kaye AJ, Rand EB, Munoz PS, et al. Effect of Kasai procedure on hepatic outcome in Alagille syndrome. J Pediatr Gastroenterol Nutr 2010;51:319–21.
11. Lykavieris P, Hadchouel M, Chardot C, et al. Outcome of liver disease in children with Alagille syndrome: a study of 163 patients. Gut 2001;49:431–5.
12. Bhadri VA, Stormon MO, Arbuckle S, et al. Hepatocellular carcinoma in children with Alagille syndrome. J Pediatr Gastroenterol Nutr 2005;41:676–8.
13. McElhinney DB, Krantz ID, Bason L, et al. Analysis of cardiovascular phenotype and genotype-phenotype correlation in individuals with JAG1 mutation and/or Alagille syndrome. Circulation 2002;106:2567–74.

14. Sanderson E, Newman V, Haigh SF, et al. Vertebral anomalies in children with Alagille syndrome: an analysis of 50 consecutive patients. Pediatr Radiol 2002;32:114–9.
15. Kamath BM, Stolle C, Bason L, et al. Craniosynostosis in Alagille syndrome. Am J Med Genet 2002;112:176–80.
16. Ryan RS, Myckatyn SO, Reid GD, et al. Alagille syndrome: case report with bilateral radio-ulnar synostosis and a literature review. Skeletal Radiol 2003;32: 489–91.
17. Bales CB, Kamath BM, Munoz PS, et al. Pathogenic lower extremity fractures in children with Alagille syndrome. J Pediatr Gastroenterol Nutr 2010;51:66–70.
18. Hingorani M, Nischal KK, Davies A, et al. Ocular abnormalities in Alagille syndrome. Ophthalmology 1999;106(2):330–7.
19. McDonald-McGinn DM, Kirschner R, Goldmuntz E, et al. The Philadelphia story: the 22q11.2 deletion: report on 250 patients. Genet Couns 1999;10(1):11–24.
20. Martin SR, Garel L, Alvarez F. Alagille's syndrome associated with cystic renal disease. Arch Dis Child 1996;74:232–5.
21. Olsen IE, Ittenbach RF, Rovner AJ, et al. Deficits in size-adjusted bone mass in children with Alagille syndrome. J Pediatr Gastroenterol Nutr 2005;40(1):76–82.
22. Rovner AJ, Schall JI, Jawad AF, et al. Rethinking growth failure in Alagille syndrome: the role of dietary intake and steatorrhea. J Pediatr Gastroenterol Nutr 2002;35:495–502.
23. Narula P, Gifford J, Steggall MA, et al. Visual loss and idiopathic intracranial hypertension in children with Alagille syndrome. J Pediatr Gastroenterol Nutr 2006;43(3):348–52.
24. Deutsch GH, Sokol RJ, Stathos TH, et al. Proliferation to paucity: evolution of bile duct abnormalities in a case of Alagille syndrome. Pediatr Dev Pathol 2001;4: 559–63.
25. Balistreri WF. Bile acid therapy in pediatric hepatobiliary disease: the role of ursodeoxycholic acid. J Pediatr Gastroenterol Nutr 1997;24(5):573–89.
26. Yerushalmi B, Sokol RJ, Narkewicz MR, et al. Use of rifampin for severe pruritus in children with chronic cholestasis. J Pediatr Gastroenterol Nutr 1999;29(4):442–7.
27. Trioche P, Samuel D, Odièvre M, et al. Ondansetron for pruritus in child with chronic cholestasis. Eur J Pediatr 1996;155(11):990.
28. Zellos A, Roy A, Schwarz KB. Use of oral naltrexone for severe pruritus due to cholestatic liver disease in children. J Pediatr Gastroenterol Nutr 2010;51(6): 787–9.
29. Neimark E, Shneider B. Novel surgical and pharmacological approaches to chronic cholestasis in children: partial external biliary diversion for intractable pruritus and xanthomas in Alagille syndrome. J Pediatr Gastroenterol Nutr 2003;36(2):296–7.
30. Hruz P, Zimmermann C, Gutmann H, et al. Adaptive regulation of the ileal apical sodium dependent bile acid transporter (ASBT) in patients with obstructive cholestasis. Gut 2006;55(3):395–402.
31. Van Mil SW, Milona A, Dixon PH, et al. Functional variants of the central bile acid sensor FXR identified in intrahepatic cholestasis of pregnancy. Gastroenterology 2007;133(2):507–16.
32. Bull LN, van Eijk MJ, Pawlikowska L, et al. A gene encoding a P-type ATPase mutated in two forms of hereditary cholestasis. Nat Genet 1998;18:219–24.
33. Paulusma CC, Folmer DE, Ho-Mok KS, et al. ATP8B1 requires an accessory protein for endoplasmic reticulum exit and plasma membrane lipid flippase activity. Hepatology 2008;47:268–78.

34. Strautnieks SS, Bull LN, Knisely AS, et al. A gene encoding a liver-specific ABC transporter is mutated in progressive familial intrahepatic cholestasis. Nat Genet 1998;20:233–8.

35. van Mil SW, van der Woerd WL, van der Brugge G, et al. Benign recurrent intrahepatic cholestasis type 2 is caused by mutations in ABCB11. Gastroenterology 2004;127:379–84.

36. Deleuze JF, Jacquemin E, Dubuisson C, et al. Defect of multidrug-resistance 3 gene expression in a subtype of progressive familial intrahepatic cholestasis. Hepatology 1996;23(4):904–8.

37. Crawford AR, Smith AJ, Hatch VC, et al. Hepatic secretion of phospholipid vesicles in the mouse critically depends on mdr2 or MDR3 P-glycoprotein expression. Visualization by electron microscopy. J Clin Invest 1997;100(10): 2562–7.

38. Groen A, Romero MR, Kunne C, et al. Complementary functions of the flippase ATP8B1 and the floppase ABCB4 in maintaining canalicular membrane integrity. Gastroenterology 2011;141(5):1927–1937.e1–4.

39. Geenes V, Williamson C. Intrahepatic cholestasis of pregnancy. World J Gastroenterol 2009;15(17):2049–66.

40. Davit-Spraul A, Fabre M, Branchereau S, et al. ATP8B1 and ABCB11 analysis in 62 children with normal gamma-glutamyl transferase progressive familial intrahepatic cholestasis (PFIC): phenotypic differences between PFIC1 and PFIC2 and natural history. Hepatology 2010;51(5):1645–55.

41. Thompson R, Strautnieks S. BSEP: function and role in progressive familial intrahepatic cholestasis. Semin Liver Dis 2001;21:545–50.

42. Knisely AS, Strautnieks SS, Meier Y, et al. Hepatocellular carcinoma in ten children under five years of age with bile salt export pump deficiency. Hepatology 2006;44(2):478–86.

43. Jacquemin E. Role of multidrug resistance 3 deficiency in pediatric and adult liver disease: one gene for three diseases. Semin Liver Dis 2001;21:551–62.

44. Knisely AS. Progressive familial intrahepatic cholestasis: a personal perspective. Pediatr Dev Pathol 2000;3:113–25.

45. Bruce CK, Smith M, Rahman F, et al. Design and validation of a metabolic disorder resequencing microarray (BRUM1). Hum Mutat 2010;31(7):858–65.

46. Lykavieris P, van Mil S, Cresteil D, et al. Progressive familial intrahepatic cholestasis type 1 and extrahepatic features: no catch-up of stature growth, exacerbation of diarrhea, and appearance of liver steatosis after liver transplantation. J Hepatol 2003;39:447–52.

47. Keitel V, Burdelski M, Vojnisek Z, et al. De novo bile salt transporter antibodies as a possible cause of recurrent graft failure after liver transplantation: a novel mechanism of cholestasis. Hepatology 2009;50(2):510–7.

48. Russell DW. The enzymes, regulation, and genetics of bile acid synthesis. Annu Rev Biochem 2003;72:137–74.

49. Clayton PT. Disorders of bile acid synthesis. J Inherit Metab Dis 2011;34(3): 593–604.

50. Buchmann MS, Kvittingen EA, Nazer H, et al. Lack of 3 beta-hydroxy-delta 5-C27-steroid dehydrogenase/isomerase in fibroblasts from a child with urinary excretion of 3 beta-hydroxy-delta 5-bile acids. A new inborn error of metabolism. J Clin Invest 1990;86(6):2034–7.

51. Akobeng AK, Clayton PT, Miller V, et al. An inborn error of bile acid synthesis (3beta-hydroxy-delta5-C27-steroid dehydrogenase deficiency) presenting as malabsorption leading to rickets. Arch Dis Child 1999;80(5):463–5.

52. Setchell KD, Suchy FJ, Welsh MB, et al. Delta 4-3-oxosteroid 5 beta-reductase deficiency described in identical twins with neonatal hepatitis. A new inborn error in bile acid synthesis. J Clin Invest 1988;82(6):2148–57.

53. Clayton PT, Casteels M, Mieli-Vergani G, et al. Familial giant cell hepatitis with low bile acid concentrations and increased urinary excretion of specific bile alcohols: a new inborn error of bile acid synthesis? Pediatr Res 1995;37(4 Pt 1): 424–31.

54. Jacquemin E, Setchell KD, O'Connell NC, et al. A new cause of progressive intrahepatic cholestasis: 3 beta-hydroxy-C27-steroid dehydrogenase/isomerase deficiency. J Pediatr 1994;125(3):379–84.

55. Naureckiene S, Sleat DE, Lackland H, et al. Identification of HE1 as the second gene of Niemann-Pick C disease. Science 2000;290(5500):2298–301.

56. Sokol J, Blanchette-Mackie J, Kruth HS, et al. Type C Niemann-Pick disease. Lysosomal accumulation and defective intracellular mobilization of low density lipoprotein cholesterol. J Biol Chem 1988;263(7):3411–7.

57. Vanier MT. Niemann-Pick disease type C. Orphanet J Rare Dis 2010;5:16.

58. Ioannou YA. The structure and function of the Niemann-Pick C1 protein. Mol Genet Metab 2000;71(1–2):175–81.

59. Ko DC, Binkley J, Sidow A, et al. The integrity of a cholesterol-binding pocket in Niemann-Pick C2 protein is necessary to control lysosome cholesterol levels. Proc Natl Acad Sci U S A 2003;100(5):2518–25.

60. Bonney DK, O'Meara A, Shabani A, et al. Successful allogeneic bone marrow transplant for Niemann-Pick disease type C2 is likely to be associated with a severe 'graft versus substrate' effect. J Inherit Metab Dis 2010. [Epub ahead of print].

61. Lloyd-Evans E, Morgan AJ, He X, et al. Niemann-Pick disease type C1 is a sphingosine storage disease that causes deregulation of lysosomal calcium. Nat Med 2008;14(11):1247–55.

62. Spiegel R, Raas-Rothschild A, Reish O, et al. The clinical spectrum of fetal Niemann-Pick type C. Am J Med Genet A 2009;149A(3):446–50.

63. Kelly DA, Portmann B, Mowat AP, et al. Niemann-Pick disease type C: diagnosis and outcome in children, with particular reference to liver disease. J Pediatr 1993;123(2):242–7.

64. Imrie J, Wraith JE. Isolated splenomegaly as the presenting feature of Niemann-Pick disease type C. Arch Dis Child 2001;84(5):427–9.

65. Garver WS, Francis GA, Jelinek D, et al. The National Niemann-Pick C1 Disease Database: report of clinical features and health problems. Am J Med Genet A 2007;143A(11):1204–11.

66. Ries M, Schaefer E, Lührs T, et al. Critical assessment of chitotriosidase analysis in the rational laboratory diagnosis of children with Gaucher disease and Niemann-Pick disease type A/B and C. J Inherit Metab Dis 2006;29(5):647–52.

67. Vanier MT, Rodriguez-Lafrasse C, Rousson R, et al. Type C Niemann-Pick disease: spectrum of phenotypic variation in disruption of intracellular LDL-derived cholesterol processing. Biochim Biophys Acta 1991;1096(4):328–37.

68. Wraith JE, Baumgartner MR, Bembi B, et al, NP-C Guidelines Working Group. Recommendations on the diagnosis and management of Niemann-Pick disease type C. Mol Genet Metab 2009;98(1–2):152–65.

69. Pineda M, Wraith JE, Mengel E, et al. Miglustat in patients with Niemann-Pick disease Type C (NP-C): a multicenter observational retrospective cohort study. Mol Genet Metab 2009;98(3):243–9.

70. Hutchin T, Preece MA, Hendriksz C, et al. Neonatal intrahepatic cholestasis caused by citrin deficiency (NICCD) as a cause of liver disease in infants in the UK. J Inherit Metab Dis 2009.

71. Kobayashi K, Sinasac DS, Iijima M, et al. The gene mutated in adult-onset type II citrullinaemia encodes a putative mitochondrial carrier protein. Nat Genet 1999; 22(2):159–63.

72. Lee NC, Chien YH, Kobayashi K, et al. Time course of acylcarnitine elevation in neonatal intrahepatic cholestasis caused by citrin deficiency. J Inherit Metab Dis 2006;29(4):551–5.

73. Kimura A, Kage M, Nagata I, et al. Histological findings in the livers of patients with neonatal intrahepatic cholestasis caused by citrin deficiency. Hepatol Res 2010;40(4):295–303.

74. Dimmock D, Kobayashi K, Iijima M, et al. Citrin deficiency: a novel cause of failure to thrive that responds to a high-protein, low-carbohydrate diet. Pediatrics 2007;119(3):e773–7.

75. Tamamori A, Okano Y, Ozaki H, et al. Neonatal intrahepatic cholestasis caused by citrin deficiency: severe hepatic dysfunction in an infant requiring liver transplantation. Eur J Pediatr 2002;161(11):609–13.

76. Takaya J, Kobayashi K, Ohashi A, et al. Variant clinical courses of 2 patients with neonatal intrahepatic cholestasis who have a novel mutation of SLC25A13. Metabolism 2005;54(12):1615–9.

77. Yazaki M, Hashikura Y, Takei Y, et al. Feasibility of auxiliary partial orthotopic liver transplantation from living donors for patients with adult-onset type II citrullinemia. Liver Transpl 2004;10(4):550–4.

78. Gissen P, Johnson CA, Morgan NV, et al. Mutations in VPS33B, encoding a regulator of SNARE-dependent membrane fusion, cause arthrogryposis-renal dysfunction-cholestasis (ARC) syndrome. Nat Genet 2004;36:400–4.

79. Cullinane AR, Straatman-Iwanowska A, Zaucker A, et al. Mutations in VIPAR cause an arthrogryposis, renal dysfunction and cholestasis syndrome phenotype with defects in epithelial polarization. Nat Genet 2010;42:303–12.

80. Smith H, Galmes R, Gogolina E, et al. Associations among genotype, clinical phenotype, and intracellular localization of trafficking proteins in ARC syndrome. Hum Mutat 2012. http://dx.doi.org/10.1002/humu.22155.

81. Jang JY, Kim KM, Kim GH, et al. Clinical characteristics and VPS33B mutations in patients with ARC syndrome. J Pediatr Gastroenterol Nutr 2009;48(3): 348–54.

82. Abu-Sa'da O, Barbar M, Al-Harbi N, et al. Arthrogryposis, renal tubular acidosis and cholestasis (ARC) syndrome: two new cases and review. Clin Dysmorphol 2005;14(4):191–6.

83. Kim SM, Chang HK, Song JW, et al, Severance Pediatric Liver Disease Research Group. Agranular platelets as a cardinal feature of ARC syndrome. J Pediatr Hematol Oncol 2010;32(4):253–8.

84. Aagenaes O, van der Hagen CD, Refsum S. Hereditary recurrent intrahepatic cholestasis from birth. Arch Dis Child 1968;43(232):646–57.

85. Drivdal M, Trydal T, Hagve TA, et al. Prognosis, with evaluation of general biochemistry, of liver disease in lymphoedema cholestasis syndrome 1 (LCS1/Aagenaes syndrome). Scand J Gastroenterol 2006;41(4):465–71.

86. Grosse B, Cassio D, Yousef N, et al. Claudin-1 involved in neonatal ichthyosis sclerosing cholangitis syndrome regulates hepatic paracellular permeability. Hepatology 2012;55(4):1249–59. http://dx.doi.org/10.1002/hep.24761.

87. Baker AJ, Portmann B, Westaby D, et al. Neonatal sclerosing cholangitis in two siblings: a category of progressive intrahepatic cholestasis. J Pediatr Gastroenterol Nutr 1993;17:317–22.

88. Paganelli M, Stephenne X, Gilis A, et al. Neonatal ichthyosis and sclerosing cholangitis syndrome: extremely variable liver disease severity from claudin-1 deficiency. J Pediatr Gastroenterol Nutr 2011;53(3):350–4.

89. Zaimidou S, van Baal S, Smith TD, et al. A1ATVar: a relational database of human SERPINA1 gene variants leading to alpha1-antitrypsin deficiency and application of the VariVis software. Hum Mutat 2009;30(3):308–13.

90. Lace B, Sveger T, Krams A, et al. Age of SERPINA1 gene PI Z mutation: Swedish and Latvian population analysis. Ann Hum Genet 2008;72(Pt 3):300–4.

91. van Hasselt PM, Kok K, Vorselaars AD, et al. Vitamin K deficiency bleeding in cholestatic infants with alpha-1-antitrypsin deficiency. Arch Dis Child Fetal Neonatal Ed 2009;94(6):F456–60.

92. Primhak RA, Tanner MS. Alpha-1 antitrypsin deficiency. Arch Dis Child 2001;85: 2–5, 1.

93. Drouin E, Russo P, Tuchweber B, et al. North American Indian cirrhosis in children: a review of 30 cases. J Pediatr Gastroenterol Nutr 2000;31(4):395–404.

94. Weber AM, Tuchweber B, Yousef I, et al. Severe familial cholestasis in North American Indian children: a clinical model of microfilament dysfunction? Gastroenterology 1981;81(4):653–62.

95. Freed EF, Prieto JL, McCann KL, et al. NOL11, implicated in the pathogenesis of North American Indian childhood cirrhosis, is required for pre-rRNA transcription and processing. PLoS Genet 2012;8(8):e1002892.

96. Yu B, Mitchell GA, Richter A. Cirhin up-regulates a canonical NF-kappaB element through strong interaction with Cirip/HIVEP1. Exp Cell Res 2009; 315(18):3086–98.

97. Waterham HR, Ebberink MS. Genetics and molecular basis of human peroxisome biogenesis disorders. Biochim Biophys Acta 2012;1822(9):1430–41.

98. Setchell KD, Bragetti P, Zimmer-Nechemias L, et al. Oral bile acid treatment and the patient with Zellweger syndrome. Hepatology 1992;15(2):198–207.

99. Badano JL, Mitsuma N, Beales PL, et al. The ciliopathies: an emerging class of human genetic disorders [review]. Annu Rev Genomics Hum Genet 2006;7: 125–48.

100. Irons M, Elias ER, Abuelo D, et al. Treatment of Smith-Lemli-Opitz syndrome: results of a multicenter trial. Am J Med Genet 1997;68(3):311–4.

Systemic Causes of Cholestasis

Andrew S. deLemos, MD[a,b], Lawrence S. Friedman, MD[a,b,c,d],*

KEYWORDS

- Amyloidosis • Cholestasis of sepsis • Congestive hepatopathy
- Granulomatous hepatitis • Lymphoma • Sarcoidosis • Sickle cell disease
- Total parenteral nutrition

KEY POINTS

- A profound systemic inflammatory response such as sepsis can disrupt the elimination of bile salts at the level of the hepatocyte and provoke cholestasis.
- A detailed clinical history, including travel, exposures, and underlying immunosuppression, is crucial when evaluating a patient with cholestasis.
- Systemic autoimmune disease in association with cholestasis should trigger an evaluation for primary autoimmune cholestatic liver disease.
- The hallmark of hepatic amyloidosis and lymphoma is a prominently increased serum alkaline phosphatase level.
- Extrahepatic biliary obstruction with subsequent cholestasis can result from a variety of systemic diseases, such as posttransplant lymphoproliferative disorder, sickle cell disease, Henoch-Schönlein purpura, and infection with cryptococcus, cytomegalovirus, or tuberculosis.

Systemic causes of cholestasis constitute a diverse group of diseases across organ systems. The pathophysiology of cholestasis in systemic disease can be a consequence of direct involvement of a disease process within the liver or extrahepatic biliary system or secondary to immune-mediated changes in bile flow (**Table 1**). Evaluating a patient with cholestasis for a systemic cause requires an understanding of the patient's risk factors, clinical setting (eg, hospitalized or immunosuppressed patient), clinical features, and pattern of laboratory abnormalities.

BACTERIAL INFECTIONS

Nearly any significant extrahepatic bacterial infection can cause cholestasis. Osler described jaundice occurring with curious irregularity in patients with pneumonia in the first edition of *The Principles and Practice of Medicine*.[1]

[a] Gastrointestinal Unit, Massachusetts General Hospital, Boston, MA 02114, USA; [b] Harvard Medical School, Boston, MA 02115, USA; [c] Tufts University School of Medicine, Boston, MA 02111, USA; [d] Department of Medicine, Newton-Wellesley Hospital, Newton, MA 02462, USA
* Corresponding author. Department of Medicine, Newton-Wellesley Hospital, 2014 Washington Street, Newton, MA 02462.
E-mail address: lfriedman@partners.org

Clin Liver Dis 17 (2013) 301–317
http://dx.doi.org/10.1016/j.cld.2012.11.001
1089-3261/13/$ – see front matter © 2013 Elsevier Inc. All rights reserved.

Table 1
Mechanisms of cholestasis in systemic disease

Mechanism	Examples
Cytokine-mediated	Graft-versus-host disease Hodgkin disease (vanishing bile duct syndrome) Sepsis and severe bacterial infections Stauffer syndrome (renal cell carcinoma)

Granulomatous hepatitis	Bacterial infections: *Yersinia enterocolitica, Brucella abortus,*
	    Mycobacterium tuberculosis infections
	Crohn disease
	Fungal infections: *Candida* species infection, coccidioidomycosis,
	    cryptococcus, histoplasmosis
	Sarcoidosis

Obstructive jaundice	Henoch-Schönlein purpura Infections: cytomegalovirus, cryptococcus Porta hepatis lymphadenopathy: posttransplant lymphoproliferative disease, *Mycobacterium tuberculosis* infection Sickle cell disease (pigment bile duct stones)
Hepatic infiltration	Amyloidosis Hemophagocytic syndrome Hepatic congestion (heart failure) Hodgkin or non-Hodgkin lymphoma Infections: miliary tuberculosis, *Mycobacterium avium* complex infection, actinomycosis Sickle cell intrahepatic cholestasis

Bacterial infections that do not necessarily involve the liver or bile ducts may lead to jaundice. Sepsis is most frequently linked to cholestasis, particularly in the intensive care unit setting (**Table 2**).[2] Both gram-positive and gram-negative organisms are potentially culpable, with *Escherichia coli* being the most common isolate in 1 retrospective analysis.[3] Jaundice develops in up to one-third of neonates and infants

Table 2
Systemic cholestasis in the intensive care unit[a]

Diagnosis	Diagnostic Tests	Treatment
Sepsis or severe bacterial infection	Blood cultures, imaging for source of infection	Antibiotics
Hepatic congestion (heart failure)	Cardiopulmonary testing (eg, echocardiography)	Measures to increase cardiac output based on cause (eg, thrombolysis for pulmonary embolism)
Progressive sclerosing cholangitis after burns or trauma	Exclusion of other causes	Aggressive volume resuscitation and treatment of underlying cause
Total parenteral nutrition	Exclusion of other causes	Initiation of enteral nutrition, cycling of parenteral nutrition, ursodeoxycholic acid

[a] Acalculous cholecystitis and drug-related cholestasis should always be excluded.

with sepsis,[4] and the incidence in adult patients is estimated to range from 6% to 54%.[5,6] Cholestasis from infections and sepsis is the second most common cause of jaundice in hospitalized patients (after malignant biliary obstruction).[7] In adults, conjugated hyperbilirubinemia, typically less than 10 mg/dL, predominates; the bilirubin level can be higher in neonates as a consequence of their underdeveloped efflux capacity. Serum alkaline phosphatase levels 2 to 3 times the upper limit of normal are typical, whereas aminotransferase levels are either normal or only modestly increased. Apart from jaundice, symptoms such as pruritus and clinical signs such as hepatomegaly are uncommon. Treatment is supportive with fluid resuscitation and antibiotics. One prospective analysis[6] did not find an association between the presence of jaundice and increased mortality.

The pathophysiology of cholestasis in sepsis is the topic of several excellent reviews.[8–10] Kupffer cells, and to a lesser extent hepatocytes and sinusoidal endothelial cells, react to bacterial endotoxins such as lipopolysaccharide by elaborating proinflammatory cytokines such as tumor necrosis factor α (TNF-α), interleukin 1 (IL-1), IL-2, IL-6, and IL-12. Endotoxemia in rats has been shown to cause downregulation of bile uptake (Na^+-taurocholate cotransporting polypeptide and organic anion-transporting polypeptide) and export (bile salt export pump and multidrug resistance protein 2) transporters for cholestasis,[11] but a posttranscriptional mechanism is favored in studies involving human liver tissues.[12] Nitric oxide and free radicals in the hepatic microvasculature can contribute to endothelial damage and the formation of fibrin microthrombi. Histologically, hepatocellular and canalicular bilirubinostasis predominates, often with nonspecific portal-based inflammation and Kupffer cell hyperplasia.[13]

A distinct cholestatic picture termed progressive sclerosing cholangitis can emerge in the setting of severe septic shock.[14] This entity may evolve as a result of biliary ischemia from systemic hypotension and has also been described after extensive trauma or burns.[15,16] The pathophysiology is poorly understood but likely involves a similar diminution in the expression of bile transporters as a result of cytokine induction as well as stasis of toxic bile salts within the ducts. Cirrhosis can result.[17]

Certain systemic bacterial organisms capable of infecting the liver directly have a predilection for cholestasis. An increase of serum alkaline phosphatase levels and jaundice frequently accompany pyogenic liver abscess. Recent case series indicate that up to 60% of liver abscesses are cryptogenic and therefore can be considered systemic.[18–21] Actinomycosis, caused by Actinomyces israelii, a filamentous gram positive rod, can present with liver involvement in rare instances. Whereas hepatic abscess is the most common presentation of actinomycosis,[22] affected patients may also follow a more indolent course of fever, abdominal pain, and anorexia associated nearly universally with increases of the serum alkaline phosphatase level.[23] Biopsies of infected tissue show characteristic sulfur granules, and treatment with penicillin or tetracycline is usually curative. Severe shigellosis can cause a cholestatic hepatitis with portal and periportal polymorphonuclear inflammatory infiltrates,[24] whereas yersiniosis can produce a granulomatous hepatitis in patients with diabetes mellitus and those predisposed to iron loading.[25]

Certain zoonotic infections, particularly brucellosis, also may lead to cholestasis, in which the development of jaundice may correlate with the severity of the illness. Necrotizing hepatic granulomas can occur in the hepatic lobules or portal tracts in association with focal mononuclear infiltrates.[26,27] Weil syndrome develops in 5% to 10% of patients with leptospirosis, a spirochetal infection acquired in warm climates from water contaminated with the urine of wild or domestic animals. Jaundice over a few weeks may denote the first phase of the illness and is followed by fever and subsequently

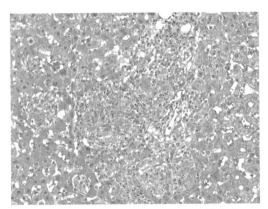

Fig. 1. Histopathology of hepatic syphilis, showing portal and lobular granulomas associated with mixed inflammation (hematoxylin-eosin, original magnification, ×10). (*Courtesy of* Joseph Misdraji, MD, Department of Pathology, Massachusetts General Hospital, Boston, MA.)

hepatic and renal injury.[28] Conjugated hyperbilirubinemia reflects intrahepatic cholestasis, which along with hypertrophy of Kupffer cells is apparent on liver biopsy specimens. Another spirochetal infection associated with cholestasis is syphilis, which can cause a lymphocytic portal triaditis with pericholangiolar inflammation and a markedly increased serum alkaline phosphatase level (**Fig. 1**). Syphilitic hepatitis in persons infected with human immunodeficiency virus (HIV) is well described, and in 1 case series of 7 patients, the average serum bilirubin level at diagnosis was 4.1 mg/dL.[29] Tickborne illnesses such as Q fever, Rocky Mountain spotted fever, and ehrlichiosis can infect the liver and cause cholestasis in rare instances, but a component of hemolysis undoubtedly contributes to the jaundice.

FUNGAL HEPATITIS

The systemic mycoses are considered opportunistic pathogens with only infrequent hepatic involvement. A high index of suspicion in the appropriate setting is crucial to expedite treatment. In the appropriate clinical context, fungal pathogens can disseminate to the liver and lead to varying degrees of cholestasis. Immunocompromised patients with hepatic candidiasis can present with suppurative granulomas, neutrophilic inflammation, and edema surrounding bile ducts.[30] High fever and an increased serum alkaline phosphatase level are typical features. Infection with the yeast *Cryptococcus neoformans* can present with several hepatic manifestations, including jaundice caused by cholangitis. Bucuvalas and colleagues[31] described a 15-year-old girl with right upper quadrant pain and jaundice in whom cryptococci were cultured from the bile duct. Tissue staining with India ink highlights the capsule, but detection of serum cryptococcal antigen is now the diagnostic test of choice. A hepatitislike picture may develop in 40% to 60% of cases of disseminated coccidioidomycosis, which is endemic in the southwest United States and can affect immunocompetent hosts. Pulmonary infiltrates with a granulomatous hepatitis, in conjunction with a markedly increased serum alkaline phosphatase level, are a classic presentation.[32] Histoplasmosis can spread from the lungs to the liver as well, generally in immunocompromised hosts. Cholestasis resulting from histoplasmosis typically occurs secondarily from development of hemophagocytic syndrome[33] (see later discussion).

MYCOBACTERIAL INFECTIONS

Hepatobiliary tuberculosis is rare, although well documented. A 10-year experience of close to 2000 patients with tuberculosis identified only 14 cases of hepatobiliary tuberculosis, of which 9 had multiorgan involvement.[34] Jaundice is classically caused by extrahepatic biliary obstruction from bulky lymphadenopathy around the porta hepatis or postinflammatory biliary strictures.[35] A characteristic granulomatous hepatitis, marked by fever, anorexia, weight loss, and night sweats with an infiltrative cholestasis, is present in 90% of patients with miliary tuberculosis. Disseminated *Mycobacterium avium* complex (MAC) infection can also present with dramatic cholestasis with only minimal increase of the serum aminotransferase levels.[36] MAC infections have become infrequent in patients with HIV infection since the availability of effective antiretroviral therapy.

SYSTEMIC VIRAL INFECTIONS

Viral diseases can occur as latent infections that reactivate in immunocompromised hosts or de novo infections in otherwise healthy persons. Epstein-Barr virus (EBV) and cytomegalovirus (CMV) are DNA viruses in the herpesvirus family that can involve the liver in either scenario. Jaundice in acute mononucleosis occurs in up to 10% of cases.[37] By contrast, EBV reactivation with subsequent development of posttransplant lymphoproliferative disorder (PTLD) is often characterized by jaundice in liver transplant recipients (see later discussion). A similar mononucleosislike illness can occur in healthy patients with acute CMV infection, which is characterized pathologically by focal hepatocyte and bile duct damage.[38] CMV infection has specific cholestatic features in certain immunocompromised settings, as in neonates, in whom obstructive biliary disease and neonatal giant cell hepatitis with cholestasis can occur.[39] Jaundice was found in 9 of 9 infants infected perinatally with CMV in a case series from Saudi Arabia.[40] CMV infection in patients with AIDS has been a cause of HIV cholangiopathy, an infectious form of sclerosing cholangitis that is rarely seen. CMV infection usually occurs 1 to 4 months after solid organ transplantation and is typically characterized by acute hepatitis with pathologic features in the liver of CMV inclusions and foci of microabscesses. Agarwal and colleagues[41] reported a case of fibrosing cholestatic hepatitis caused by CMV infection in a renal transplant recipient. After solid organ transplantation, CMV-positive recipients or recipients of CMV-positive donor organs should receive prophylaxis with valganciclovir.

Severe viral infections such as influenza and severe acute respiratory syndrome are believed to be associated with immune-mediated liver damage as a result of cytokine activation; neither infection generally leads to cholestasis. By contrast, measles (rubeola) may result in 1 of 2 patterns of hepatic dysfunction: most commonly, asymptomatic increase of the serum aminotransferase levels and rarely, prolonged jaundice and cholestasis, which develop as the usual symptoms of measles resolve.[42]

HEPATIC SARCOIDOSIS

Typically, sarcoidosis presents with noncaseating granulomas in the lungs and lymph nodes. The liver is an occasional extrapulmonary site of disease. In 1 retrospective series,[43] liver biochemical test abnormalities were found in 204 of 837 (24.4%) patients with sarcoidosis, of whom 15.2% were believed to have hepatic sarcoidosis. Prevalence rates are highest among African American and Scandinavian persons between the ages of 20 and 40 years. Liver involvement in sarcoidosis is usually clinically silent.

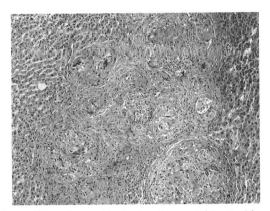

Fig. 2. Histopathology of hepatic sarcoidosis, showing portal tract with multiple noncaseating epithelioid granulomas encased in fibrosis characteristic of hepatic sarcoid (hematoxylin-eosin, original magnification, ×10). (*Courtesy of* Joseph Misdraji, MD, Department of Pathology, Massachusetts General Hospital, Boston, MA.)

A few patients (4%–7%) experience symptoms such as nausea, vomiting, and abdominal pain or signs such as hepatomegaly, jaundice, and portal hypertension. Abnormal liver biochemical test levels were identified in 58 of 100 patients who underwent a liver biopsy in 1 case series.[44] The serum alkaline phosphatase level is disproportionately high. In addition, 75% of untreated patients with sarcoidosis have an increase in the serum angiotensin-converting enzyme level. The pathognomonic lesion is the noncaseating granuloma, which results from a helper T cell type 1 response to an as-yet-unidentified antigen. Pathologically, hepatic sarcoidosis can be indistinguishable from primary biliary cirrhosis or primary sclerosing cholangitis. Although granulomas can be seen within the hepatic lobule, the principal findings are in the portal tracts and include a variety of bile duct lesions, such as acute or chronic cholangitis,[45] periductal fibrosis, and bile duct loss (**Fig. 2**).[46] Presinusoidal portal hypertension can develop from scarring of portal venules. In general, treatment is not recommended in patients with asymptomatic hepatic disease but is advised when symptoms of portal hypertension or severe cholestasis are apparent. Although patients may improve symptomatically with glucocorticoids and ursodeoxycholic acid,[47] structural changes to the bile ducts can progress to biliary cirrhosis, resulting in some cases in the need for liver transplantation.[48]

HEPATIC AMYLOIDOSIS

Systemic amyloidosis may be primary (AL) or secondary (AA). The precipitation of immunoglobulin light chains characterizes AL amyloid and develops in the context of plasma cell dyscrasias such as Waldenstrom macroglobulinemia or multiple myeloma. Although the heart, kidney, and peripheral nerves are the most commonly affected organs, 1 autopsy series of primary amyloidosis reported liver involvement in 70% of cases. A Mayo Clinic study reported on the natural history of 98 patients with liver biopsy-proven AL amyloid over a 20-year period.[49] Unintentional weight loss, with hepatomegaly on examination, was the most frequent presenting symptom. Serum alkaline phosphatase levels were strikingly increased, with a median value of 657 U/L (normal level <250 U/L), and were more than normal in 86% of patients. The median survival was 5.4 months in patients with an alkaline phosphatase level

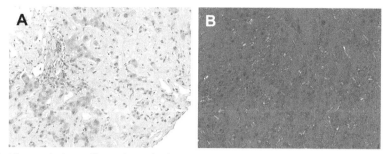

Fig. 3. Histopathology of hepatic amyloidosis. (*A*) Liver biopsy specimen showing massive sinu-soidal infiltration by waxy pink amyloid deposits (hematoxylin-eosin, original magnification, ×20). (*B*) Congo Red stain of the same biopsy specimen viewed under polarized light shows apple-green birefringence, confirming amyloid (original magnification, ×20). (*Courtesy of Joseph Misdraji, MD, Department of Pathology, Massachusetts General Hospital, Boston, MA.*)

greater than 500 U/L and 1 month in those with a total bilirubin level greater than 34 μmol/L (2 mg/dL). Most patients (82%) had amyloid deposits detected in biopsy specimens from extrahepatic tissue as well. The treatment of choice for primary amyloidosis is chemotherapy and, when possible, hematopoietic stem-cell transplantation.

Secondary, or AA, amyloidosis develops in the setting of systemic inflammatory disorders such as rheumatoid arthritis or chronic infections such as osteomyelitis or tuberculosis. The pathologic protein involved is serum amyloid A, which is an acute-phase reactant produced perpetually in the liver in response to inflammatory cytokines, such as TNF-α, IL-1, and IL-6. Amyloidogenic proteins deposit in the extracellular matrices of various organs, as in AL disease. Preventing this process from occurring by identifying and treating the underlying inflammatory condition is paramount in the management of affected patients. AA amyloidosis is less common than AL amyloid-osis, but the histopathologic findings are similar, with protein deposition in the space of Disse, portal tracts, and vessel walls causing architectural distortion and cholestasis (**Fig. 3**). Congo Red staining continues to be the mainstay of identifying tissue-based amyloid.

HEMOPHAGOCYTIC SYNDROME

Hemophagocytic syndrome, or hemophagocytic lymphohistiocytosis (HLH), is a rare condition involving the proliferation of macrophages responsible for phagocytosis of blood cells in hematopoietic organs. Hematologic malignancies, infections (histoplas-mosis, tuberculosis, CMV infection, HIV infection), or autoimmune diseases (rheuma-toid arthritis, systemic lupus erythematosus, Still disease) provoke a sustained immune activation of histiocytes, natural killer (NK) cells, and cytotoxic lymphocytes. Germline mutations in perforin have been found in familial cases of HLH.[50] Perforin is a cytolytic protein expressed by NK cells and cytotoxic T cells that is critical for inducing apoptosis of infected cells. Clinically, the features of HLH include fever, hep-atosplenomegaly, cytopenias in at least 2 cell lines, hypertriglyceridemia or hypofibri-nogenemia (or both), and a high serum ferritin level. In a case series from France of 30 patients with hepatic HLH,[51] 22 had a previous diagnosis of lymphoma or leukemia. Nineteen of the 30 patients were admitted to the hospital because of hepatic manifes-tations of the disease, including 50% with jaundice. Liver biopsies were performed in

25 patients and in all cases showed hemophagocytosis, Kupffer cell hyperplasia, and sinusoidal dilatation. Of the original cohort, there were 12 deaths caused by multiorgan failure or sepsis. Fifteen of 21 patients who could be treated achieved a complete remission. A high serum bilirubin or alkaline phosphatase level was associated with a poorer prognosis. HLH is a glucocorticoid-responsive disease, and current therapy combines dexamethasone with etoposide followed by an allogeneic hematopoietic stem-cell transplant in cases of genetic HLH or in the context of hematologic malignancy.

SICKLE CELL DISEASE

Cholestasis caused by sickle cell disease results from 1 of 2 processes (or both): extrahepatic or intrahepatic.[52] Extrahepatic cholestasis can be caused by choledocholithiasis. Pigment gallstones develop in roughly one-half of patients with sickle cell disease. In 1 series of 65 patients with sickle cell disease who underwent cholecystectomy, bile duct stones were found in 18%.[53] In 7% to 10% of patients hospitalized for sickle cell crisis, hepatic complications caused by sickling are found. Hepatic crisis can mimic acute cholecystitis or cholangitis, with right upper quadrant pain, jaundice, hepatomegaly, and fever. As much as 50% of the hyperbilirubinemia is attributable to conjugated bilirubin, and the total bilirubin level is relatively more increased than the aminotransferase levels. Sickle cell intrahepatic cholestasis (SCIC) is a term used in the literature to describe acute hepatic failure from sickle cell disease.[54] Bilirubinostasis identified pathologically in the liver is a consequence of sinusoidal distension from erythrocyte sickling. Erythrophagocytosis and hemosiderosis are also characteristic histologic findings. SCIC is associated with profound hyperbilirubinemia and has been treated successfully in occasional cases with exchange transfusion[55] and by liver transplantation.[56]

LYMPHOMAS

Important oncologic causes of cholestasis include Hodgkin lymphoma (HL) and non-Hodgkin lymphoma (NHL). Liver involvement is less frequent in HL than in NHL and typically occurs with disease above and below the diaphragm (stage III) or disseminated extranodal disease (stage IV). Five percent of patients with HL have liver involvement at the time of diagnosis, and Reed-Sternberg cells are pathognomonic. Forty percent of patients have an increased serum alkaline phosphatase level. Intrahepatic tumor infiltration has been seen in 45% of jaundiced patients with HL at autopsy.[57,58] Several investigators have reported intrahepatic cholestasis caused by a vanishing bile duct syndrome in HL in the absence of tumor infiltration.[59] Ballonoff and colleagues[60] reviewed 37 cases described in the literature and found an association between an improvement in cholestasis and complete response to chemotherapy or radiation therapy (or both). Acute liver failure is a potential complication of HL, either directly caused by hepatic infiltration or secondarily caused by a paraneoplastic process.

Liver involvement in NHL has pathologic characteristics similar to those in HL, including a nodular tumor infiltrate in portal tracts and epithelioid granulomas. However, primary hepatic lymphoma (PHL) is rare, accounting for less than 1% of cases of NHL.[61] PHL is defined by an absence of lymphoma involvement in the spleen, lymph nodes, and bone marrow at the time of diagnosis. B symptoms of fever and weight loss occur in one-third of patients. The most common presentation is with abdominal pain caused by hepatomegaly. Serum alkaline phosphatase and bilirubin levels are increased in 70% of cases. A solitary lesion is the most frequent finding radiographically and is encountered in 50% to 60% of cases. Estimating the prognosis of PHL is difficult because the condition is rare. Nodular as opposed to diffusely infiltrative disease may have a more favorable outcome with chemotherapy, with 3-year survival rates of 57% and 18%, respectively. Although there are some case reports of hepatitis C–associated PHL, an increased risk of NHL (diffuse large B-cell lymphoma, marginal zone lymphoma, and lymphoplasmocytic lymphoma) in patients with chronic hepatitis C is not specifically associated with an increased risk of PHL.

Both solid organ and hematopoietic stem-cell transplant recipients are at risk for PTLD, a type of NHL driven in most cases by EBV infection (see earlier discussion). PTLD complicates approximately 4% of liver transplantations. Liver and spleen involvement in PTLD is not unusual, occurring in 16% of patients in a 20-year experience at the University of Pittsburgh.[62] If present in the liver, PTLD can cause intrahepatic cholestasis or extrahepatic cholestasis from bulky lymphadenopathy around the porta hepatis.

Hepatosplenic T-cell lymphoma (HSTCL) is a rare, aggressive lymphoma that infiltrates the hepatic sinusoids. Male patients younger than 35 years with inflammatory bowel disease (IBD) and at least a 2-year history of exposure to combined thiopurine and biologic therapy may be at increased risk for developing HSTCL.[63]

SOLID ORGAN MALIGNANCIES

Stauffer syndrome, originally termed nephrogenic hepatic dysfunction, refers to a rare paraneoplastic complication of renal cell carcinoma.[64] Overexpression of IL-6 by the tumor is believed to play a role in the pathophysiology. Cholestasis typically resolves within 1 to 2 months after surgical resection of the primary tumor. Hepatic dysfunction after resection may portend tumor recurrence. The presentation is with cholestasis, sometimes with jaundice, and usually with right upper quadrant pain caused by hepatomegaly. Liver biopsy specimens show nonspecific changes, including steatosis, portal lymphocytic inflammation, and Kupffer cell hyperplasia. Renal cell carcinoma can also metastasize to the pancreas and cause obstructive jaundice. Biliary obstruction caused by primary or metastatic cancer in the head of the pancreas, ampulla, or bile duct are more common causes of obstructive jaundice.

HEPATIC GRAFT-VERSUS-HOST DISEASE

The gastrointestinal tract and liver are often affected by acute graft-versus-host disease (GVHD).[65] Acute hepatic GVHD occurs in the first 100 days after allogeneic stem-cell transplantation. GVHD arises from expansion of the population of donor T cells in the transplant recipient. Risk factors for developing GVHD include an HLA mismatch, gender mismatch, and high number of T cells transfused from the donor. Liver involvement typically follows skin and gastrointestinal involvement. When profound cholestasis develops, the prognosis is poor. A serum bilirubin level greater than 6.1 mg/dL establishes a diagnosis of severe GVHD.[66] The pathophysiology is complex and likely involves a constellation of immune-mediated features, including cytokine activation, endothelial damage from conditioning regimens, and many antigen-presenting cells in target organs. Histologically, lymphocytes are seen infiltrating small bile ducts, and epithelial cells undergo apoptosis. Ursodeoxycholic acid is effective in preventing hepatic GVHD and is administered as prophylaxis for the first 80 days after hematopoietic stem-cell transplantation.[67] Immunosuppression is the foundation of therapy for GVHD. When chronic liver GVHD occurs, destructive bile duct damage is also characteristic, but progressive fibrosis is unusual except in cases of concomitant chronic liver disease such as hepatitis C.

ENDOCRINE DYSFUNCTION

Thyroid disease may affect hepatic dysfunction in a few distinct circumstances. Primary biliary cirrhosis and hypothyroidism may occur together because of their shared autoimmune pathogenesis. Jaundice in patients with myxedema coma is typically caused by acute hepatic congestion from heart failure.[68] Several reports in the adult and pediatric literature describe cholestatic hepatitis occurring in patients with Graves disease.[69,70] A mild increase in the serum alkaline phosphatase level occurs in 65% of patients with hyperthyroidism, although the increase can also arise from bone. Simultaneous heart failure may complicate the recognition of hepatic dysfunction caused by thyrotoxic crisis, which can eventuate in acute liver failure.

The liver can be affected in patients with diabetes mellitus, most commonly by nonalcoholic fatty liver disease. Harrison and colleagues[71] coined the term diabetic hepatosclerosis (DHS) in 2006, after reviewing liver biopsy specimens from patients with long-standing diabetes mellitus. Salient features included an absence of steatosis and dense perisinusoidal fibrosis. The original description included 14 patients with diabetes mellitus, most of whom had a normal body mass index (calculated as weight in kilograms divided by the square of height in meters), evidence of microvascular complications, and increased serum alkaline phosphatase level. A larger follow-up autopsy series from the same investigators did not find an association with cholestasis.[72] Nevertheless, DHS is believed to represent a hepatic form of microvascular disease in patients with diabetes mellitus.

CARDIAC DISEASE

Heart failure can cause a variety of hepatic manifestations, from asymptomatic increases of liver biochemical test levels to cirrhosis and acute hepatic failure.[73] Acute and chronic hepatic congestion are associated with a modest hyperbilirubinemia in 1.2% to 20% of patients, respectively. In a retrospective cohort study of 661 patients from the Royal Cornwall Hospital in England who were referred over a 4-year to 5-year period to a jaundice hotline, 8 of the 661 (1.2%) were found to have a primary cardiac cause of cholestasis.[74] The hyperbilirubinemia of heart failure is typically unconjugated, with a serum bilirubin level of less than 3 mg/dL, but it can be conjugated and associated with higher bilirubin levels. Jaundice may become worse with repeated episodes of heart failure, often in association with a cardiac index less than 1.5 L/min/m^2. Pathologically, the low-flow state of heart failure and resulting reduced oxygen tension cause zone 3 hepatic necrosis and ischemic biliary changes with cholestasis from bile thrombi formation. Bilirubinostasis is also postulated to occur as a result of extrinsic compression from sinusoidal and hepatic venule dilatation. Ischemic hepatitis (shock liver), which can result from myocardial infarction, massive pulmonary embolus, arrhythmia, or cardiac tamponade, is a distinct entity characterized by increased serum aminotransferase levels of at least 20 times the upper limit of normal and a rapid return to normal. Similarly high serum lactate dehydrogenase levels are characteristic. Seeto and colleagues[75] compared 31 patients with ischemic hepatitis with 31 patients with hypovolemic shock secondary to trauma and found an average total bilirubin level of 2.8 mg/dL in the ischemic hepatitis cohort compared with 0.8 mg/dL in the traumatic shock group. Classically, the peak in serum bilirubin occurs as the aminotransferase levels are declining.

SYSTEMIC AUTOIMMUNE DISEASES

Cholestasis may occur during the course of several autoimmune diseases. Autoimmune sclerosing cholangitis and IgG4-related disease are discussed elsewhere in this issue by Dr Marina Silveira. Several systemic autoimmune conditions may be associated with primary autoimmune liver disease; in particular, Sjögren syndrome and systemic sclerosis may coexist with primary biliary cirrhosis. The serum alkaline phosphatase level may be increased in systemic lupus erythematosus and rheumatoid arthritis, but cholestasis is uncommon. Concomitant pharmacologic therapy and joint and bone involvement in both diseases may have led to misinterpretation of increased alkaline phosphatase levels as cholestasis in older case series.

Henoch-Schönlein purpura (HSP) is clearly associated with cholestasis. HSP is a common systemic vasculitis of childhood characterized by palpable purpura and at least 1 of the following: abdominal pain, IgA deposits in biopsy specimens, arthritis, or renal involvement. The disease typically evolves in the setting of a viral infection (parvovirus B19, upper respiratory infection) or bacterial infection (group A *Streptococcus*, *Salmonella*, *Shigella*, *Campylobacter* spp). A predisposing malignancy, such as nonsmall cell lung cancer or lymphoma, is often noted in adults. The leukocytoclastic vasculitis can involve the gallbladder and cause acute acalculous cholecystitis.[76] The peribiliary vessels may be affected, thereby resulting in biliary ischemia, stenosis of the bile ducts, and obstructive jaundice.[77]

IBD may be associated with a primary autoimmune cholestatic liver disease (primary sclerosing cholangitis or IgG4-related disease). In addition, granulomatous hepatitis, characterized by an increased serum alkaline phosphatase level, is well described in patients with Crohn disease.[78] Bile salt malabsorption after ileal resection for Crohn disease increases the risk of cholelithiasis, which can cause biliary obstruction because of bile duct stones. Celiac disease has been associated with increased aminotransferase levels in many cases and occasionally with advanced liver disease.[79] Increase of the alkaline phosphatase level is less common and may be caused by bone involvement from secondary hyperparathyroidism.

TOTAL PARENTERAL NUTRITION

The consequences of parenteral nutrition on the development of cholestatic liver disease are reviewed in detail elsewhere. Cholestasis in neonates is especially problematic and can progress to life-threatening liver dysfunction. The incidence of parenteral nutrition-associated liver complications has decreased in neonates over time.[80] The duration of parenteral nutrition in infants correlates with the risk of developing more progressive cholestatic jaundice. After 10 days of parenteral nutrition, canalicular cholestasis was present in 84.2% of infants, and after 3 weeks, bile duct proliferation was found in 63.6% of infants.[81] The pathogenesis of parenteral nutrition-associated cholestasis is multifactorial. The neonatal liver is immature and unable to excrete bile salts at a normal rate, thereby leading to bile acid toxicity, particularly from the secondary bile acid lithocholate. Bacterial translocation across an underdeveloped or unused segment of intestine causes systemic endotoxemia and contributes to cholestasis in the context of altered postsurgical anatomy (eg, bypass, short bowel, absent ileocecal valve). Enteral intake stimulates bile flow as a result of cholecystokinin (CCK) release, and in the absence of CCK, gallbladder dysmotility occurs and can result in biliary sludge, gallstones, and even acalculous cholecystitis. Hepatic steatosis is a more common manifestation in adult patients on parenteral nutrition, but cholestasis from biliary sludge and gallstones is also encountered. Early resumption of oral intake is critical to preventing the development of parenteral nutrition-associated cholestasis, as

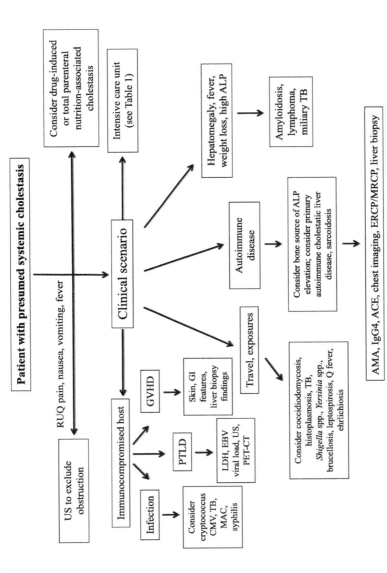

Fig. 4. Algorithm for the evaluation of the patient with systemic cholestasis. ACE, angiotensin-converting enzyme level; ALP, alkaline phosphatase level; AMA, antimitochondrial antibodies; CMV, cytomegalovirus; EBV, Epstein-Barr virus; ERCP, endoscopic retrograde cholangiopancreatography; GI, gastrointestinal; GVHD, graft-versus-host disease; LDH, lactate dehydrogenase level; MAC, *Mycobacterium avium* complex; MRCP, magnetic resonance cholangiopancreatography; MRI, magnetic resonance imaging; PET-CT, positron emission tomography with computed tomography; PTLD, posttransplant lymphoproliferative disorder; TB, tuberculosis; US, ultrasonography.

is cycling of the parenteral nutrition infusion to allow for normalization of insulin and counterregulatory hormone levels. Ursodeoxycholic acid is effective for the prevention of cholestasis in patients with short bowel syndrome on long-term parenteral nutrition.[82]

SUMMARY

The evaluation of a patient with systemic cholestasis requires careful attention to the clinical circumstances (**Fig. 4**). In general, exclusion of drug-induced cholestasis, parenteral nutrition-induced cholestasis, and biliary obstruction is a useful first step in both inpatients and outpatients. Cholestasis in the intensive care unit should raise suspicion for sepsis syndrome, particularly in the pediatric patient population. Severe hypovolemic shock can cause ischemic cholangiopathy characterized by pronounced cholestasis. In adult inpatients with mild hyperbilirubinemia, a detailed cardiopulmonary physical examination and transthoracic echocardiography are useful to exclude heart failure; marked increase in serum aminotransferase levels accompanying jaundice suggests ischemic hepatitis. Cholestasis in immunocompromised patients should prompt a detailed clinical history for evidence of an infectious exposure. A comprehensive workup for infectious organisms should follow. Transplant recipients should be evaluated for PTLD; evaluation should include a serum lactate dehydrogenase level and an EBV viral load. Often, cross-sectional imaging with positron emission tomography and evaluation for obstructive lymphadenopathy with ultrasonography are warranted. Hepatic sarcoidosis is typically a histologic diagnosis, but chest imaging and a serum angiotensin-converting enzyme level are usually helpful. Striking cholestasis in the setting of weight loss and hepatosplenomegaly are highly suggestive of systemic malignancy with hepatic involvement, especially lymphoma, as well as amyloidosis. In either case, pursuing a tissue diagnosis is necessary, although liver tissue specifically is not essential. Cholestasis in the setting of a systemic autoimmune disease should prompt evaluation for a primary autoimmune cholestatic liver disease such as primary biliary cirrhosis or primary sclerosing cholangitis. An extrahepatic source of alkaline phosphatase should be excluded if the only evidence of cholestasis is an increased alkaline phosphatase level. Liver biopsy is usually definitive and the procedure of choice when the diagnosis remains uncertain after a comprehensive noninvasive evaluation. The evaluation of a patient with systemic cholestasis requires a meticulous approach, with treatment directed toward the underlying cause.

REFERENCES

1. Osler W. The principles and practice of medicine: designed for the use of practitioners and students of medicine. New York: D. Appleton; 1892.
2. Moseley RH. Sepsis and cholestasis. Clin Liver Dis 1999;3:465–75.
3. Tung CB, Tung CF, Yang DY, et al. Extremely high levels of alkaline phosphatase in adult patients as a manifestation of bacteremia. Hepatogastroenterology 2005; 52:1347–50.
4. Hamilton JR, Sass-Kortsak A. Jaundice associated with severe bacterial infection in young infants. J Pediatr 1963;63:121–32.
5. Franson TR, Hierholzer WJ Jr, LaBrecque DR. Frequency and characteristics of hyperbilirubinemia associated with bacteremia. Rev Infect Dis 1985;7:1–9.
6. Sikuler E, Guetta V, Keynan A, et al. Abnormalities in bilirubin and liver enzyme levels in adult patients with bacteremia. A prospective study. Arch Intern Med 1989;149:2246–8.

7. Whitehead MW, Hainsworth I, Kingham JG. The causes of obvious jaundice in South West Wales: perceptions versus reality. Gut 2001;48:409–13.

8. Fuchs M, Sanyal AJ. Sepsis and cholestasis. Clin Liver Dis 2008;12:151–72, ix.

9. Geier A, Fickert P, Trauner M. Mechanisms of disease: mechanisms and clinical implications of cholestasis in sepsis. Nat Clin Pract Gastroenterol Hepatol 2006;3: 574–85.

10. Chand N, Sanyal AJ. Sepsis-induced cholestasis. Hepatology 2007;45:230–41.

11. Wagner M, Zollner G, Trauner M. New molecular insights into the mechanisms of cholestasis. J Hepatol 2009;51:565–80.

12. Zollner G, Fickert P, Zenz R, et al. Hepatobiliary transporter expression in percutaneous liver biopsies of patients with cholestatic liver diseases. Hepatology 2001;33:633–46.

13. Fahrlaender H, Huber F, Gloor F. Intrahepatic retention of bile in severe bacterial infections. Gastroenterology 1964;47:590–9.

14. Engler S, Elsing C, Flechtenmacher C, et al. Progressive sclerosing cholangitis after septic shock: a new variant of vanishing bile duct disorders. Gut 2003;52: 688–93.

15. Benninger J, Grobholz R, Oeztuerk Y, et al. Sclerosing cholangitis following severe trauma: description of a remarkable disease entity with emphasis on possible pathophysiologic mechanisms. World J Gastroenterol 2005;11: 4199–205.

16. Schmitt M, Kolbel CB, Muller MK, et al. Sclerosing cholangitis after burn injury. Z Gastroenterol 1997;35:929–34 [in German].

17. Scheppach W, Druge G, Wittenberg G, et al. Sclerosing cholangitis and liver cirrhosis after extrabiliary infections: report on three cases. Crit Care Med 2001;29:438–41.

18. Seeto RK, Rockey DC. Pyogenic liver abscess. Changes in etiology, management, and outcome. Medicine (Baltimore) 1996;75:99–113.

19. Zhu X, Wang S, Jacob R, et al. A 10-year retrospective analysis of clinical profiles, laboratory characteristics and management of pyogenic liver abscesses in a Chinese hospital. Gut Liver 2011;5:221–7.

20. Chou FF, Sheen-Chen SM, Chen YS, et al. Single and multiple pyogenic liver abscesses: clinical course, etiology, and results of treatment. World J Surg 1997;21:384–8 [discussion: 388–9].

21. Cheng HC, Chang WL, Chen WY, et al. Long-term outcome of pyogenic liver abscess: factors related with abscess recurrence. J Clin Gastroenterol 2008; 42:1110–5.

22. Joshi V, Koulaouzidis A, McGoldrick S, et al. Actinomycotic liver abscess: a rare complication of colonic diverticular disease. Ann Hepatol 2010;9:96–8.

23. Sharma M, Briski LE, Khatib R. Hepatic actinomycosis: an overview of salient features and outcome of therapy. Scand J Infect Dis 2002;34:386–91.

24. Stern MS, Gitnick GL. Shigella hepatitis. JAMA 1976;235:2628.

25. Saebo A, Lassen J. Acute and chronic liver disease associated with *Yersinia enterocolitica* infection: a Norwegian 10-year follow-up study of 458 hospitalized patients. J Intern Med 1992;231:531–5.

26. Cervantes F, Bruguera M, Carbonell J, et al. Liver disease in brucellosis. A clinical and pathological study of 40 cases. Postgrad Med J 1982;58:346–50.

27. Janbon F. The liver and brucellosis. Gastroenterol Clin Biol 1999;23:431–2 [in French].

28. den Haan PJ, van Vliet AC, Hazenberg BP. Weil's disease as a cause of jaundice. Neth J Med 1993;42:171–4.

29. Mullick CJ, Liappis AP, Benator DA, et al. Syphilitic hepatitis in HIV-infected patients: a report of 7 cases and review of the literature. Clin Infect Dis 2004; 39:e100–5.

30. Johnson TL, Barnett JL, Appelman HD, et al. *Candida* hepatitis. Histopathologic diagnosis. Am J Surg Pathol 1988;12:716–20.

31. Bucuvalas JC, Bove KE, Kaufman RA, et al. Cholangitis associated with *Cryptococcus neoformans*. Gastroenterology 1985;88:1055–9.

32. Zangerl B, Edel G, von Manitius J, et al. Coccidioidomycosis as the cause of granulomatous hepatitis. Med Klin (Munich) 1998;93:170–3 [in German].

33. Kumar N, Jain S, Singh ZN. Disseminated histoplasmosis with reactive hemophagocytosis: aspiration cytology findings in two cases. Diagn Cytopathol 2000;23: 422–4.

34. Chong VH. Hepatobiliary tuberculosis: a review of presentations and outcomes. South Med J 2008;101:356–61.

35. Chong VH, Lim KS. Hepatobiliary tuberculosis. Singapore Med J 2010;51: 744–51.

36. Young LS. *Mycobacterium avium* complex infection. J Infect Dis 1988;157:863–7.

37. Hinedi TB, Koff RS. Cholestatic hepatitis induced by Epstein-Barr virus infection in an adult. Dig Dis Sci 2003;48:539–41.

38. Snover DC, Horwitz CA. Liver disease in cytomegalovirus mononucleosis: a light microscopical and immunoperoxidase study of six cases. Hepatology 1984;4: 408–12.

39. Finegold MJ, Carpenter RJ. Obliterative cholangitis due to cytomegalovirus: a possible precursor of paucity of intrahepatic bile ducts. Hum Pathol 1982;13: 662–5.

40. Hasosah MY, Kutbi SY, Al-Amri AW, et al. Perinatal cytomegalovirus hepatitis in Saudi infants: a case series. Saudi J Gastroenterol 2012;18:208–13.

41. Agarwal SK, Kalra V, Dinda A, et al. Fibrosing cholestatic hepatitis in renal transplant recipient with CMV infection: a case report. Int Urol Nephrol 2004;36:433–5.

42. Khatib R, Siddique M, Abbass M. Measles associated hepatobiliary disease: an overview. Infection 1993;21:112–4.

43. Cremers J, Drent M, Driessen A, et al. Liver-test abnormalities in sarcoidosis. Eur J Gastroenterol Hepatol 2012;24:17–24.

44. Devaney K, Goodman ZD, Epstein MS, et al. Hepatic sarcoidosis. Clinicopathologic features in 100 patients. Am J Surg Pathol 1993;17:1272–80.

45. Alam I, Levenson SD, Ferrell LD, et al. Diffuse intrahepatic biliary strictures in sarcoidosis resembling sclerosing cholangitis. Case report and review of the literature. Dig Dis Sci 1997;42:1295–301.

46. Nakanuma Y, Kouda W, Harada K, et al. Hepatic sarcoidosis with vanishing bile duct syndrome, cirrhosis, and portal phlebosclerosis. Report of an autopsy case. J Clin Gastroenterol 2001;32:181–4.

47. Alenezi B, Lamoureux E, Alpert L, et al. Effect of ursodeoxycholic acid on granulomatous liver disease due to sarcoidosis. Dig Dis Sci 2005;50:196–200.

48. Ishak KG. Sarcoidosis of the liver and bile ducts. Mayo Clin Proc 1998;73:467–72.

49. Park MA, Mueller PS, Kyle RA, et al. Primary (AL) hepatic amyloidosis: clinical features and natural history in 98 patients. Medicine (Baltimore) 2003;82:291–8.

50. Molleran Lee S, Villanueva J, Sumegi J, et al. Characterisation of diverse PRF1 mutations leading to decreased natural killer cell activity in North American families with haemophagocytic lymphohistiocytosis. J Med Genet 2004;41:137–44.

51. de Kerguenec C, Hillaire S, Molinie V, et al. Hepatic manifestations of hemophagocytic syndrome: a study of 30 cases. Am J Gastroenterol 2001;96:852–7.

52. Ebert EC, Nagar M, Hagspiel KD. Gastrointestinal and hepatic complications of sickle cell disease. Clin Gastroenterol Hepatol 2010;8:483–9 [quiz: e70].

53. Schubert TT. Hepatobiliary system in sickle cell disease. Gastroenterology 1986; 90:2013–21.

54. Lacaille F, Lesage F, de Montalembert M. Acute hepatic crisis in children with sickle cell disease. J Pediatr Gastroenterol Nutr 2004;39:200–2.

55. Brunetta DM, Silva-Pinto AC, do Carmo Favarin de Macedo M, et al. Intrahepatic cholestasis in sickle cell disease: a case report. Anemia 2011;2011:975731.

56. Friedman LS. Liver transplantation for sickle cell hepatopathy. Liver Transpl 2007; 13:483–5.

57. Birrer MJ, Young RC. Differential diagnosis of jaundice in lymphoma patients. Semin Liver Dis 1987;7:269–77.

58. Perera DR, Greene ML, Fenster LF. Cholestasis associated with extrabiliary Hodgkin's disease. Report of three cases and review of four others. Gastroenterology 1974;67:680–5.

59. Hubscher SG, Lumley MA, Elias E. Vanishing bile duct syndrome: a possible mechanism for intrahepatic cholestasis in Hodgkin's lymphoma. Hepatology 1993;17:70–7.

60. Ballonoff A, Kavanagh B, Nash R, et al. Hodgkin lymphoma-related vanishing bile duct syndrome and idiopathic cholestasis: statistical analysis of all published cases and literature review. Acta Oncol 2008;47:962–70.

61. Noronha V, Shafi NQ, Obando JA, et al. Primary non-Hodgkin's lymphoma of the liver. Crit Rev Oncol Hematol 2005;53:199–207.

62. Jain A, Nalesnik M, Reyes J, et al. Posttransplant lymphoproliferative disorders in liver transplantation: a 20-year experience. Ann Surg 2002;236:429–36 [discussion: 436–7].

63. Kotlyar DS, Osterman MT, Diamond RH, et al. A systematic review of factors that contribute to hepatosplenic T-cell lymphoma in patients with inflammatory bowel disease. Clin Gastroenterol Hepatol 2011;9:36–41.e1.

64. Morla D, Alazemi S, Lichtstein D. Stauffer's syndrome variant with cholestatic jaundice: a case report. J Gen Intern Med 2006;21:C11–3.

65. Tuncer HH, Rana N, Milani C, et al. Gastrointestinal and hepatic complications of hematopoietic stem cell transplantation. World J Gastroenterol 2012;18: 1851–60.

66. Przepiorka D, Weisdorf D, Martin P, et al. 1994 consensus conference on acute GVHD grading. Bone Marrow Transplant 1995;15:825–8.

67. Tay J, Tinmouth A, Fergusson D, et al. Systematic review of controlled clinical trials on the use of ursodeoxycholic acid for the prevention of hepatic veno-occlusive disease in hematopoietic stem cell transplantation. Biol Blood Marrow Transplant 2007;13:206–17.

68. Huang MJ, Liaw YF. Clinical associations between thyroid and liver diseases. J Gastroenterol Hepatol 1995;10:344–50.

69. Regelmann MO, Miloh T, Arnon R, et al. Graves' disease presenting with severe cholestasis. Thyroid 2012;22:437–9.

70. Abdel Khalek M, Abd ElMageed Z, Khan A, et al. Cholestatic hepatitis in a patient with Graves' disease resolved with total thyroidectomy. Trop Gastroenterol 2011; 32:328–30.

71. Harrison SA, Brunt EM, Goodman ZD, et al. Diabetic hepatosclerosis: diabetic microangiopathy of the liver. Arch Pathol Lab Med 2006;130:27–32.

72. Chen G, Brunt EM. Diabetic hepatosclerosis: a 10-year autopsy series. Liver Int 2009;29:1044–50.

73. Giallourakis CC, Rosenberg PM, Friedman LS. The liver in heart failure. Clin Liver Dis 2002;6:947–67, viii–ix.
74. van Lingen R, Warshow U, Dalton HR, et al. Jaundice as a presentation of heart failure. J R Soc Med 2005;98:357–9.
75. Seeto RK, Fenn B, Rockey DC. Ischemic hepatitis: clinical presentation and pathogenesis. Am J Med 2000;109:109–13.
76. McCrindle BW, Wood RA, Nussbaum AR. Henoch-Schönlein syndrome. Unusual manifestations with hydrops of the gallbladder. Clin Pediatr (Phila) 1988;27:254–6.
77. Viola S, Meyer M, Fabre M, et al. Ischemic necrosis of bile ducts complicating Schönlein-Henoch purpura. Gastroenterology 1999;117:211–4.
78. Navaneethan U, Shen B. Hepatopancreatobiliary manifestations and complications associated with inflammatory bowel disease. Inflamm Bowel Dis 2010;16:1598–619.
79. Rubio-Tapia A, Murray JA. The liver in celiac disease. Hepatology 2007;46:1650–8.
80. Kubota A, Yonekura T, Hoki M, et al. Total parenteral nutrition-associated intrahepatic cholestasis in infants: 25 years' experience. J Pediatr Surg 2000;35:1049–51.
81. Cohen C, Olsen MM. Pediatric total parenteral nutrition. Liver histopathology. Arch Pathol Lab Med 1981;105:152–6.
82. Cowles RA, Ventura KA, Martinez M, et al. Reversal of intestinal failure-associated liver disease in infants and children on parenteral nutrition: experience with 93 patients at a referral center for intestinal rehabilitation. J Pediatr Surg 2010;45:84–7 [discussion: 87–8].

Advances in Pathogenesis and Treatment of Pruritus

Ruth Bolier, MD, Ronald P.J. Oude Elferink, PhD,
Ulrich Beuers, PhD, MD*

KEYWORDS

- Cholestasis • Itch • Autotaxin • Lysophosphatidate • Pruriception • Bile salts

KEY POINTS

- The pathogenesis of itch in cholestatic hepatobiliary disorders remains unclear. Proposed pruritogenic factors include increased serum autotaxin activity and subsequent lysophosphatidate formation, hyperexcitability of sensory neurons, female steroid hormones, and altered enterohepatic pruritogen (biotrans)formation.
- Stepwise treatment of cholestatic pruritus with anion exchanger resins (cholestyramine), pregnane X receptor agonists (rifampicin), opioid antagonists (naltrexone, naloxone), and serotonin reuptake inhibitors (sertraline) is recommended in guidelines.
- In patients with severe pruritus, unresponsive to standard treatment, experimental approaches including UV-B phototherapy, extracorporeal albumin dialysis, and nasobiliary drainage need to be considered. Liver transplantation represents the last option in the most desperate cases.

INTRODUCTION

Pruritus is a common symptom in patients suffering from various hepatobiliary disorders. The common denominator, cholestasis, can have its origin at different levels of the biliary tree: (1) hepatocellular secretory failure (eg, in intrahepatic cholestasis of pregnancy (ICP), progressive familiar intrahepatic cholestasis, benign recurrent intrahepatic cholestasis, and various examples of drug-induced cholestasis); (2) intrahepatic bile duct abnormalities (eg, in primary biliary cirrhosis [PBC], primary sclerosing cholangitis [PSC], Alagille syndrome); as well as (3) extrahepatic, obstructive cholestasis caused by gallstones, benign strictures (eg, primary or secondary sclerosing cholangitis) or tumor growth (eg, cholangiocarcinoma, pancreatic carcinoma, or hilar lymph node metastasis). Itch is also reported in some patients with (4) chronic hepatitis C.[1,2]

Conflict of interest: None.
Tytgat Institute for Liver and Intestinal Research, Department of Gastroenterology and Hepatology, Academic Medical Center, University of Amsterdam, G4-216, PO Box 22600, Amsterdam NL-1100 DD, The Netherlands
* Corresponding author.
E-mail address: u.h.beuers@amc.nl

Clin Liver Dis 17 (2013) 319–329
http://dx.doi.org/10.1016/j.cld.2012.11.006
1089-3261/13/$ – see front matter © 2013 Elsevier Inc. All rights reserved.

Generalized pruritus determines quality of life of patients to a great extent, leading to sleep deprivation, depression, and, anecdotally, suicidal ideation.[3] The pathogenesis of this intruding symptom has been under investigation for decades, but the molecular mechanism is still largely unclear. Concordantly, treatment options proposed in current evidence-based guidelines (**Table 1**) do not yet provide relief for all patients. Consequently, experimental therapeutic approaches are increasingly applied, broadening insight in the possible molecular targets involved in cholestatic itch. However, desperate cases of severe cholestatic pruritus, refractory to any treatment modalities mentioned earlier, represent an indication for liver transplantation often performed in the precirrhotic stage.[4]

STUDYING ITCH IN CHOLESTASIS

In the clinical setting, itch intensity is mostly evaluated in cholestatic patients by visual analogue scales (VAS) or comparable scores.[5,6] Two decades ago, devices to objectify scratching activity were proposed to evaluate itch intensity in an objective manner and were regarded as a golden diagnostic standard to prove efficacy of novel therapies.[7] However, limited availability and the considerable costs of these devices as well as the undervalued subjective component of the symptom itch have questioned these devices as a golden diagnostic standard in the community. Therefore, use of VAS together with validated quality-of-life questionnaires has become an accepted method to adequately evaluate novel therapeutic approaches. However, it remains essential to include adequate placebo controls in all therapeutic trials because placebo treatment alone has consistently improved pruritus in about 30% of tested patients in various trials.[5]

Cholestatic experimental animals barely develop itch. Thus, animal studies are being severely hampered by the ongoing search for a proper rodent model of cholestatic pruritus. Estradiol-induced cholestasis in rats may be an exception.[8] In general, animal itch studies describe acute models, in which intracutaneous injection of pruritogens

---

Table 1
Stepwise treatment of itch in cholestatic liver disease according to current guidelines.[16] Ursodeoxycholic acid (UDCA) is regarded as standard treatment of ICP and PBC,[16] but consistently alleviates pruritus only in ICP.[16] A comparable antipruritic effect of UDCA has not been reported in other cholestatic disorders

Step	Intervention	Remarks
1	Cholestyramine (up to 4 times 4 g daily)	Alternate with intake of other oral medication with time intervals of at least 4 h; monitor fat-soluble vitamins
2	Rifampicin (150 mg, increase up to 600 mg daily)	Monitor serum liver tests because of risk of hepatotoxicity
3	Naltrexone (25 mg, increase up to 50 mg daily)	Possible withdrawallike symptoms at initiation
4	Sertraline (50 mg, increase up to 75 mg daily)	
5	Experimental approaches (eg, UV-B therapy, extracorporeal albumin dialysis, nasobiliary drainage)	Refer to specialized center
6	Liver transplantation	

From European Association for the Study of the Liver. EASL Clinical Practice Guidelines: management of cholestatic liver diseases. J Hepatol 2009;51(2):259; with permission.

elicits transient scratch responses. Quantification of scratching in rodents ranges from videorecording and counting by the naked eye to oscillographic registration of the typical 10-Hz to 20-Hz scratch movements by use of magnets implanted subcutaneously in the hind paws.[9,10] Altered nociception has also been reported as a symptom of cholestasis in experimental animal models, but its relation with itch is complex.[11,12]

In vitro, properties of (potential) pruritogens have been tested on neuronal cell lines,[10] unraveling putative receptors involved in development of pruritus. Transcriptional and translational modulation of expression of proposed pruritogens by physiologic and medicinal conditions is under investigation.[13,14]

PATHOGENESIS OF PRURITUS

Impaired bile formation or stasis of bile leads to the accumulation of biliary compounds in the systemic circulation and peripheral tissues. Bile salts are potent signaling molecules in liver, bile ducts, and intestine. Their reduced intraluminal presence during cholestasis causes a range of effects in involved abdominal organs. For example, disturbed digestion of lipids, deficient uptake of fat-soluble vitamins,[15] and disturbance of intestinal flora homeostasis and of intestinal defense against bacterial overgrowth may affect the metabolism of cholestatic patients. Several potential pathogenetic factors for development of pruritus have been discussed in the past, some of which are reviewed in the following sections.

Histamine

Although a well-recognized pruritogen in allergic reactions, histamine seems not to be involved in pruritus of cholestasis. Pruritus of cholestasis was not alleviated by blocking histamine 1 receptors.[16,17] An initial observation that serum histamine levels are increased in cholestatic pruritus[18] was not supported by subsequent observations.[10] Also, the classic signs accompanying histamine-induced itch (such as edema and erythema) are lacking in pruritus of cholestasis,[19] just as any other primary skin lesions. However, secondary scratch lesions can be extensive.

Bile Salts

The efficacy of anion exchange resins such as cholestyramine in some patients suffering from cholestatic itch has been attributed by some investigators to disruption of the enterohepatic circulation of bile salts and the subsequent induction of hepato biliary bile salt secretion. Similarly, nasobiliary drainage, which quickly resolves severe pruritus in these patients, is a more drastic approach to interrupting the enterohepatic circulation of bile salts (and also of many other bile components).[10,20–22] Although one of the main components in bile, bile salt accumulation in the circulation does not seem to directly cause itch, because total serum bile salts before and after treatment do not correlate with itch relief in these studies, and many patients with severe itch do not have highly increased bile salt levels in serum and skin. A recent trial comparing colesevelam and placebo in treatment of cholestatic pruritus showed no significant difference between the two, whereas colesevelam did significantly decrease serum total bile salts.[5] However, these comparably safe agents give some relief in pruritus caused by other systemic diseases such as uremia and polycythemia vera[23] and are assigned as first-line agents by guidelines on cholestatic pruritus.[16] In **Table 2**, the arguments in favor of and against a causative role of bile salts in the pruritus of cholestasis are outlined. We and others are trying to identify a biliary component different from bile salts as the factor X that would be the missing molecular link for the development of pruritus in chronic cholangiopathies.[24]

Table 2
Arguments in favor of and against a causal role of increased serum bile salt levels in cholestatic pruritus

In Favor	References	Against	References
Bile salts induce itch when applied onto blister bases	77	No correlation between itch intensity and serum bile salts in cholestatic patients	13
Increased serum bile salt levels and some effectiveness of anion exchange resins in pruritus caused by liver disease, uremia, and pruritus of unknown origin	23,78	Pruritus observed in patients with normal bile salt levels	79
		Anion exchange resin colesevelam does not exceed placebo effect in treating cholestatic itch	5
Administration of ursodeoxycholic acid (UDCA) improves pruritus in ICP (but not other cholestatic liver diseases)	6,32,80,81	Women with ICP by definition suffer from itch, although bile salt levels are often only mildly increased	80
		Increased serum bile salt levels are also found in asymptomatic pregnant controls	82
		Itch relief after rifampicin, nasobiliary drainage, and extracorporeal albumin dialysis treatment does not correlate with serum bile salt concentration	13,21,34,83

Lysophosphatidate

Recently, we identified lysophosphatidate (LPA) as a possible pruritogen in cholestasis. Injected intracutaneously, LPA elicits a dose-dependent scratch response in mice.[10,25] Serum autotaxin (ATX), a lysophospholipase D, is the enzyme responsible for LPA formation in blood. Determination of serum ATX activity is reliable and serum ATX protein is stable, whereas serum LPA levels are unstable and highly dependent on adequate handling of serum samples. ATX activity is the only serum parameter found to correlate with itch intensity in cholestatic patients.[10] Increased serum ATX activity correlates with pruritus in cholestasis, but not pruritus during uremia or Hodgkin disease.[13] Neither ATX activity nor the ATX protein was detected in bile, although serum ATX activity rapidly decreased during nasobiliary drainage.[10] Thus, a bile-derived factor X might modulate ATX expression and, thereby, intensity of pruritus in cholestasis.[24]

The Pregnane X Receptor

The pregnane X receptor (PXR) agonist rifampicin effectively alleviates pruritus in cholestatic patients and is considered as second-line treatment of cholestatic itch.[16] Its mechanism of action is unclear. Our recent observation in vitro that rifampicin markedly reduced ATX expression at the transcriptional level in a PXR-dependent manner in human hepatoma cells may indicate the underlying molecular mechanism of the antipruritogenic action of rifampicin in cholestatic, but not other forms of itch.[13] However, additional effects cannot be excluded, because rifampicin, an antibiotic agent successfully applied for decades for treatment of tuberculosis, may affect the composition of the intestinal microbiota and, thereby, alter the microbial metabolism of potential pruritogens.

Genetic Factors

The interindividual differences in susceptibility for pruritus during cholestasis are striking and support the notion that genetic factors play a key role in the development of itch during cholestasis. The genetic background of ICP has in part been unraveled.[26–29] ICP is defined by the presence of itch, increased fasted serum bile salt and serum alanine transaminase levels during the second to third trimester of pregnancy and rapid normalization after delivery, together with the quick amelioration of itch complaints. ICP represents a model disease of hepatocellular secretory failure, with heterozygous loss-of-function mutations in the hepatocellular phospholipid transporter ABCB4 (MDR3) in up to 15% of patients, and mutations in ABCB11 (BSEP),[30] ATP8B1 (FIC1),[31] and the nuclear bile salt receptor, farnesoid X receptor in some others. Additional biliary and placental transport defects are still under investigation.[32,33]

Genome-wide association studies will soon provide information about risk genes for development of pruritus in chronic cholangiopathies such as PBC and PSC.

Environmental and Dietary Factors

Because some patients experience aggravation of itch after consumption of specific foods, environmental and dietary factors have to be taken into consideration in the efforts to unravel the pathogenesis of cholestatic itch.

Pruritogen Accumulation in the Circulation

Extracorporeal albumin dialysis, initially proposed for use in liver failure to bridge patients to transplantation, appeared to improve itch complaints impressively in two-thirds of patients.[13,34–39] During extracorporeal albumin dialysis (eg, Molecular Adsorbents Recirculating System [Gambro, Germany], The Prometheus system [Fresenius Medical Care, Germany]), the patient's blood is dialyzed against an albumin-rich fluid compartment and passes charcoal and anion exchange filters. Again, serum bile salt levels do not seem to correlate with itch relief.[13,35,37,40] In contrast, serum ATX correlated with the difference in itch intensity before and after albumin dialysis.[13,34] As a 125-kDa protein, ATX is not filtered out during the procedure. Thus, a modulator of ATX expression rather than ATX itself seems to be removed during extracorporeal albumin dialysis. Studies are under way to identify this potential factor or factors, removed from the systemic circulation of cholestatic patients suffering from severe itch by albumin dialysis, which either act as a direct pruritogen or as a modulator of ATX expression.[36]

Pruritogen Accumulation in the Skin

No topical agents have proven efficacy in pruritus of cholestasis.[16] Inspired by a phototherapeutic approach of uremic patients with resistant pruritus,[41] broad-band UV-B therapy has been applied in patients with cholestatic pruritus with some success.[19] The wavelength spectrum seems to matter here, because in a UV-A–controlled trial in uremic patients, narrow-band UV-B rays did not show additional benefit.[43] However, controlled studies are highly warranted for UV-B application in cholestatic pruritus before any conclusions can be drawn.

Because patients report a circadian rhythm of itch intensity, which is worse during late evening and night, the retinothalamic neuronal pathway has also been targeted by bright light therapy directed at the retina.[44] A trend toward itch improvement in a small patient cohort was reported, but this study was never followed up.

Pain as an Inhibitor of Itch

It has been proposed that pain and itch are sensed via the same sensory neurons, and that mild stimuli giving itch can be overruled by a stronger pain stimulus, such as scratching. This view is outdated because more and more experimental evidence has arisen indicating that specific itch neurons exist.[45] Instead, the inhibitory effect of pain on itch is proposed to take place at the interneuron levels in the dorsal horn of the spinal cord. Mice lacking this interneuronal inhibition show significantly enhanced scratch responses to pruritic agents and even develop self-inflicted skin lesions caused by excessive licking and scratching.[46] Proposed central and peripheral signaling pathways include opioidergic, serotonergic, and cannabinoid circuits.

Opioidergic Tone

Opioid antagonists, such as naltrexone and naloxone, are considered as third-line treatment in cholestatic pruritic patients.[16,47,48] The first clue for involvement of the opioidergic system in cholestatic itch was that intrathecal administration of opioids, such as morphine, was reported to give rise to itchy sensations in the anesthetized area.[49–51] Decreased nociception in bile duct–ligated rats was reversed by the opioid antagonist naloxone, whereas healthy rats showed no alterations.[52] Under cholestatic conditions in man and rodents, increased concentrations of 1 or more of 10 plasma opioidergic peptides have been reported.[53] Besides, the antinociceptive effect in cholestatic rats occurs at cutaneous nerve endings rather than centrally.[54]

Several observations argue against a key role of endogenous opioids in the development of itch in cholestasis. In cholestatic patients, the highest concentrations of opioidergic peptides are found during late-stage disease, whereas most severe pruritus is often observed at earlier stages of chronic cholangiopathies such as PBC and PSC. Furthermore, a correlation of serum opioidergic peptides with itch intensity is absent.[10,55] Nevertheless, the opioid withdrawallike symptoms observed on oral naltrexone administration in these patients[56] are believed to occur as a result of sudden inhibition of the chronically enhanced opioidergic tone during cholestasis. A careful administration of opioid antagonists in cholestatic pruritus with only slowly increasing doses is advocated to prevent the development of an opioid withdrawallike syndrome.[57]

Serotoninergic Tone

Sertraline, a serotonin reuptake inhibitor, is recommended as a fourth-line treatment of pruritus in cholestasis.[16,58] In contrast, guidelines discourage the use of the serotonin receptor antagonist ondansetron, from which some cases have been reported to have a minor benefit.[59] Similarly, based on 1 case report and some animal studies,[3,11,60,61] cannabinoid receptor agonists may enhance the increased nociception threshold during cholestasis, but are not generally recommended as therapeutic agents in pruritus of cholestasis.

As mentioned earlier, serum ATX activity and serum LPA levels are increased during cholestasis.[10] LPA receptors are involved in neuropathic pain in mice.[62,63] The scratch response on intradermal LPA injection[10] seems to be dependent on both transient receptor potential vanilloid subtype 1 (TRPV1) and histamine 1 receptors,[25] and LPA has recently been shown to be a ligand for TRPV1.[64] Thus, LPA may affect nociception and itch perception via different receptor-dependent signaling pathways.

Female Steroid Hormones

Female sex hormones may have an aggravating role in pruritus of cholestasis. During pregnancy, estrogen levels increase to 100 to 200 times the levels outside pregnancy.

Itch related to ICP quickly resolves after delivery, when female sex hormones normalize.[65] Itch was also observed more frequently in female than male patients with PBC,[66] and de novo pruritus may occur during pregnancy in patients with PBC and PSC.[67] In addition, hormone replacement therapy can give rise to recurrence of pruritus in patients with former ICP.[68,69] Ursodeoxycholic acid was found to decrease urinary excretion of progesterone disulfates.[70] Serum ATX activity is higher during administration of oral contraceptives (Kremer and colleagues, submitted) and hippocampal ATX expression is modified by estrogens in rats.[71] Thus, estrogens might modify itch intensity in an ATX-dependent fashion.

Similar to sex differences in analgesia observed in humans,[72,73] female mice show a stronger scratch response on pruritogen injection compared with males.[74] Several endogenous steroid hormones show neuromodulating properties, potentiating steroid metabolism to regulate (itch) nerve activation.[75] Here too, one of the neuroactive steroids (pregnenolone sulfate) acts via TRPV1 in rat dorsal root ganglia to modulate nociception.[76] Further research aims to therapeutically target this complex interplay of steroid hormone metabolites and itch in cholestasis.

SUMMARY

For the cholestatic patient, pruritus can markedly affect quality of life. Next to adequate treatment of the underlying disease, standard treatment of pruritus in cholestasis includes, in a stepwise manner: anion exchanger resins (eg, cholestyramine), the PXR-agonizing antibiotic rifampicin, opioid antagonists such as naltrexone and the serotonin reuptake inhibitor sertraline. Experimental approaches such as UV-B phototherapy, extracorporeal albumin dialysis, and nasobiliary drainage can be considered in experienced centers when standard treatment has failed to alleviate severe itch. New insight into the pathogenesis of pruritus is emerging, with the recent identification of potential pruritogens such as LPA formed by the lysophospholipase ATX. However, the complete pathogenetic concept for pruritus in cholestasis is lacking. This situation is in part a result of the lack of proper animal models for cholestatic itch. A biliary factor X possibly modulating ATX expression remains to be identified. Novel therapeutic approaches are to be expected once the pathogenesis of itch has been further elucidated.

REFERENCES

1. Lebovics E, Seif F, Kim D, et al. Pruritus in chronic hepatitis C: association with high serum bile acids, advanced pathology, and bile duct abnormalities. Dig Dis Sci 1997;42(5):1094–9.
2. Chia SC, Bergasa NV, Kleiner DE, et al. Pruritus as a presenting symptom of chronic hepatitis C. Dig Dis Sci 1998;43(10):2177–83.
3. Neff GW, O'Brien CB, Reddy KR, et al. Preliminary observation with dronabinol in patients with intractable pruritus secondary to cholestatic liver disease. Am J Gastroenterol 2002;97(8):2117–9.
4. Abraham SC, Kamath PS, Eghtesad B, et al. Liver transplantation in precirrhotic biliary tract disease: portal hypertension is frequently associated with nodular regenerative hyperplasia and obliterative portal venopathy. Am J Surg Pathol 2006;30(11):1454–61.
5. Kuiper EM, van Erpecum KJ, Beuers U, et al. The potent bile acid sequestrant colesevelam is not effective in cholestatic pruritus: results of a double-blind, randomized, placebo-controlled trial. Hepatology 2010;52(4):1334–40.

6. Chappell LC, Gurung V, Seed PT, et al. Ursodeoxycholic acid versus placebo, and early term delivery versus expectant management, in women with intrahepatic cholestasis of pregnancy: semifactorial randomised clinical trial. BMJ 2012;344:e3799.
7. Molenaar HA, Oosting J, Jones EA. Improved device for measuring scratching activity in patients with pruritus. Med Biol Eng Comput 1998;36(2):220–4.
8. Inan S, Cowan A. Nalfurafine, a kappa opioid receptor agonist, inhibits scratching behavior secondary to cholestasis induced by chronic ethynylestradiol injections in rats. Pharmacol Biochem Behav 2006;85(1):39–43.
9. Inagaki N, Igeta K, Shiraishi N, et al. Evaluation and characterization of mouse scratching behavior by a new apparatus, MicroAct. Skin Pharmacol Appl Skin Physiol 2003;16(3):165–75.
10. Kremer AE, Martens JJ, Kulik W, et al. Lysophosphatidic acid is a potential mediator of cholestatic pruritus. Gastroenterology 2010;139(3):1008–18, 1018.e1.
11. Gingold AR, Bergasa NV. The cannabinoid agonist WIN 55, 212-2 increases nociception threshold in cholestatic rats: implications for the treatment of the pruritus of cholestasis. Life Sci 2003;73(21):2741–7.
12. Hasanein P, Parviz M, Keshavarz M, et al. Modulation of cholestasis-induced antinociception in rats by two NMDA receptor antagonists: MK-801 and magnesium sulfate. Eur J Pharmacol 2007;554(2–3):123–7.
13. Kremer AE, van Dijk R, Leckie P, et al. Serum autotaxin is increased in pruritus of cholestasis, but not of other origin, and responds to therapeutic interventions. Hepatology 2012;56(4):1391–400.
14. Gonzalez R, Cruz A, Ferrin G, et al. Cytoprotective properties of rifampicin are related to the regulation of detoxification system and bile acid transporter expression during hepatocellular injury induced by hydrophobic bile acids. J Hepatobiliary Pancreat Sci 2011;18(5):740–50.
15. Maillette de Buy Wenniger L, Beuers U. Bile salts and cholestasis. Dig Liver Dis 2010;42(6):409–18.
16. European Association for the Study of the Liver. EASL Clinical Practice Guidelines: management of cholestatic liver diseases. J Hepatol 2009;51(2):237–67.
17. Jones EA, Bergasa NV. Evolving concepts of the pathogenesis and treatment of the pruritus of cholestasis. Can J Gastroenterol 2000;14(1):33–40.
18. Gittlen SD, Schulman ES, Maddrey WC. Raised histamine concentrations in chronic cholestatic liver disease. Gut 1990;31(1):96–9.
19. Bergasa NV. An approach to the management of the pruritus of cholestasis. Clin Liver Dis 2004;8(1):55–66, vi.
20. Singh V, Bhalla A, Sharma N, et al. Nasobiliary drainage in acute cholestatic hepatitis with pruritus. Dig Liver Dis 2009;41(6):442–5.
21. Stapelbroek JM, van Erpecum KJ, Klomp LW, et al. Nasobiliary drainage induces long-lasting remission in benign recurrent intrahepatic cholestasis. Hepatology 2006;43(1):51–3.
22. Toros AB, Ozerdenen F, Bektas H, et al. A case report: nasobiliary drainage inducing remission in benign recurrent intrahepatic cholestasis. Turk J Gastroenterol 2012;23(1):75–8.
23. Eisendle K, Muller H, Ortner E, et al. Pruritus of unknown origin and elevated total serum bile acid levels in patients without clinically apparent liver disease. J Gastroenterol Hepatol 2011;26(4):716–21.
24. Jones DE. Pathogenesis of cholestatic itch: old questions, new answers, and future opportunities. Hepatology 2012;56(4):1194–6.

25. Hashimoto T, Ohata H, Momose K. Itch-scratch responses induced by lysophosphatidic acid in mice. Pharmacology 2004;72(1):51–6.
26. Reyes H, Ribalta J, Gonzalez-Ceron M. Idiopathic cholestasis of pregnancy in a large kindred. Gut 1976;17(9):709–13.
27. Holzbach RT, Sivak DA, Braun WE. Familial recurrent intrahepatic cholestasis of pregnancy: a genetic study providing evidence for transmission of a sex-limited, dominant trait. Gastroenterology 1983;85(1):175–9.
28. Hirvioja ML, Kivinen S. Inheritance of intrahepatic cholestasis of pregnancy in one kindred. Clin Genet 1993;43(6):315–7.
29. Eloranta ML, Heinonen S, Mononen T, et al. Risk of obstetric cholestasis in sisters of index patients. Clin Genet 2001;60(1):42–5.
30. Pauli-Magnus C, Lang T, Meier Y, et al. Sequence analysis of bile salt export pump (ABCB11) and multidrug resistance p-glycoprotein 3 (ABCB4, MDR3) in patients with intrahepatic cholestasis of pregnancy. Pharmacogenetics 2004;14(2):91–102.
31. Mullenbach R, Bennett A, Tetlow N, et al. ATP8B1 mutations in British cases with intrahepatic cholestasis of pregnancy. Gut 2005;54(6):829–34.
32. Pusl T, Beuers U. Intrahepatic cholestasis of pregnancy. Orphanet J Rare Dis 2007;2:26.
33. Geenes VL, Lim YH, Bowman N, et al. A placental phenotype for intrahepatic cholestasis of pregnancy. Placenta 2011;32(12):1026–32.
34. Leckie P, Tritto G, Mookerjee R, et al. 'Out-patient' albumin dialysis for cholestatic patients with intractable pruritus. Aliment Pharmacol Ther 2012;35(6):696–704.
35. Pares A, Herrera M, Aviles J, et al. Treatment of resistant pruritus from cholestasis with albumin dialysis: combined analysis of patients from three centers. J Hepatol 2010;53(2):307–12.
36. Gay M, Pares A, Carrascal M, et al. Proteomic analysis of polypeptides captured from blood during extracorporeal albumin dialysis in patients with cholestasis and resistant pruritus. PLoS One 2011;6(7):e21850.
37. Schaefer B, Schaefer F, Wittmer D, et al. Molecular Adsorbents Recirculating System dialysis in children with cholestatic pruritus. Pediatr Nephrol 2012;27(5):829–34.
38. Bellmann R, Graziadei IW, Feistritzer C, et al. Treatment of refractory cholestatic pruritus after liver transplantation with albumin dialysis. Liver Transpl 2004;10(1):107–14.
39. Pares A, Cisneros L, Salmeron JM, et al. Extracorporeal albumin dialysis: a procedure for prolonged relief of intractable pruritus in patients with primary biliary cirrhosis. Am J Gastroenterol 2004;99(6):1105–10.
40. Huster D, Schubert C, Achenbach H, et al. Successful clinical application of extracorporal albumin dialysis in a patient with benign recurrent intrahepatic cholestasis (BRIC). Z Gastroenterol 2001;39(Suppl 2):13–4.
41. Gilchrest BA, Rowe JW, Brown RS, et al. Ultraviolet phototherapy of uremic pruritus. Long-term results and possible mechanism of action. Ann Intern Med 1979;91(1):17–21.
42. Decock S, Roelandts R, Steenbergen WV, et al. Cholestasis-induced pruritus treated with ultraviolet B phototherapy: an observational case series study. J Hepatol 2012;57(3):637–41.
43. Ko MJ, Yang JY, Wu HY, et al. Narrowband ultraviolet B phototherapy for patients with refractory uraemic pruritus: a randomized controlled trial. Br J Dermatol 2011;165(3):633–9.
44. Bergasa NV, Link MJ, Keogh M, et al. Pilot study of bright-light therapy reflected toward the eyes for the pruritus of chronic liver disease. Am J Gastroenterol 2001;96(5):1563–70.

45. Schmelz M, Schmidt R, Bickel A, et al. Specific C-receptors for itch in human skin. J Neurosci 1997;17(20):8003 8.

46. Ross SE, Mardinly AR, McCord AE, et al. Loss of inhibitory interneurons in the dorsal spinal cord and elevated itch in Bhlhb5 mutant mice. Neuron 2010; 65(6):886–98.

47. Wolfhagen FH, Sternieri E, Hop WC, et al. Oral naltrexone treatment for cholestatic pruritus: a double-blind, placebo-controlled study. Gastroenterology 1997;113(4):1264–9.

48. Terg R, Coronel E, Sorda J, et al. Efficacy and safety of oral naltrexone treatment for pruritus of cholestasis, a crossover, double blind, placebo-controlled study. J Hepatol 2002;37(6):717–22.

49. Wu Z, Kong M, Wang N, et al. Intravenous butorphanol administration reduces intrathecal morphine-induced pruritus after cesarean delivery: a randomized, double-blind, placebo-controlled study. J Anesth 2012;26(5):752–7.

50. Reich A, Szepietowski JC. Non-analgesic effects of opioids: peripheral opioid receptors as promising targets for future anti-pruritic therapies. Curr Pharm Des 2012. [Epub ahead of print].

51. Angst MS, Lazzeroni LC, Phillips NG, et al. Aversive and reinforcing opioid effects: a pharmacogenomic twin study. Anesthesiology 2012;117(1):22–37.

52. Bergasa NV, Alling DW, Vergalla J, et al. Cholestasis in the male rat is associated with naloxone-reversible antinociception. J Hepatol 1994;20(1):85–90.

53. Thornton JR, Losowsky MS. Methionine enkephalin is increased in plasma in acute liver disease and is present in bile and urine. J Hepatol 1989;8(1):53–9.

54. Nelson L, Vergnolle N, D'Mello C, et al. Endogenous opioid-mediated antinociception in cholestatic mice is peripherally, not centrally, mediated. J Hepatol 2006;44(6):1141–9.

55. Spivey JR, Jorgensen RA, Gores GJ, et al. Methionine-enkephalin concentrations correlate with stage of disease but not pruritus in patients with primary biliary cirrhosis. Am J Gastroenterol 1994;89(11):2028–32.

56. Tandon P, Rowe BH, Vandermeer B, et al. The efficacy and safety of bile acid binding agents, opioid antagonists, or rifampin in the treatment of cholestasis-associated pruritus. Am J Gastroenterol 2007;102(7):1528–36.

57. Jones EA, Neuberger J, Bergasa NV. Opiate antagonist therapy for the pruritus of cholestasis: the avoidance of opioid withdrawal-like reactions. QJM 2002;95(8): 547–52.

58. Mayo MJ, Handem I, Saldana S, et al. Sertraline as a first-line treatment for cholestatic pruritus. Hepatology 2007;45(3):666–74.

59. Muller C, Pongratz S, Pidlich J, et al. Treatment of pruritus in chronic liver disease with the 5-hydroxytryptamine receptor type 3 antagonist ondansetron: a randomized, placebo-controlled, double-blind cross-over trial. Eur J Gastroenterol Hepatol 1998;10(10):865–70.

60. Hasanein P. The endocannabinoid transport inhibitor AM404 modulates nociception in cholestasis. Neurosci Lett 2009;462(3):230–4.

61. Cichewicz DL, Martin ZL, Smith FL, et al. Enhancement mu opioid antinociception by oral delta9-tetrahydrocannabinol: dose-response analysis and receptor identification. J Pharmacol Exp Ther 1999;289(2):859–67.

62. Inoue M, Rashid MH, Fujita R, et al. Initiation of neuropathic pain requires lysophosphatidic acid receptor signaling. Nat Med 2004;10(7):712–8.

63. Lin ME, Rivera RR, Chun J. Targeted deletion of LPA5 identifies novel roles for lysophosphatidic acid signaling in development of neuropathic pain. J Biol Chem 2012;287(21):17608–17.

64. Nieto-Posadas A, Picazo-Juarez G, Llorente I, et al. Lysophosphatidic acid directly activates TRPV1 through a C-terminal binding site. Nat Chem Biol 2012;8(1):78–85.

65. Van Mil SW, Milona A, Dixon PH, et al. Functional variants of the central bile acid sensor FXR identified in intrahepatic cholestasis of pregnancy. Gastroenterology 2007;133(2):507–16.

66. Lucey MR, Neuberger JM, Williams R. Primary biliary cirrhosis in men. Gut 1986; 27(11):1373–6.

67. Chapman R, Fevery J, Kalloo A, et al. Diagnosis and management of primary sclerosing cholangitis. Hepatology 2010;51(2):660–78.

68. Kremer AE, Maillette de Buy WL, Oude Elferink RP, et al. Pruritus in liver disease. Pathogenesis and treatment. Ned Tijdschr Geneeskd 2011;155(52):A4045 [in Dutch].

69. Kunzmann S, Kullak-Ublick GA, Greiner A, et al. Effective opiate-receptor antagonist therapy of cholestatic pruritus induced by an oral contraceptive. J Pediatr Gastroenterol Nutr 2005;40(5):596–9.

70. Glantz A, Reilly SJ, Benthin L, et al. Intrahepatic cholestasis of pregnancy: amelioration of pruritus by UDCA is associated with decreased progesterone disulphates in urine. Hepatology 2008;47(2):544–51.

71. Takeo C, Ikeda K, Horie-Inoue K, et al. Identification of Igf2, Igfbp2 and Enpp2 as estrogen-responsive genes in rat hippocampus. Endocr J 2009;56(1):113–20.

72. Sun LS. Gender differences in pain sensitivity and responses to analgesia. J Gend Specif Med 1998;1(1):28–30.

73. Lawson KP, Nag S, Thompson AD, et al. Sex-specificity and estrogen-dependence of kappa opioid receptor-mediated antinociception and antihyperalgesia. Pain 2010;151(3):806–15.

74. Green AD, Young KK, Lehto SG, et al. Influence of genotype, dose and sex on pruritogen-induced scratching behavior in the mouse. Pain 2006;124(1–2):50–8.

75. Kremer AE, Beuers U, Oude-Elferink RP, et al. Pathogenesis and treatment of pruritus in cholestasis. Drugs 2008;68(15):2163–82.

76. Chen SC, Liu BC, Chen CW, et al. Intradermal pregnenolone sulfate attenuates capsaicin-induced nociception in rats. Biochem Biophys Res Commun 2006; 349(2):626–33.

77. Kirby J, Heaton KW, Burton JL. Pruritic effect of bile salts. Br Med J 1974;4(5946): 693–5.

78. Di PC, Tritapepe R, Rovagnati P, et al. Double-blind placebo-controlled clinical trial of microporous cholestyramine in the treatment of intra- and extra-hepatic cholestasis. relationship between itching and serum bile acids. Methods Find Exp Clin Pharmacol 1984;6(12):773 6.

79. Ghent CN, Bloomer JR. Itch in liver disease: facts and speculations. Yale J Biol Med 1979;52(1):77–82.

80. Geenes V, Williamson C. Intrahepatic cholestasis of pregnancy. World J Gastroenterol 2009;15(17):2049–66.

81. Hohenester S, Oude-Elferink RP, Beuers U. Primary biliary cirrhosis. Semin Immunopathol 2009;31(3):283 307.

82. Pascual MJ, Serrano MA, El-Mir MY, et al. Relationship between asymptomatic hypercholanaemia of pregnancy and progesterone metabolism. Clin Sci (Lond) 2002;102(5):587–93.

83. Ghent CN, Carruthers SG. Treatment of pruritus in primary biliary cirrhosis with rifampin. Results of a double-blind, crossover, randomized trial. Gastroenterology 1988;94(2):488–93.

Care of the Cholestatic Patient

Andrea A. Gossard, MS, CNP

KEYWORDS

- Cholestasis • Biliary tract disease • Bile duct obstruction • Primary biliary cirrhosis
- Primary sclerosing cholangitis • Cholestatic liver disease

KEY POINTS

- Cholestasis may be identified through blood work or may be clinically evident.
- Causes of cholestasis require a thorough review of the patient's medical and surgical history, medication list, and symptomatology.
- Initial evaluation of the patient with cholestasis should include imaging of the liver and biliary tree.
- Management of reversible conditions may require endoscopic or surgical intervention.
- Chronic cholestatic liver disease may contribute to fatigue, pruritus, fat-soluble vitamin deficiencies, and bone loss.

INTRODUCTION

Cholestasis is defined as impairment of bile formation or bile flow. Care of the patient with cholestatic features is dependent on identifying the cause of the cholestasis, initiating appropriate treatment of reversible conditions, and the recognition and management of cholestasis-specific complications. Cholestasis may include extrahepatic ducts and intrahepatic bile ducts, or may be limited to one or the other. Jaundice and pruritus are the hallmarks of cholestasis clinically but biochemical evidence may, and often does, precede the clinical manifestations.

DIAGNOSIS
Clinical Presentation

Patients with cholestasis may present with pruritus, fatigue, or jaundice. Dark urine and acholic stools are also symptoms of cholestasis. Many patients, however, are entirely asymptomatic and are diagnosed only after the discovery of liver test abnormalities on routine blood work.

Clinically, a cholestatic disorder can often be differentiated from a primarily hepatocellular disorder by the enzyme pattern. If there is a greater elevation proportionally in

Cholestatic Liver Disease Study Group, Division of Gastroenterology and Hepatology, Mayo Clinic, 200 First Street SW, Rochester, MN 55901, USA
E-mail address: Gossard.Andrea@mayo.edu

Clin Liver Dis 17 (2013) 331–344
http://dx.doi.org/10.1016/j.cld.2012.11.005
1089-3261/13/$ – see front matter © 2013 Elsevier Inc. All rights reserved.

the alkaline phosphatase when compared with the aminotransferases, the profile is more consistent with cholestasis. The increased serum levels of alkaline phosphatase are thought to be caused by the damaging effect of high concentrations of bile acids on intracellular and biliary membranes.[1] If an alkaline phosphatase is elevated in isolation, isoenzyme fractionation may be warranted. The gamma glutamyltranspeptidase is also often elevated in cholestasis.

Patients who are cholestatic may present with conjugated hyperbilirubinemia. Extrahepatic biliary obstruction causes conjugated hyperbilirubinemia in 80% of patients. Serum bile acids are the most sensitive test for cholestasis but testing is usually not readily available in the clinical setting.

Cholestasis is considered chronic when present for greater than 6 months. It may be further defined as primarily intrahepatic or extrahepatic, and many cases are acute on chronic. Most chronic cases of cholestasis are intrahepatic and approximately 50% of these patients demonstrate conjugated hyperbilirubinemia.

Evaluation

Obtaining a thorough patient history is essential to the diagnostic process. First, a patient's medication list should be thoroughly reviewed for potentially offending agents. Any medicines taken within the previous 6 weeks should be considered. The list of possible medicines to consider is extensive but may include estrogens, oral contraceptives, anabolic steroids, phenytoin, cyclosporin, dapsone, and erythromycin (**Box 1**). Use of herbal medicines or teas, vitamins, and other supplements should be reviewed and discontinued when possible. Total parenteral nutrition may also cause cholestasis. A history of fever, especially when accompanied by rigors or right upper quadrant abdominal pain, is more suggestive of cholangitis caused by obstructive processes, such as choledocholithiasis. These symptoms may be seen in alcoholic disease, however, and rarely in the setting of viral hepatitis.[1] Recent surgery in the region of the biliary system may have resulted in an inadvertent injury to a bile duct and should also be considered as a possible cause.

Abdominal ultrasound (US) is often the initial imaging performed when evaluating cholestasis. Advantages of US include relatively low cost, noninvasiveness, and the absence of radiation. US can effectively evaluate for intrahepatic and extrahepatic bile duct dilation and the presence of mass lesions; however, operator variability can be an issue. US is highly dependent on the skill of the sonographer and the experience of the interpreter. In addition, technical limitations include the inability to penetrate bone, and bowel gas obstructing the view. Ultrasound can differentiate between intrahepatic and extrahepatic causes of biliary tract disease, however, and can readily identify gallbladder pathology.[2]

Computed tomography is less operator dependent than US, is more effective when imaging obese patients, and is less susceptible to bowel gas when evaluating the distal bile ducts. Computed tomography is more accurate than US at identifying the level (88%–97% vs 23%–95%) and the cause (70%–94% vs 38%–94%) of biliary obstruction if present.[3] It is not as able to identify choledocholithiasis, however, and exposes the patient to radiation.[4] Computed tomography is reserved for equivocal US findings rather than for first-line imaging.

Magnetic resonance imaging is useful in the diagnosis of chronic versus acute causes of cholestasis. Use of magnetic resonance cholangiopancreatogram (MRCP) is considered a safe, noninvasive tool for evaluating the biliary tree. Advantages include the lack of radiation and sharp contrast resolution between normal and abnormal tissues. The accuracy of MRCP is comparable with endoscopic cholangiography. A review of 67 studies found that MRCP sensitivity and specificity to

Box 1
Common agents that may cause cholestasis

Anabolic steroids and androgens

Antifungals

Amoxicillin-clavulanic acid

Azathioprine

Captopril

Carbamazepine

Chlorpromazine

Chlordiazepoxide

Cyclosporin

Dapsone

Diltiazem

Erythromycin

Green tea extract

Gold salts

Imipramine

Lycopodium serratum (Jin Bu Huan)

Nitrofurantoin

Nonsteroidal anti-inflammatory drugs

Oral contraceptives and estrogen

Phenytoin

Teucrium chamaedrys (Germander)

5-Fluorouracil or floxuridine

diagnose biliary obstruction to be 95% and 97%, respectively.[5,6] Because the bile ducts are visualized in their normal physiologic state, MRCP may be a better indicator of their true caliber than endoscopic cholangiogram. However, the sensitivity for biliary strictures is lower.[6]

When suspicion is high or signs on cross-sectional imaging point to mechanical obstruction, direct cholangiography either endoscopically or percutaneously may be necessary. The primary advantage of endoscopic retrograde cholangiopancreatography (ERCP) is the ability to diagnose and intervene therapeutically when indicated. Unfortunately, 3% to 5% of all patients who undergo ERCP experience complications, such as pancreatitis.[7] Percutaneous transhepatic cholangiography should be reserved for patients in whom ERCP is precluded for anatomic reasons.

In certain diseases, such as primary sclerosing cholangitis (PSC), cholangiography is essential to making the diagnosis. In the setting of chronic cholestasis detected in a middle-aged woman with positive antimitochondrial antibodies (AMA), however, cholangiography is seldom needed because this presentation points more toward primary biliary cirrhosis (PBC).

Many of the conditions in the differential diagnosis may be excluded by history, basic laboratory studies, and imaging studies. A liver biopsy is useful when suspecting unusual conditions, such as autoimmune cholangitis, overlap syndromes, or in patients with suspected sarcoidosis.

DIFFERENTIAL DIAGNOSIS

Prescription medicines, over-the-counter drugs, and herbal supplements are some of the most common causes of cholestasis in adults. A thorough history should be obtained to rule out a potentially offending agent. In addition, a family history of cholestasis is important to note because it may suggest a hereditary disorder, such as progressive familial intrahepatic cholestasis.

The differential diagnosis beyond medicines includes the most common cause of extrahepatic cholestasis, which is choledocholithiasis.[8,9] Other causes to consider include extrabiliary tumors, cysts, parasites, and lymphoma (**Box 2**). Diseases that cause intrahepatic cholestasis include immune-mediated diseases, such as PBC, PSC, and sarcoidosis (**Box 3**).

Extrahepatic causes of chronic cholestatic liver disease should be excluded early because they are potentially reversible and failure to do so may result in complications, such as recurrent cholangitis or secondary biliary cirrhosis. Hepatocellular diseases that may cause intrahepatic cholestatic liver disease include viral hepatitis B and C. Hepatitis C has been associated with chronic cholestasis, although the usual biochemical abnormalities reflect hepatocellular damage. Alcoholic hepatitis may present with clinical and biochemical features of cholestatic liver disease. This type of hepatocellular disease may also coexist with other liver diseases, so a detailed history is imperative.

Autoimmune hepatitis (AIH) may present similarly to PBC and some degree of overlap is not uncommon.[10] The precise prevalence is unknown but perhaps 10% of patients could be classified in this overlap category.[11-13] Most patients with AIH have antinuclear antibodies and anti–smooth muscle antibodies in the serum, however, and histologically there is rarely destruction of the bile ducts. Pruritus is less common in AIH, and the serum alkaline phosphatase level is typically only

---

Box 2
Extrahepatic biliary obstruction

Intraductal obstruction and abnormalities

    Gallstones

    Cysts

    Strictures

    IgG4-related disease

    Malignancy of bile ducts

    Malformation

    AIDS cholangiopathy (rare in North America)

    Parasites

Extrinsic compression

    Extrabiliary malignancies

    Pancreatitis

    Lymphoma

| Box 3 |
Intrahepatic cholestasis
Primary biliary cirrhosis
Primary sclerosing cholangitis
Hepatocellular disease
Alcoholic hepatitis
Hepatitis B
Hepatitis C
Autoimmune hepatitis
Miscellaneous causes
Sarcoidosis
Idiopathic adult ductopenia
Benign recurrent intrahepatic cholestasis
Cystic fibrosis
Drug-induced cholestasis
Sepsis
Amyloidosis
Total parenteral nutrition
Malignancy

minimally elevated. In some cases differentiating between AIH and PBC is difficult, but under these circumstances patients with AIH experience a dramatic response to immunosuppressive therapy, whereas patients with PBC do not.

Chronic cholestatic sarcoidosis, a disease most common in young African American men, can present with features that are histologically similar to PBC and in some cases PSC. Granulomatous destruction of small ducts is the hallmark of this condition. The granulomas are typically large and well defined, in contrast to the small and poorly defined granulomas seen in PBC. Most of these patients have hilar adenopathy on chest roentgenograms and other features of sarcoidosis, and do not have AMA.

Benign recurrent intrahepatic cholestasis is a rare syndrome characterized by recurrent attacks of pruritus and jaundice. During the attack, serum alkaline phosphatase levels are elevated and cholestasis is noted histologically. The cholangiogram is normal, however, and all cases eventually go into remission. Cirrhosis does not develop and the prognosis is excellent.[14]

Patients with cystic fibrosis may have neonatal jaundice that resolves yet recurs later in life.[15] Histologic examination of the liver reveals mucus-plugged cholangioles without significant parenchymal damage; consequently, portal hypertension is a prominent manifestation, whereas liver failure is rare. Approximately one-third of patients have abnormalities of the gallbladder or cystic duct. Prognosis is largely determined by the status of the pulmonary disease.

The most common cause of chronic intrahepatic cholestatic liver disease in adults is PBC.[16] It is estimated that in the United States the prevalence of PBC is about 150 to 400 cases per million individuals. PSC is the second most common and is characterized by an inflammatory and fibrotic process that damages the intrahepatic and extrahepatic ducts.[17] The prevalence of PSC is estimated to range from 50 to 70 cases per million individuals. PSC is a progressive disorder that eventually leads to cirrhosis. PBC is also considered progressive although seemingly at a slower pace.

PBC may have a very long natural history. The presence of AMA is noted in more than 95% of patients with PBC and is helpful in making the diagnosis. The specificity of AMA for PBC is 95%.[18] More than 80% of patients with PBC are female. The terms "autoimmune cholangitis" and "AMA-negative PBC" have been used for patients who have clinical and histologic features of PBC but are AMA negative. These patients are generally positive for antinuclear or anti–smooth muscle antibodies. Autoimmune cholangitis and PBC seem to be part of a disease spectrum with very similar clinical and histologic features and a similar response to therapy. Liver biopsy is helpful in confirmation of this disease, but in patients who have prominent cholestatic liver biochemistries and a strongly positive AMA, the diagnosis of PBC is highly likely and liver biopsy is usually unnecessary.

The natural history of PSC is less well defined and seemingly more variable. Patients may be asymptomatic, but as the disease progresses, complications including dominant strictures often develop. PSC is more common in men with a 2:1 male to female ratio. The disease is strongly associated with inflammatory bowel disease (IBD) with about 80% of patients having concurrent colitis. Of those with PSC and IBD, approximately 80% have chronic ulcerative colitis, 10% Crohn colitis, and another 10% mixed features or indeterminate colitis.[19] Patients with both PSC and IBD are at an increased risk of developing colorectal cancer compared with those with IBD alone. AMA are typically absent in patients who have PSC. Other antibodies, such as antinuclear antibodies and antineutrophil cytoplasmic antibodies, are frequently found.

Bile duct imaging with magnetic resonance cholangiography is very helpful in confirming the diagnosis of PSC. It is a noninvasive test that does not require administration of contrast or use of radiation. Classic cholangiographic features of PSC include multifocal stricturing with and sacular segmental dilatation causing a beaded appearance.[20] Usually the intrahepatic and extrahepatic ducts are involved but perhaps up to 20% of patients have only intrahepatic duct disease. Involvement of only the extrahepatic ducts is rare. Liver biopsy is useful for histologic confirmation and in staging the disease but it is not always necessary.

Occasionally patients present with histologic features of PSC in the setting of chronic colitis but have normal cholangiograms. These patients are considered to have small-duct PSC and comprise approximately 5% of all patients with PSC.[21] Small-duct PSC may develop into cholangiographically evident disease over time but the natural history is less well known.

MANAGEMENT
Primary Biliary Cirrhosis

The most common cause of intrahepatic cholestasis is PBC. Multiple clinical trials have studied ursodeoxycholic acid (UDCA) as treatment of PBC at doses of 13 to 15 mg/kg/day and have found it to be safe and well-tolerated. UDCA has been shown to improve liver biochemistries and survival free of transplantation, particularly in those patients with early stage disease.[22,23]

Primary Sclerosing Cholangitis

Unfortunately, there is no effective therapy for PSC. UDCA is the most studied but the role remains unclear in regard to ability to slow disease progression.[24–29] The use of UDCA at doses of 28 to 30 mg/kg/day is not advised after a large study by Lindor and colleagues[29,30] revealed that UDCA was found to increase the risk of esophageal varices and need to liver transplantation.

Patients with PSC are at risk for biliary obstruction secondary to strictures. If there is evidence of a dominant biliary stricture on imaging, ERCP may be indicated. Often strictures may be readily managed endoscopically with balloon dilation. Biliary stenting may also be performed but is not clearly superior to balloon dilation.[31]

Pruritus

Arguably the most problematic symptom of cholestasis is pruritus. The cause remains poorly understood but may be from the accumulation of hydrophobic bile acids or endogenous opioids. This symptom is difficult to manage, and intractable pruritus has led to liver transplantation.

In the absence of bile duct obstruction amenable to treatment, management of pruritus typically involves oral therapies (**Box 4**). Topical treatments have not demonstrated efficacy in improving pruritus.

Cholestyramine, an anion-exchange resin, at doses of 4 g twice daily is considered as first-line therapy for pruritus.[32] Cholestyramine improves itching in 80% of patients with cholestasis but palatability can be an issue. If deemed ineffective or not well tolerated by the patient, then use of rifampin, typically at doses of 150 to 300 mg twice a day, should be considered.[33–36] Rifampin is effective in approximately 50% of patients. Patients should be monitored for rare complications including hepatitis, hemolytic anemia, and renal dysfunction. In case series, drug-induced hepatic dysfunction has been reported in up to 12% of patients with cholestasis.[37]

Opioid antagonists, such as naltrexone, have been studied as treatment of cholestatic pruritus.[38–43] Naltrexone may be used at a dose of 50 mg/day or nalmefene, 4 to 240 mg/day. Problems with opiate withdrawal-type reactions have been noted, however, and this risk should be reviewed with the patient.

There is also evidence to support use of sertraline, 75 to 100 mg/day, as therapy for pruritus, although many clinicians experience disappointing results with this choice.[44] Initial studies of ondansetron demonstrated efficacy; however, subsequent placebo-controlled evidence suggested there was no benefit.[45,46]

Fatigue

Fatigue is a complex and potentially debilitating symptom associated with cholestatic liver disease. Fatigue may be described as a pervasive sense of exhaustion with an inability to complete normal daily activities or engage in physical or mental work.[47] Studies of patients with PBC have found fatigue is present in 68% to 81% of patients.[48–53] It is nearly as prevalent in patients with PSC or drug-induced cholestasis.[50,54,55] For many with cholestasis, it is identified as the most problematic symptom.

Box 4
Management of pruritus

Cholestyramine, 4 g twice daily

Rifampin, 150–300 mg twice daily

Naltrexone, 50 mg/day, or nalmefene, 4–240 mg/day

Sertraline, 75–100 mg/day

The pathogenesis of fatigue in cholestasis is not well understood. It seems to involve changes in central neurotransmission, which result from signaling between the diseased liver and the brain.[56] There is poor correlation with degree of fatigue and stage of cholestatic disease.

The initial step in managing fatigue is ruling out potentially contributing factors, such as depression, anemia, thyroid dysfunction, renal dysfunction, and sleep disturbances. For those patients with depression, treatment with antidepressants may improve fatigue.

To date, management options for fatigue are limited and no therapies have been identified as clearly beneficial. In PBC, fluoxetine was studied and was not helpful.[57] Modafinil has also been evaluated at doses of 100 to 200 mg/day and in one study of 42 patients provided benefit to 73% of those who took it.[58,59] However, in another study evaluating 40 patients who were randomized to modafinil at doses of up to 200 mg/day for 12 weeks or placebo,[60] modafinil was not associated with improvement in fatigue. Additional studies are warranted. Emphasis on stress reduction, healthy lifestyle, avoidance of alcohol and caffeine, regular exercise, and adequate sleep may help.[61,62]

Osteoporosis

Osteoporosis occurs in cirrhosis of all etiologies.[63] Increased resorption and decreased formation of bone contribute to the development of osteoporosis in patients with cholestasis.[64] Patients who smoke, are inactive, have low body weight, and are female are at greater risk of osteoporosis. Screening for bone loss in PBC should be performed with bone mineral density assessment (DEXA) at baseline with follow-up at between 1 and 5 years depending on outcome and general osteoporosis risk.[65]

Use of calcium, 600 mg twice daily, with 400 IU of vitamin D and weight-bearing activities should be considered as initial prophylaxis, although this does not reliably improve bone density in patients with PBC.[66] Hormone-replacement therapy has been shown to improve bone mass in postmenopausal patients with PBC. However, the potential risks associated with this therapy should be reviewed because oral use has been associated with increased risk of breast cancer, stroke, and myocardial infarction.[67–69] Use of testosterone is not recommended. Raloxifene is a selective estrogen receptor modulator that works by reducing bone resorption and may be considered.[70]

Bisphosphonate therapy has proved beneficial in patients with PBC and osteoporosis and should be considered as first-line treatment in those patients with significant or progressive bone loss.[71–73] Use of oral bisphosphonates in the setting of esophageal varices, however, is not advised. These medicines may cause esophagitis and esophageal erosions increasing the risk of variceal bleeding. Use of intravenous forms of bisphosphonates, such as pamidronate, should be considered as an alternative to oral therapy for these patients. In addition, use of teriparatide subcutaneously or zolendronic acid intravenously may be an option for some patients.

Vitamin Deficiency

Patients with cholestatic liver disease rarely present with fat-soluble vitamin deficiencies. In a randomized, placebo-controlled trial of 180 patients with PBC, the proportion of patients with vitamin A, D, E, and K deficiencies was 33.5%, 13.2%, 1.9%, and 7.8%, respectively.[74] Patients with chronic cholestatic liver disease are at increased risk for fat-soluble vitamin deficiencies and malabsorption of nutrients because of the decreased availability of bile salts necessary for absorption in the intestinal lumen.

Patients with early stage disease could consider using a daily multivitamin. Vitamin D deficiency can be confirmed by measuring serum vitamin D levels and should be performed at the time of diagnosis and then annually. When encountered, 50,000 units of water-soluble vitamin D given once or twice per week for 8 to 12 weeks are usually sufficient to correct the deficiency. Ongoing use of vitamin D at doses of 800 to 1200 units indefinitely thereafter is reasonable. Vitamin A deficiency is uncommon and may present clinically with night blindness. Vitamin A levels can be measured, and when low, replacement with 25,000 to 50,000 units two to three times per week should be instituted, starting at the lower levels. The adequacy of replacement therapy should be assessed by repeat serum assays because excessive vitamin A has been associated with hepatotoxicity. Vitamin E deficiency has been reported in a few cases of PBC. Typically, vitamin E deficiency causes a neurologic abnormality primarily affecting the posterior columns and characterized by areflexia or loss of proprioception and ataxia. Replacement of vitamin E in these patients has been disappointing. However, patients with low serum levels of vitamin E should be started on replacement therapy, usually 100 mg twice daily.

Celiac sprue has been reported in patients with PBC and PSC. Furthermore, because of the association of PBC and scleroderma, wide-mouth diverticula and bacterial overgrowth seen in scleroderma can complicate PBC. In addition, PBC and PSC have been associated with pancreatic insufficiency, and this must be considered when dealing with patients who have either of these two disorders and evidence of malabsorption.

Dyslipidemia

Approximately 75% of patients with PBC have a total cholesterol level higher than 200 mg/dL. A cross-sectional study showed that patients with early stage PBC histologically tend to have low levels of low-density lipoproteins and marked increases in high-density lipoproteins. When the disease is advanced, patients are more likely to have marked elevations of low-density lipoproteins with the presence of lipoprotein-X and a significant decrease in high-density lipoproteins.[75] For patients with cholesterol deposits in the form of xanthomas or xanthelasma, therapy with UDCA or cholestyramine may stabilize and even decrease the size of these cutaneous deposits.

Treatment of hyperlipidemia in PBC is controversial because the data suggest there is not necessarily an increased risk of cardiovascular events in patients with PBC and elevated cholesterol levels. If therapy is deemed appropriate for a particular patient given personal or family risk factors, use of statins may be considered. Similarly, patients with PSC often have lipid levels that are elevated but there does not seem to be an increased incidence risk of cardiovascular events.[76]

Portal Hypertension

Varices can occur in cholestatic liver disease as with other forms of liver disease and are associated with an impaired prognosis.[77,70] Appropriate screening, prophylaxis, and treatment of varices should be used as with other liver diseases.[79–81] First-line therapy for moderate to large varices is typically nonselective β-blockade. If large varices with high-risk stigmata are noted or if the patient has evidence of decompensated liver disease, variceal band ligation may be indicated as primary prophylaxis. If the varices are small but there is evidence of decompensation, use of β-blockers may be considered.

Up to 20% of patients with PBC and PSC may have precirrhotic portal hypertension. Use of noninvasive measures, such as Mayo risk score of greater than 4.5 or platelet level of less than 150,000 to predict risk of esophageal varices, may be particularly helpful for these patients.[82]

Malignancy

The risk of developing hepatocellular carcinoma and cholangiocarcinoma is increased in the setting of chronic cholestatic liver disease. The risk of hepatocellular carcinoma in PBC is increased particularly in males of advanced age and those with evidence of portal hypertension.[83] Interventions including radiofrequency ablation, alcohol injection, chemoembolization, and orthotopic liver transplantation may increase survival.[84]

The cumulative lifetime risk of cholangiocarcinoma in PSC is 10% to 15%.[85] Interestingly, up to 50% of cholangiocarcinoma is diagnosed within the first year of PSC diagnosis. After that, the yearly incidence is 0.5% to 1.5%. Ongoing surveillance for malignant transformation with serial imaging for patients with chronic cholestatic liver disease is recommended.

SUMMARY

The care of the patient with cholestasis hinges on identifying the cause, treating reversible causes, and managing chronic cholestatic processes. PBC and PSC are important causes of chronic cholestasis and are the most common causes of cholestatic liver disease. Effective therapy is available for patients with PBC, whereas none exists for patients with PSC. Awareness of the complications that may be associated with cholestasis and implementing appropriate management is essential.

REFERENCES

1. Heathcote EJ. Diagnosis and management of cholestatic liver disease. Clin Gastroenterol Hepatol 2007;5(7):776–82.
2. Bennett WF, Bova JG. Review of hepatic imaging and a problem-oriented approach to liver masses. Hepatology 1990;12(4 Pt 1):761–75.
3. Reddy SI, Grace ND. Liver imaging. A hepatologist's perspective. Clin Liver Dis 2002;6(1):297–310, ix.
4. Saini S. Imaging of the hepatobiliary tract. N Engl J Med 1997;336(26):1889–94.
5. Romagnuolo J, Bardou M, Rahme E, et al. Magnetic resonance cholangiopancreatography: a meta-analysis of test performance in suspected biliary disease. Ann Intern Med 2003;139(7):547–57.
6. Varghese JC, Liddell RP, Farrell MA, et al. The diagnostic accuracy of magnetic resonance cholangiopancreatography and ultrasound compared with direct cholangiography in the detection of choledocholithiasis. Clin Radiol 1999;54(9):604–14.
7. Freeman ML, Nelson DB, Sherman S, et al. Complications of endoscopic biliary sphincterotomy. N Engl J Med 1996;335(13):909–18.
8. Mark DH, Flamm CR, Aronson N. Evidence-based assessment of diagnostic modalities for common bile duct stones. Gastrointest Endosc 2002;56(Suppl 6):S190–4.
9. Baillie J, Paulson EK, Vitellas KM. Biliary imaging: a review. Gastroenterology 2003;124(6):1686–99.
10. Heathcote EJ. Overlap of autoimmune hepatitis and primary biliary cirrhosis: an evaluation of a modified scoring system. Am J Gastroenterol 2002;97(5):1090–2.
11. Poupon R, Chazouilleres O, Corpechot C, et al. Development of autoimmune hepatitis in patients with typical primary biliary cirrhosis. Hepatology 2006;44(1):85–90.

12. Rust C, Beuers U. Overlap syndromes among autoimmune liver diseases. World J Gastroenterol 2008;14(21):3368–73.
13. Czaja AJ. The variant forms of autoimmune hepatitis. Ann Intern Med 1996; 125(7):588–98.
14. Nakamuta M, Sakamoto S, Miyata Y, et al. Benign recurrent intrahepatic cholestasis: a long-term follow-up. Hepatogastroenterology 1994;41(3):287–9.
15. Colombo C, Battezzati PM, Crosignani A, et al. Liver disease in cystic fibrosis: a prospective study on incidence, risk factors, and outcome. Hepatology 2002; 36(6):1374–82.
16. Ludwig J. Idiopathic adulthood ductopenia: an update. Mayo Clin Proc 1998; 73(3):285–91.
17. Maggs JR, Chapman RW. An update on primary sclerosing cholangitis. Curr Opin Gastroenterol 2008;24(3):377–83.
18. Invernizzi P, Lleo A, Podda M. Interpreting serological tests in diagnosing autoimmune liver diseases. Semin Liver Dis 2007;27(2):161–72.
19. Loftus EV Jr, Harewood GC, Loftus CG, et al. PSC-IBD: a unique form of inflammatory bowel disease associated with primary sclerosing cholangitis. Gut 2005; 54(1):91–6.
20. MacCarty RL, LaRusso NF, Wiesner RH, et al. Primary sclerosing cholangitis: findings on cholangiography and pancreatography. Radiology 1983;149(1):39–44.
21. Bjornsson E, Olsson R, Bergquist A, et al. The natural history of small-duct primary sclerosing cholangitis. Gastroenterology 2008;134(4):975–80.
22. Lindor KD, Poupon R, Heathcote EJ, et al. Ursodeoxycholic acid for primary biliary cirrhosis. Lancet 2000;355(9204):657–8.
23. Corpechot C, Carrat F, Bahr A, et al. The effect of ursodeoxycholic acid therapy on the natural course of primary biliary cirrhosis. Gastroenterology 2005;128(2): 297–303.
24. Beuers U, Spengler U, Kruis W, et al. Ursodeoxycholic acid for treatment of primary sclerosing cholangitis: a placebo-controlled trial. Hepatology 1992; 16(3):707–14.
25. Stiehl A. Ursodeoxycholic acid in the treatment of primary sclerosing cholangitis. Ann Med 1994;26(5):345–9.
26. Lindor KD. Ursodiol for primary sclerosing cholangitis. Mayo primary sclerosing cholangitis-ursodeoxycholic acid study group. N Engl J Med 1997;336(10): 691–5.
27. Cullen SN, Rust C, Fleming K, et al. High dose ursodeoxycholic acid for the treatment of primary sclerosing cholangitis is safe and effective. J Hepatol 2008;48(5): 792–800.
28. Olsson R, Boberg KM, de Muckadell OS, et al. High-dose ursodeoxycholic acid in primary sclerosing cholangitis: a 5-year multicenter, randomized, controlled study. Gastroenterology 2005;129(5):1464–72.
29. Lindor KD, Kowdley KV, Luketic VA, et al. High-dose ursodeoxycholic acid for the treatment of primary sclerosing cholangitis. Hepatology 2009;50(3):808–14.
30. Imam MH, Sinakos E, Gossard AA, et al. High-dose ursodeoxycholic acid increases risk of adverse outcomes in patients with early stage primary sclerosing cholangitis. Aliment Pharmacol Ther 2011;34(10):1185–92.
31. Kaya M, Petersen BT, Angulo P, et al. Balloon dilation compared to stenting of dominant strictures in primary sclerosing cholangitis. Am J Gastroenterol 2001; 96(4):1059–66.
32. Imam MH, Gossard AA, Sinakos E, et al. Pathogenesis and management of pruritus in cholestatic liver disease. J Gastroenterol Hepatol 2012;27(7):1150–8.

33. Ghent CN, Carruthers SG. Treatment of pruritus in primary biliary cirrhosis with rifampin. Results of a double-blind, crossover, randomized trial. Gastroenterology 1988;94(2):488–93.

34. Heathcote EJ. Is rifampin a safe and effective treatment for pruritus caused by chronic cholestasis? Nat Clin Pract Gastroenterol Hepatol 2007;4(4):200–1.

35. Bachs L, Pares A, Elena M, et al. Effects of long-term rifampicin administration in primary biliary cirrhosis. Gastroenterology 1992;102(6):2077–80.

36. Podesta A, Lopez P, Terg R, et al. Treatment of pruritus of primary biliary cirrhosis with rifampin. Dig Dis Sci 1991;36(2):216–20.

37. Prince MI, Burt AD, Jones DE. Hepatitis and liver dysfunction with rifampicin therapy for pruritus in primary biliary cirrhosis. Gut 2002;50(3):436–9.

38. Heathcote J. The pruritus of cholestasis is relieved by an opiate antagonist: is this pruritus a centrally mediated phenomenon? Hepatology 1996;23(5): 1280–2.

39. Bergasa NV, Alling DW, Talbot TL, et al. Oral nalmefene therapy reduces scratching activity due to the pruritus of cholestasis: a controlled study. J Am Acad Dermatol 1999;41(3 Pt 1):431–4.

40. Thornton JR, Losowsky MS. Opioid peptides and primary biliary cirrhosis. BMJ 1988;297(6662):1501–4.

41. Bergasa NV, Alling DW, Talbot TL, et al. Effects of naloxone infusions in patients with the pruritus of cholestasis. A double-blind, randomized, controlled trial. Ann Intern Med 1995;123(3):161–7.

42. Bergasa NV, Jones EA. The pruritus of cholestasis: potential pathogenic and therapeutic implications of opioids. Gastroenterology 1995;108(5):1582–8.

43. Wolfhagen FH, Sternieri E, Hop WC, et al. Oral naltrexone treatment for cholestatic pruritus: a double-blind, placebo-controlled study. Gastroenterology 1997;113(4):1264–9.

44. Mayo MJ, Handem I, Saldana S, et al. Sertraline as a first-line treatment for cholestatic pruritus. Hepatology 2007;45(3):666–74.

45. Muller C, Pongratz S, Pidlich J, et al. Treatment of pruritus in chronic liver disease with the 5-hydroxytryptamine receptor type 3 antagonist ondansetron: a randomized, placebo-controlled, double-blind cross-over trial. Eur J Gastroenterol Hepatol 1998;10(10):865–70.

46. O'Donohue JW, Pereira SP, Ashdown AC, et al. A controlled trial of ondansetron in the pruritus of cholestasis. Aliment Pharmacol Ther 2005;21(8):1041–5.

47. Barofsky I, Legro MW. Definition and measurement of fatigue. Rev Infect Dis 1991;13(Suppl 1):S94–7.

48. Witt-Sullivan H, Heathcote J, Cauch K, et al. The demography of primary biliary cirrhosis in Ontario, Canada. Hepatology 1990;12(1):98–105.

49. Cauch-Dudek K, Abbey S, Stewart DE, et al. Fatigue in primary biliary cirrhosis. Gut 1998;43(5):705–10.

50. Huet PM, Deslauriers J, Tran A, et al. Impact of fatigue on the quality of life of patients with primary biliary cirrhosis. Am J Gastroenterol 2000;95(3):760–7.

51. Vuoristo M, Farkkila M, Karvonen AL, et al. A placebo-controlled trial of primary biliary cirrhosis treatment with colchicine and ursodeoxycholic acid. Gastroenterology 1995;108(5):1470–8.

52. Lindor KD, Dickson ER, Baldus WP, et al. Ursodeoxycholic acid in the treatment of primary biliary cirrhosis. Gastroenterology 1994;106(5):1284–90.

53. Heathcote EJ, Cauch-Dudek K, Walker V, et al. The Canadian multicenter double-blind randomized controlled trial of ursodeoxycholic acid in primary biliary cirrhosis. Hepatology 1994;19(5):1149–56.

54. Gross CR, Malinchoc M, Kim WR, et al. Quality of life before and after liver transplantation for cholestatic liver disease. Hepatology 1999;29(2):356–64.

55. Katsinelos P, Vasiliadis T, Xiarchos P, et al. Ursodeoxycholic acid (UDCA) for the treatment of amoxycillin-clavulanate potassium (Augmentin)-induced intrahepatic cholestasis: report of two cases. Eur J Gastroenterol Hepatol 2000; 12(3):365–8.

56. Swain MG. Fatigue in liver disease: pathophysiology and clinical management. Can J Gastroenterol 2006;20(3):181–8.

57. Talwalkar JA, Donlinger JJ, Gossard AA, et al. Fluoxetine for the treatment of fatigue in primary biliary cirrhosis: a randomized, double-blind controlled trial. Dig Dis Sci 2006;51(11):1985–91.

58. Abbas G, Jorgensen RA, Lindor KD. Fatigue in primary biliary cirrhosis. Nat Rev Gastroenterol Hepatol 2010;7(6):313–9.

59. Ian Gan S, de Jongh M, Kaplan MM. Modafinil in the treatment of debilitating fatigue in primary biliary cirrhosis: a clinical experience. Dig Dis Sci 2009; 54(10):2242–6.

60. Silveira MG, DeCook AA, Keach AC, et al. Modafinil in the treatment of fatigue in patients with primary biliary cirrhosis. Hepatology 2011;54(Suppl 4):1211A.

61. Swain MG. Fatigue in chronic disease. Clin Sci (Lond) 2000;99(1):1–8.

62. Bergasa NV, Mehlman JK, Jones EA. Pruritus and fatigue in primary biliary cirrhosis. Baillieres Best Pract Res Clin Gastroenterol 2000;14(4):643–55.

63. Sokhi RP, Anantharaju A, Kondaveeti R, et al. Bone mineral density among cirrhotic patients awaiting liver transplantation. Liver Transpl 2004;10(5): 648–53.

64. Guichelaar MM, Malinchoc M, Sibonga J, et al. Bone metabolism in advanced cholestatic liver disease: analysis by bone histomorphometry. Hepatology 2002;36(4 Pt 1):895–903.

65. Newton J, Francis R, Prince M, et al. Osteoporosis in primary biliary cirrhosis revisited. Gut 2001;49(2):282–7.

66. Crippin JS, Jorgensen RA, Dickson ER, et al. Hepatic osteodystrophy in primary biliary cirrhosis: effects of medical treatment. Am J Gastroenterol 1994;89(1): 47–50.

67. Pereira SP, O'Donohue J, Moniz C, et al. Transdermal hormone replacement therapy improves vertebral bone density in primary biliary cirrhosis: results of a 1-year controlled trial. Aliment Pharmacol Ther 2004;19(5):563–70.

68. Boone RH, Cheung AM, Girlan LM, et al. Osteoporosis in primary biliary cirrhosis: a randomized trial of the efficacy and feasibility of estrogen/progestin. Dig Dis Sci 2006;51(6):1103–12.

69. Hulley S, Grady D, Bush T, et al. Randomized trial of estrogen plus progestin for secondary prevention of coronary heart disease in postmenopausal women. Heart and Estrogen/progestin Replacement Study (HERS) Research Group. JAMA 1998;280(7):605–13.

70. Lowy C, Harnoie DM, Angulo P, et al. Raloxifene improves bone mass in osteopenic women with primary biliary cirrhosis: results of a pilot study. Liver Int 2005;25(1):117–21.

71. Guanabens N, Pares A, Ros I, et al. Alendronate is more effective than etidronate for increasing bone mass in osteopenic patients with primary biliary cirrhosis. Am J Gastroenterol 2003;98(10):2268–74.

72. Musialik J, Petelenz M, Gonciarz Z. Effects of alendronate on bone mass in patients with primary biliary cirrhosis and osteoporosis: preliminary results after one year. Scand J Gastroenterol 2005;40(7):873–4.

73. Zein CO, Jorgensen RA, Clarke B, et al. Alendronate improves bone mineral density in primary biliary cirrhosis: a randomized placebo-controlled trial. Hepatology 2005;42(4):762–71.

74. Phillips JR, Angulo P, Petterson T, et al. Fat-soluble vitamin levels in patients with primary biliary cirrhosis. Am J Gastroenterol 2001;96(9):2745–50.

75. Jahn CE, Schaefer EJ, Taam LA, et al. Lipoprotein abnormalities in primary biliary cirrhosis. Association with hepatic lipase inhibition as well as altered cholesterol esterification. Gastroenterology 1985;89(6):1266–78.

76. Sinakos E, Abbas G, Jorgensen RA, et al. Serum lipids in primary sclerosing cholangitis. Dig Liver Dis 2012;44(1):44–8.

77. Gores GJ, Wiesner RH, Dickson ER, et al. Prospective evaluation of esophageal varices in primary biliary cirrhosis: development, natural history, and influence on survival. Gastroenterology 1989;96(6):1552–9.

78. Jones DE, Metcalf JV, Collier JD, et al. Hepatocellular carcinoma in primary biliary cirrhosis and its impact on outcomes. Hepatology 1997;26(5):1138–42.

79. Garcia-Tsao G, Sanyal AJ, Grace ND, et al. Prevention and management of gastroesophageal varices and variceal hemorrhage in cirrhosis. Hepatology 2007;46(3):922–38.

80. Bressler B, Pinto R, El-Ashry D, et al. Which patients with primary biliary cirrhosis or primary sclerosing cholangitis should undergo endoscopic screening for oesophageal varices detection? Gut 2005;54(3):407–10.

81. Bruix J, Sherman M. Management of hepatocellular carcinoma. Hepatology 2005; 42(5):1208–36.

82. Levy C, Zein CO, Gomez J, et al. Prevalence and predictors of esophageal varices in patients with primary biliary cirrhosis. Clin Gastroenterol Hepatol 2007;5(7): 803–8.

83. Suzuki A, Lymp J, Donlinger J, et al. Clinical predictors for hepatocellular carcinoma in patients with primary biliary cirrhosis. Clin Gastroenterol Hepatol 2007; 5(2):259–64.

84. Imam MH, Silveira MG, Sinakos E, et al. Long-term outcomes of patients with primary biliary cirrhosis and hepatocellular carcinoma. Clin Gastroenterol Hepatol 2012;10(2):182–5.

85. Lazaridis KN, Gores GJ. Primary sclerosing cholangitis and cholangiocarcinoma. Semin Liver Dis 2006;26(1):42–51.

Liver Transplant for Cholestatic Liver Diseases

Andres F. Carrion, MD[a], Kalyan Ram Bhamidimarri, MD, MPH[b],*

KEYWORDS

- Cholestatic liver disease • Primary sclerosing cholangitis • Primary biliary cirrhosis
- Liver transplantation • Recurrence • Outcomes

KEY POINTS

- Cholestatic liver diseases are a heterogeneous of group of disorders that can progress to biliary cirrhosis.
- Disease-specific manifestations in each of these cholestatic liver diseases pose specific risks that significantly affect the morbidity and mortality of affected patients.
- Liver transplant (LT) is the only definitive therapy for patients in whom the condition has progressed to end-stage liver disease.
- In general, cholestatic liver diseases have the best posttransplant outcomes when compared with other indications of LT.
- Disease recurrence and extrahepatic manifestations of cholestatic liver diseases can significantly affect the quality of life, and long-term studies are needed to understand the natural history after LT.

PRIMARY SCLEROSING CHOLANGITIS

Primary sclerosing cholangitis (PSC) is considered a rare disease, but the average annual percentage incidence of PSC has increased by 5%.[1] The estimated 10-year survival is approximately 65%.[2] Despite the modest increase in incidence, the number of transplants has remained stable between 1995 and 2006.[3] PSC is the fifth most common indication for LT in the United States and the number one indication in Scandinavian countries.[4] PSC accounts for approximately 250 LTs or 5% of all LTs per year in the United States (United Network for Organ Sharing [UNOS]). The rates of LT in Europe, especially in the Scandinavian and Nordic regions, are higher than that in the United States (8%–16% per year) because of the lower incidence of viral and

[a] Division of Gastroenterology, Department of Medicine, University of Miami Miller School of Medicine, 1120 Northwest 14th Street, Suite 310E, Miami, FL 33136, USA; [b] Division of Hepatology, Department of Medicine, University of Miami Miller School of Medicine, 1500 Northwest 12th Avenue, Suite 1101, Miami, FL 33136, USA
* Corresponding author.
E-mail address: kbhamidimari@med.miami.edu

Clin Liver Dis 17 (2013) 345–359
http://dx.doi.org/10.1016/j.cld.2012.12.005
1089-3261/13/$ – see front matter © 2013 Elsevier Inc. All rights reserved.

alcoholic liver disease and expanded selection criteria, which additionally include patients with PSC with high grade biliary dysplasia and early cholangiocarcinoma (CCA). At present, there is no effective therapy for the management of PSC except for LT.[4–7]

LT Evaluation

Organ allocation for PSC is similar to that for other indications in the United States and is prioritized by the Model for End-stage Liver Disease (MELD) score, which is cause independent. Several prognostic models specific for PSC have been developed by combining demographic, serologic, and radiologic variables known to independently affect survival of patients with PSC. Nevertheless, these models are imprecise in predicting outcomes for individual patients, and no consensus exists about the optimal model. Thus, the American Association for the Study of Liver Disease recommends against using disease-specific models for predicting clinical outcomes in individual patients.[4]

Additional MELD (exception) points can be requested from the regional transplant review boards for specific manifestations of PSC such as intractable pruritus, recurrent or refractory bacterial cholangitis, and carefully selected limited-stage CCA,[4] which are granted on a case-by-case basis by determining risk of waitlist mortality, waitlist removal, and non–liver-related comorbidities.[5] According to current consensus recommendations, exception points are granted to patients with PSC with either 2 or more episodes of culture-proven bacteremia within a 6-month period or noniatrogenic septic complications of cholangitis with positive result of blood cultures, no identifiable correctable structural lesion, and the absence of biliary stents.[6] Data from the UNOS show that 12.2% of patients with PSC listed for LT between 2002 and 2011 received exception points and an overwhelming majority of them did not conform to established consensus recommendations.[7]

LT Evaluation for PSC with Cholangiocarcinoma

CCA is the second most common primary hepatic malignancy with a reported incidence 0.6% to 1.5% per year and a lifetime risk 7% to 17% in patients with PSC.[8,9] The prognosis of CCA is extremely poor with an average 5-year survival of 5% to 10%.[10] Surgical resection provides the only possibility of cure for localized CCA, and adjuvant chemoradiation should be considered in all cases.[11] LT for unresectable CCA is not considered a standard therapy at present, and some transplant centers even consider CCA as a contraindication for LT. Nevertheless, dismal survival rates initially reported (0%–20% at 5 years post-LT) have been challenged by more recent reports describing an improved 5-year survival rate of 30% to 55% after LT for unresectable CCA.[12,13] MELD exception points may be obtained only in selected patients with early unresectable hilar CCA who complete standardized protocols with neoadjuvant chemoradiation by an individual written petition, which must be approved by regional transplant review boards.[14] The Mayo Clinic protocol is one of the commonly followed protocols, which consists of external beam radiotherapy or brachytherapy plus chemotherapy and staging laparotomy.[14] Under this protocol, only patients with confirmed stage I or II disease are eligible for LT. Palliative options include biliary stenting, chemotherapy, chemoembolization, photodynamic therapy, and radiofrequency ablation.[15]

Post-LT Outcomes

Survival of patients with PSC after LT has increased markedly in the past few decades and is approximately 80% at 5 years.[16] Living donor LT (LDLT) and deceased donor LT

(DDLT) fare well for PSC and show similar graft and patient survival outcomes.[17] The 1-, 3-, and 5-year graft survival rates among LDLT and DDLT recipients were 89.6%, 87.1%, and 87.1% and 87%, 79.7%, and 79.2%, respectively, and the 1-, 3-, and 5-year patient survival rates among LDLT and DDLT recipients were 97.2%, 95.4%, and 95.4% and 93%, 87.5%, 87.5%, respectively. Similarly, longer-term outcomes are also favorable with 10-year patient and graft survival rates of 69.8% and 60.5%, respectively.[18,19] Such encouraging survival rates have shifted the focus to analyze outcomes related to disease recurrence and morbidity from extrahepatic manifestations of PSC.

Acute cellular rejection (ACR) occurs in more than 50% of patients with PSC in the immediate posttransplant period, and although some data suggest that steroid-resistant ACR or ACR needing intense immunosuppression may have significant influence on the risk of recurrent PSC, the role of ACR as a significant risk factor for recurrent PSC and the cause-effect relation of ACR to recurrent PSC is still debatable.[16,20,21] Despite the seemingly increased rates of acute and chronic allograft rejection noted in patients who underwent transplant for PSC, the use of modern immunosuppressive agents has resulted in successful management of these complications.[18]

Clinically active inflammatory bowel disease (IBD) occurs in a variable proportion of patients with PSC after LT with some reports describing quiescent or relatively mild form and others describing an aggressive form of ulcerative colitis.[22,23] It is hypothesized that gut-derived long-lived memory lymphocytes play an important role in predisposing to biliary tract inflammation and injury, and there is accumulating evidence that concurrent IBD is strongly linked to recurrent PSC.[24] Recent studies reported that colectomy before LT or at the time of LT protects against the risk of recurrent PSC, but the protective effect disappears if colectomy is performed after LT.[16] Most retrospective data had variable definitions of IBD activity and included different immunosuppressive regimens. Combined effects of longstanding colitis and posttransplant immunosuppression could play a role in the development of colon cancer, and increased incidence of colon cancer has also been reported after LT.[25,26] Therefore, current guidelines endorse annual surveillance for colon cancer in patients with PSC after LT.[4]

Patients who underwent transplant for CCA and were managed per Mayo protocol had 1-, 3-, and 5-year post-LT survival rates of 92%, 82%, and 82%, respectively. Management per such protocol also resulted in lower incidence of tumor recurrence when compared with surgical resection (10% vs 27%).[14]

Similar to other cholestatic liver diseases, patients with PSC have a higher prevalence of metabolic bone disease after LT and thus warrant surveillance and treatment of this complication.[27]

Disease Recurrence

Recurrence of PSC after LT is 6-fold higher than that of primary biliary cirrhosis (PBC).[28] The risk of recurrent PBC during the first year posttransplant is low (2%); nevertheless, it has been reported in 20% to 37% of patients followed up for 3 to 10 years[29,30] and even higher rates of up to 59.1% have been reported in some individual studies.[16] Retrospective data suggest that the presence of CCA, steroid-resistant ACR, and donor or recipient human leukocyte antigen (HLA)-DRB1*08 are predictive variables for posttransplant recurrence of PSC.[20,30] Interestingly, other variables previously considered to be predictors of recurrence such as recipient age, male gender, coexistent IBD, presence of an intact colon before transplant, use of different immunosuppressive regimen, or use of ursodeoxycholic acid (UDCA) were not found to be significant predictors of disease recurrence in a large series.[30] The diagnosis of recurrent PSC after LT may be difficult to establish because it is frequently confounded by the development of secondary sclerosing cholangitis (SSC) due to ischemia/reperfusion injury of the biliary tree and/or recurrent infectious cholangitis.[31] Recurrent PSC can be established in patients who meet the criteria described in **Box 1**.[18] Incidence of recurrent PSC based on cholangiography alone is reported to be 15.7%, developing after a mean time of 21 months after transplant,[21] but the actual recurrence rate ranges from 8.6% to 12.5% if all the biochemical, cholangiographic, and histologic criteria are taken into account.[32,33] There is no established medical therapy for recurrent PSC post-LT.[4]

Retransplant is a viable option in patients who have recurrent PSC and graft loss, and rates as high as 24% and 43% were reported in the previous years.[34,35] A large retrospective analysis from the UNOS database shows that retransplant rates were significantly higher in patients with PSC than in those with PBC (12.4% vs 8.5%).[36] Recurrence of the disease seems to significantly affect graft survival approximately after 7 years from the time of first LT and is associated with poorer patient survival rates after retransplant compared with patients who underwent retransplant and did not have recurrent PSC. Retransplant is a more complex procedure than primary LT, and the complexity increases with the number of retransplants. Perioperative mortality for primary LT and retransplant is 5% and 20%, respectively, and the average 5-year survival after a second retransplant is 40%. Although disease-specific survival rates are absent, the 5- and 10-year survival rates after retransplant in general are 57% and 47%, respectively.[37,38]

PRIMARY BILIARY CIRRHOSIS

PBC is the sixth leading indication for LT in the United States with an incidence of 2.7 per 100,000 person-years. Despite the steady increase in the incidence of PBC, there is a decline in the absolute number of LTs performed per year by about 20% as per UNOS data and a similar declining trend by 5-fold as per European database (1988–2006), which parallels the increased use of UDCA.[39] Early diagnosis and the efficacy of pharmacologic treatment in delaying the progression may account for the decreasing numbers of LT.[39]

LT Evaluation

Indications for LT in PBC are similar to those in other chronic liver diseases, and apart from complications of portal hypertension, intractable pruritus in patients with PBC

Box 1
Criteria for diagnosis of recurrent PSC

PSC diagnosed before LT

and

Exclusion of other causes of biliary strictures after LT (ie, hepatic artery thrombosis/stenosis, anastomotic stricture, chronic ductopenic rejection, ABO blood group incompatibility, viral/bacterial cholangitis)

and any one of the following:

1. Cholangiography: Evidence of nonanastomotic strictures of the intrahepatic and extrahepatic bile ducts with beading and irregularities after 90 days of transplant
2. Histology: Fibrous cholangitis and/or fibro-obliterative lesions with or without ductopenia

merits consideration for early LT. The Mayo model is the most widely used prognostic model to estimate short-term and long-term survival in patients with PBC, and LT should be considered when bilirubin levels increase over 6 mg/dL, Mayo risk score is greater than 7.8, or the MELD score is greater than 12.[40,41]

Post-LT Outcomes

Post-LT outcomes for patients with PBC are excellent with data from Europe showing 5-year patient and graft survival rates of 78% and 75%, respectively, and 10-year patient and graft survival rates of 67% and 61%, respectively.[42] LDLT also has similar outcomes as DDLT as per the analysis from UNOS database from 2002 to 2006.[17] Patient survival rates at 1, 3, and 5 years among LDLT and DDLT recipients were 92.8%, 90.1%, 86.4% and 89.6%, 87%, and 85.1%, respectively. Graft survival rates at 1, 3, and 5 years among LDLT and DDLT recipients were 85.6%, 80.9%, and 77.4% and 85.2%, 82.5%, and 80.7%, respectively.

LT in patients with PBC improves some symptoms rapidly in the immediate weeks after transplant, including pruritus and fatigue; nevertheless, ascites, jaundice, and splenomegaly slowly improve over a longer period.[39] Hepatic osteodystrophy typically worsens during the initial 6 months after LT (the mean rate of lumbar spine bone mineral density loss is 18.1% per year), but the bone mineral density returns to baseline by 12 to 18 months posttransplant and improves thereafter.[43]

Disease Recurrence

Recurrent PBC rates post-LT were underestimated previously, but with the use of protocol biopsies post-LT, current reports suggest an incidence rate of 21% to 37% at 10 years and 43% at 15 years[3,44,45] and the median time for its development ranges between 3 and 5.5 years.[3] The gold standard for the diagnosis of recurrent PBC post-LT is liver biopsy with characteristic histologic findings and the absence of alternate causes. Serum antimitochondrial antibodies may persist or reappear post-transplant but do not necessarily indicate recurrent PBC.[39] There are several reports suggesting that HLA mismatch,[3] choice of calcineurin inhibitors (tacrolimus is associated with an earlier and increased likelihood of recurrent PBC when compared with cyclosporine),[46] and other immunosuppressive agents (glucocorticoids, azathioprine, mycophenolate mofetil) could be associated with increased recurrence, but none of the data showed any conclusive evidence in predicting the risk of PBC recurrence.[47] Furthermore, there was no significant impact on patient or graft survival due to recurrent PBC or due to the use of any of the immunosuppressive agents.[44,45] In one study, recurrent PBC resulted in a graft loss of 5.4% in a median time of 7.8 years from the time of recurrence.[28] Therapy with UDCA can improve biochemical tests, but there is no evidence to support its beneficial role in improving patient or graft survival or in altering the natural course of recurrent PBC.[44,48] Although there are several reports of retransplant in patients with PBC, none of them are due to graft loss from recurrent PBC. Furthermore, patients who underwent retransplant had higher rates of adverse outcomes as expected.[49]

CHOLESTASIS ASSOCIATED WITH TOTAL PARENTERAL NUTRITION

Liver disease induced by total parenteral nutrition (TPN) is potentially reversible if enteral feeding is resumed and TPN is discontinued before development of severe fibrosis or cirrhosis,[50] but the only effective treatment for patients with intestinal failure that progressed to end-stage liver disease is LT, which is often performed in combination with small bowel transplant or multivisceral transplant.[51]

LT Evaluation

Isolated LT is proposed as an alternative option in select cases because it can improve the waitlist mortality for patients who need multivisceral transplant, as it provides adequate time for gut adaptation and has a theoretical advantage of adult liver graft that might be resistant to TPN-induced cholestasis. However, patients requiring continuous TPN after isolated LT have rapid recurrence of cholestatic liver disease and the outcomes are poor. Therefore, although there are no standard guidelines, the consensus criteria used for consideration of isolated LT are selection of patients with a residual small bowel length of at least 25 cm and who can tolerate more than 50% of goal of enteral calories.[51,52] This approach results in normalization of hepatic function and resolution of portal hypertension, which may allow for continued intestinal adaptation and enteral autonomy. Nevertheless, this procedure should only be performed at specialized centers because the mortality remains high. Sequential small bowel transplant after isolated LT has also been proposed for patients who fail intestinal adaptation post-LT,[53] and this approach requires careful assessment to exclude underlying gastrointestinal motility disorders and structural abnormalities, which may impair intestinal adaptation post-LT.[53]

Post-LT Outcomes

Although there are no large studies available, disease-specific mortality rates of 43% and 40% have been reported among recipients of isolated LT or multivisceral transplant, respectively.[51] Patient and graft survival rates for intestinal transplant and multivisceral transplant were 65% and 60%, respectively, at the end of 1 year, and the overall survival rate was 57% at the end of 2 years.[51,54] Recurrence of intestinal failure requiring TPN, TPN-induced cholestatic liver disease, sepsis, and surgical complications are some of the major risk factors for mortality in the posttransplant period, and it is interesting to note that most of the deaths occurred when the patients are at home.[51]

In summary, isolated LT should be considered only in patients with adequate residual enteral function but not as a bridge for sequential small bowel transplant or multivisceral transplant. Further research on nontransplant modalities such as bowel lengthening procedures (Bianchi procedure), serial transverse enteroplasty, and pharmacotherapy to modulate gut function and motility might decrease the need for transplant and optimize survival in these patients.

BILIARY ATRESIA

Biliary atresia (BA) is the most common cause of congenital neonatal cholestasis and is also the most common indication accounting for more than 50% of the volume of LT in children.[55] This condition is found in 1 in 10,000 to 15,000 live births.[56] Approximately 10% to 35% of patients with BA can have concomitant anomalies especially congenital heart disease. Untreated BA typically results in cirrhosis, liver failure, and death within the first 12 to 18 months of life. As per data from the European Liver Transplant Registry (2005), 76% of children with BA undergo LT by the age of 2 years.

Patient survival rates at 5 and 10 years after the Kasai procedure alone are 48% to 64.5% and 52.8%, respectively.[57,58] Furthermore, 2 large series show that long-term survival rates are not significantly different between patients who underwent the Kasai procedure versus those who did not, even if adequate bile flow is achieved and cholestasis resolves with the Kasai procedure.[59,60] Although most patients with BA including 58% to 60% of those who undergo the Kasai procedure eventually require LT, the Kasai procedure may delay the need for LT.[61] This sequential therapeutic approach with an initial Kasai procedure and reserving LT for older children who develop postprocedure progressive liver disease has been favored because it is safe and successful.[62]

LT Evaluation

Indications for LT in patients with BA include refractory failure to thrive despite aggressive nutritional support (including nasogastric tube feedings), primary failure of the Kasai procedure (absent bile drainage), complications of portal hypertension, and progressive liver dysfunction.[63]

Post-LT Outcomes

Analysis of the UNOS database demonstrates an overall good prognosis after LT with 1-, 5-, and 10-year patient survival rates of 92.1%, 87.2%, and 85.8%, respectively, and 10-year graft survival rate of 72.7%.[63] LDLT has effectively increased the donor pool and the number of transplants for BA. Retrospective data suggest that in children younger than 2 years, LDLT results in superior graft survival (50% lower risk of graft failure) compared with DDLT full size or split size allografts.[64] LDLT, however, is associated with increased rates of vascular complications such as thrombosis of hepatic artery, hepatic vein, and portal vein or biliary complications, and the rates of such complication improved with the center's experience. In contrast, older children do not seem to have additional benefit from LDLT and either split or full size allografts from deceased donors should be used.[65]

ALAGILLE SYNDROME

Alagille syndrome is an autosomal dominant disorder (rarely autosomal recessive) caused by the variable expression of JAG1/NOTCH2 gene mutations resulting in defective vasculogenesis in the embryo/fetus. It is estimated that 21% to 31% of patients with Alagille syndrome will require LT, accounting for 5% of all LTs in pediatrics.[66] The median age of LT in children with Alagille syndrome is between 3.5 and 7.8 years, and there is no existing data on LT for adult patients with Alagille syndrome.

LT Evaluation

An aggressive pretransplant evaluation needs to be performed to address cardiac, renal, and vascular disorders that are often associated with this syndrome. Cardiac testing protocols developed by the King's college and Brussels' group include pharmacologic stress tests and cardiac catheterization to estimate cardiac reserve.[67] Patients who were deemed to have inadequate cardiac reserve would then undergo aggressive interventional or surgical procedures to correct the underlying cardiac defects before LT. Patients can also be evaluated for combined heart-liver transplant or heart-lung-liver transplant if feasible, but it can be technically very challenging. Although the inheritance is autosomal dominant, most related kin may have variable penetrance or sporadic mutations. Thus, living related donors should be carefully assessed, preferably with a liver biopsy, and should not be deemed as donors if they harbor stigmata for Alagille syndrome based on their biopsies or if the test results are positive for JAG1 mutation.[68]

Post-LT Outcomes

Mortality within the first month post-LT is high in patients with Alagille syndrome, which seems to be due to the systemic involvement that could have been missed or suboptimally addressed during the pretransplant evaluation. Survival rates at 1 year post-LT are reported between 57% and 100%, but the median survival rate is around 79%.[68] Similar survival rate of 80% at 1 year post-LT was also reported among recipients of LDLT.[66] Structural and functional renal disorders are frequently encountered in patients with Alagllle syndrome and often complicate the posttransplant course. Aggressive renal evaluation before LT and minimized use of calcineurin inhibitors post-LT are proposed strategies to reduce the risk of renal dysfunction. Patients with Alagille syndrome are also at increased risk for vascular complications such as fatal intracranial hemorrhages, hepatic artery thrombosis, and so forth. Approximately 21% of patients had vascular complications post-LT that required an intervention/surgery compared with only 9% in patients with BA.[69] Finally, LT may treat the cholestasis, nutritional deficiencies, and bone disease but does not have any impact on growth or height of patients with Alagille syndrome.

MISCELLANEOUS CHOLESTATIC LIVER DISEASES
Progressive Familial Intrahepatic Cholestasis

Progressive familial intrahepatic cholestasis (PFIC) is an autosomal recessive disorder of infancy because of gene defects involved in bile acid secretion. The incidence of this condition is about 1 in 50,000 to 100,000 births and accounts for 10% to 15% of the total LTs in pediatrics.[70] Approximately 50% of patients with PFIC will need LT by the mean age of 7.5 years. Indications for LT include cirrhosis and development of complications related to portal hypertension. Three types of PFIC have been described based on gene mutations, and although they have variable phenotypic presentation and variable severity of liver disease, they are all associated with progressive cholestasis and liver failure in childhood.

PFIC type I or Byler disease (ATP8B1 mutation) is a systemic disorder, and there are several extrahepatic manifestations such as growth retardation, diarrhea, and pancreatitis, which may not resolve with LT. Severe graft steatosis and graft dysfunction can ultimately result in retransplant especially in patients with PFIC type I, and thus the role of LT in these patients is debatable.

PFIC type II (ABCB11 mutation, bile salt export pump [BSEP] gene defect) is a liver-specific disorder and is associated with severe cholestasis, liver failure, and uniquely increased risk of hepatocellular carcinoma or CCA in early life. Screening for hepatic malignancy should thus begin by the end of infancy (1 year). Most patients require LT before adolescence. Unlike PFIC type I, this disease is not associated with extrahepatic manifestations, and thus LT results in resolution of most symptoms. Patients with PFIC type II can develop recurrent cholestasis post-LT because of the development of alloimmunity to graft BSEP proteins.

PFIC type III (MDR3/ABCB4 mutation) is also a liver-specific disorder resulting in hepatobiliary injury from the production of phospholipid-deficient bile. Such bile is lithogenic, and medical therapy with bile chelators seems to be effective. Similar to patients with PFIC type II, patients with PFIC type III do not have any extrahepatic manifestations and the prognosis after LT is often excellent.[71]

Overlap Syndromes

Post-LT outcomes in patients with overlap syndromes seem to be similar to those seen in patients with PBC who undergo LT. Increased rates of rejection are seen in patients with autoimmune hepatitis (AIH) compared with those without AIH. There is no strong post-LT data available in overlap syndromes, but inconsistent evidence from small case series suggest that long-term steroid maintenance and tacrolimus-based immunosuppression had lower rejection and recurrence rates and overall better outcomes. Post-LT survival at 5 years in patients with autoimmune sclerosing cholangiopathy, an overlap of AIH and PSC in children, is 80%.[72]

Secondary Sclerosing Cholangitis

Transplant-free survival of patients with secondary sclerosing cholangitis (SSC) seems to be lower than that of PSC. Sclerosing cholangitis occuring in critically ill patients is a separate entity which may be seen in patients who have recovered from severe life-threatening illness requiring aggressive intensive care. SSC is associated with ischemic type cholangiopathy and bile plugs and can rapidly progress to cirrhosis. Survival without transplant is poor, and survival after LT is similarly poor with a median survival of 13 months posttransplant.[73] In summary, although there are very limited data, patients with SSC seem to have poor outcomes with or without LT.

Sarcoidosis

This disorder predominantly affects adults and mortality due to liver disease is rare. The incidence of cirrhosis and portal hypertension in patients with sarcoidosis is 6% to 8% and 3 to 18%, respectively. Sarcoidosis is a rare indication for LT in adults, accounting for 0.12% of all the LTs performed between 1987 and 2007.[74] Although the number of LTs for sarcoidosis did not show any annual increase, an increased number of patients with sarcoidosis were wait-listed during that period, which could be the result of increased recognition, referrals, and increased access to health care (and specifically to transplant centers) among African Americans.

Previous reports from small case series showed an excellent patient survival at 1 and 5 years, which could be the result of selection bias in these studies.[75,76] However, recent analysis of 20-year data from UNOS shows post-LT patient and graft survival rates at 1, 3, and 5-years of 78%, 67%, and 61% and 78%, 66%, and 60%, respectively, which are significantly worse than those observed in their matched PSC/PBC cohorts.[74] Retransplant was performed in 4.9% of the patients, and 2% of them underwent a third LT because of vascular thrombosis, biliary complications, and recurrent sarcoidosis. Donor risk index was the only variable that correlated with poor outcome in the study. Although outcomes of LT in patients with sarcoidosis are similar to those of other indications of LT, they are significantly worse when compared with those of other cholestatic diseases such as PSC or PBC.

Cystic-Fibrosis-Associated Liver Disease (CFALD)

Cystic-fibrosis-associated liver disease CFALD affects approximately one-third of patients with cystic fibrosis, and cirrhosis is almost always diagnosed before the age of 20 years,[77] which is the second most common cause of disease-related death in patients with cystic fibrosis.[40] Such patients should be considered for LT as long as their pulmonary function is not severely compromised.[78] Furthermore, it is important to carefully evaluate the nutritional status and history of multidrug-resistant infections before LT.[79] Outcomes of LT for CFALD are comparable to those for other causes of end-stage liver disease.[40] Reported posttransplant 1- and 5-year survival rates for patients with CFALD are 91.6% and 75%, respectively.[80] Although technically difficult and only offered in a small number of specialized centers, simultaneous lung-liver transplant seems to be an effective therapeutic option for patients with end-stage lung disease and advanced liver disease.[81] Actuarial survival after combined lung-liver transplant has been reported to be 75% to 85% at 1 year without significant change at 3 years of follow-up.[81,82]

Sickle Cell Hepatopathy

Sickle cell disease (SCD) represents a group of hemoglobinopathies (HbSS, HbSC, and HbSβ thalassemia) and affects 0.2% (homozygous) and 6% to 10% (heterozygous) of African American newborns.[83] Liver is almost universally affected, and a spectrum of hepatic manifestations is seen ranging from asymptomatic biochemical abnormalities, acute sickle hepatic crisis, sickle cell intrahepatic cholestasis, to cirrhosis.[84,85] Acute sickle hepatic crisis may be observed in up to 10% of patients with SCD and typically resolves spontaneously within 3 to 14 days with supportive treatment only.[86] Sickle cell intrahepatic cholestasis is a rare but severe complication of SCD, associated with an ominous prognosis.[87]

LT for SCD hepatopathy has been infrequently reported in isolated case reports, and thus there are no data on efficacy and outcomes of LT for this disorder. Experience from reported cases, however, suggests that LT for SCD hepatopathy may be a feasible option but vascular complications, including graft thrombosis, are important concerns.[88]

Fibropolycystic Disease of Liver

Fibropolycystic disease of the liver is a rare congenital disease characterized by multifocal, segmental saccular dilatation of large intrahepatic bile ducts.[89] There are 2 variants of this disease; first is the Caroli syndrome, characterized by dilatation of the bile ducts in association with congenital hepatic fibrosis, and the second is Caroli disease (less common), characterized by bile duct ectasia without apparent hepatic abnormalities.[90] The prevalence of fibropolycystic disease of the liver is 1 in 1,000,000.[91] Apart from medical management, partial hepatectomy is the treatment of choice for patients with disease confined to a single hepatic lobe. LT is the only therapeutic option for patients with extensive or refractory disease.[92] The most common indication for LT in patients with fibropolycystic disease of the liver is recurrent cholangitis.[91] Analysis of data from the UNOS database shows excellent outcomes after LT with 1-year patient and graft survival rates of 86.3% and 79.9%, respectively, and 5-year patient and graft survival rates of 77% and 72.4%, respectively.[91] Unfortunately, data from 2 different series show retransplant rates as high as 14% to 25% for patients with fibropolycystic disease.[93,94]

SUMMARY

Cholestatic liver diseases are a heterogeneous group of diseases that are increasing in incidence and result in significant morbidity and mortality. At present, there are no definitive medical therapies that can provide curative options to the affected patients. LT is the only definitive therapy in patients who have progressed to end-stage liver disease. This review summarizes several aspects of cholestatic liver disease including current trends of LT, pretransplant evaluation, and posttransplant outcomes and provides a comprehensive review of the most common and rare cholestatic liver diseases. Short-term outcomes posttransplant are excellent; however, studies regarding long-term outcomes need to be done to better understand the natural history of this heterogeneous and complex group of liver diseases.

REFERENCES

1. Molodecky NA, Kareemi H, Parab R, et al. Incidence of primary sclerosing cholangitis: a systematic review and meta-analysis. Hepatology 2011;53(5):1590–9.

2. Tischendorf JJ, Hecker H, Kruger M, et al. Characterization, outcome, and prognosis in 273 patients with primary sclerosing cholangitis: a single center study. Am J Gastroenterol 2007;102(1):107–14.
3. Carbone M, Neuberger J. Liver transplantation in PBC and PSC: indications and disease recurrence. Clin Res Hepatol Gastroenterol 2011;35(6–7):446–54.
4. Chapman R, Fevery J, Kalloo A, et al. Diagnosis and management of primary sclerosing cholangitis. Hepatology 2010;51(2):660–78.
5. Freeman RB Jr, Gish RG, Harper A, et al. Model for end-stage liver disease (MELD) exception guidelines: results and recommendations from the MELD Exception Study Group and Conference (MESSAGE) for the approval of patients who need liver transplantation with diseases not considered by the standard MELD formula. Liver Transpl 2006;12(12 Suppl 3):S128–36.
6. Gores GJ, Gish RG, Shrestha R, et al. Model for end-stage liver disease (MELD) exception for bacterial cholangitis. Liver Transpl 2006;12(12 Suppl 3):S91–2.
7. Goldberg D, Bittermann T, Makar G. Lack of standardization in exception points for patients with primary sclerosing cholangitis and bacterial cholangitis. Am J Transplant 2012;12(6):1603–9.
8. Burak K, Angulo P, Pasha TM, et al. Incidence and risk factors for cholangiocarcinoma in primary sclerosing cholangitis. Am J Gastroenterol 2004;99(3): 523–6.
9. Bergquist A, Ekbom A, Olsson R, et al. Hepatic and extrahepatic malignancies in primary sclerosing cholangitis. J Hepatol 2002;36(3):321–7.
10. Nakeeb A, Pitt HA, Sohn TA, et al. Cholangiocarcinoma. A spectrum of intrahepatic, perihilar, and distal tumors. Ann Surg 1996;224(4):463–73 [discussion: 473–5].
11. Eckel F, Jelic S. Biliary cancer: ESMO clinical recommendation for diagnosis, treatment and follow-up. Ann Oncol 2009;20(Suppl 4):46–8.
12. Rosen CB, Heimbach JK, Gores GJ. Surgery for cholangiocarcinoma: the role of liver transplantation. HPB (Oxford) 2008;10(3):186–9.
13. Friman S, Foss A, Isoniemi H, et al. Liver transplantation for cholangiocarcinoma: selection is essential for acceptable results. Scand J Gastroenterol 2011;46(3): 370–5.
14. Rea DJ, Heimbach JK, Rosen CB, et al. Liver transplantation with neoadjuvant chemoradiation is more effective than resection for hilar cholangiocarcinoma. Ann Surg 2005;242(3):451–8 [discussion: 458–61].
15. Ibrahim SM, Mulcahy MF, Lowandowski RJ, et al. Treatment of unresectable cholangiocarcinoma using yttrium-90 microspheres: results from a pilot study. Cancer 2008;113(8):2119–28.
16. Fosby B, Karlsen TH, Melum E. Recurrence and rejection in liver transplantation for primary sclerosing cholangitis. World J Gastroenterol 2012;18(1):1–15.
17. Kashyap R, Safadjou S, Chen R, et al. Living donor and deceased donor liver transplantation for autoimmune and cholestatic liver diseases–an analysis of the UNOS database. J Gastrointest Surg 2010;14(9):1362–9.
18. Graziadei IW, Wiesner RH, Marotta PJ, et al. Long-term results of patients undergoing liver transplantation for primary sclerosing cholangitis. Hepatology 1999; 30(5):1121–7.
19. Brandsaeter B, Friman S, Broome U, et al. Outcome following liver transplantation for primary sclerosing cholangitis in the Nordic countries. Scand J Gastroenterol 2003;38(11):1176–83.
20. Alexander J, Lord JD, Yeh MM, et al. Risk factors for recurrence of primary sclerosing cholangitis after liver transplantation. Liver Transpl 2008;14(2):245–51.

21. Jeyarajah DR, Netto GJ, Lee SP, et al. Recurrent primary sclerosing cholangitis after orthotopic liver transplantation: is chronic rejection part of the disease process? Transplantation 1998;66(10):1300–6.

22. Papatheodoridis GV, Hamilton M, Mistry PK, et al. Ulcerative colitis has an aggressive course after orthotopic liver transplantation for primary sclerosing cholangitis. Gut 1998;43(5):639–44.

23. Navaneethan U, Venkatesh PG, Mukewar S, et al. Progressive primary sclerosing cholangitis requiring liver transplantation is associated with reduced need for colectomy in patients with ulcerative colitis. Clin Gastroenterol Hepatol 2012;10(5): 540–6.

24. Adams DH, Eksteen B. Aberrant homing of mucosal T cells and extra-intestinal manifestations of inflammatory bowel disease. Nat Rev Immunol 2006;6(3): 244–51.

25. Loftus EV Jr, Aguilar HI, Sandborn WJ, et al. Risk of colorectal neoplasia in patients with primary sclerosing cholangitis and ulcerative colitis following orthotopic liver transplantation. Hepatology 1998;27(3):685–90.

26. Vera A, Gunson BK, Ussatoff V, et al. Colorectal cancer in patients with inflammatory bowel disease after liver transplantation for primary sclerosing cholangitis. Transplantation 2003;75(12):1983–8.

27. Trautwein C, Possienke M, Schlitt HJ, et al. Bone density and metabolism in patients with viral hepatitis and cholestatic liver diseases before and after liver transplantation. Am J Gastroenterol 2000;95(9):2343–51.

28. Rowe IA, Webb K, Gunson BK, et al. The impact of disease recurrence on graft survival following liver transplantation: a single centre experience. Transpl Int 2008;21(5):459–65.

29. Vera A, Moledina S, Gunson B, et al. Risk factors for recurrence of primary sclerosing cholangitis of liver allograft. Lancet 2002;360(9349):1943–4.

30. Campsen J, Zimmerman MA, Trotter JF, et al. Clinically recurrent primary sclerosing cholangitis following liver transplantation: a time course. Liver Transpl 2008;14(2):181–5.

31. Harrison RF, Davies MH, Neuberger JM, et al. Fibrous and obliterative cholangitis in liver allografts: evidence of recurrent primary sclerosing cholangitis? Hepatology 1994;20(2):356–61.

32. Narumi S, Roberts JP, Emond JC, et al. Liver transplantation for sclerosing cholangitis. Hepatology 1995;22(2):451–7.

33. Goss JA, Shackleton CR, Farmer DG, et al. Orthotopic liver transplantation for primary sclerosing cholangitis. A 12-year single center experience. Ann Surg 1997;225(5):472–81 [discussion: 481–3].

34. Alabraba E, Nightingale P, Gunson B, et al. A re-evaluation of the risk factors for the recurrence of primary sclerosing cholangitis in liver allografts. Liver Transpl 2009;15(3):330–40.

35. Cholongitas E, Shusang V, Papatheodoridis GV, et al. Risk factors for recurrence of primary sclerosing cholangitis after liver transplantation. Liver Transpl 2008; 14(2):138–43.

36. Maheshwari A, Yoo HY, Thuluvath PJ. Long-term outcome of liver transplantation in patients with PSC: a comparative analysis with PBC. Am J Gastroenterol 2004; 99(3):538–42.

37. Reese PP, Yeh H, Thomasson AM, et al. Transplant center volume and outcomes after liver retransplantation. Am J Transplant 2009;9(2):309–17.

38. Akpinar E, Selvaggi G, Levi D, et al. Liver retransplantation of more than two grafts for recurrent failure. Transplantation 2009;88(7):884–90.

39. Lindor KD, Gershwin ME, Poupon R, et al. Primary biliary cirrhosis. Hepatology 2009;50(1):291–308.
40. European Association for the Study of the Liver. EASL Clinical Practice Guidelines: management of cholestatic liver diseases. J Hepatol 2009;51(2): 237–67.
41. Gong Y, Huang ZB, Christensen E, et al. Ursodeoxycholic acid for primary biliary cirrhosis. Cochrane Database Syst Rev 2008;(3):CD000551.
42. Liermann Garcia RF, Evangelista Garcia C, McMaster P, et al. Transplantation for primary biliary cirrhosis: retrospective analysis of 400 patients in a single center. Hepatology 2001;33(1):22–7.
43. Eastell R, Dickson ER, Hodgson SF, et al. Rates of vertebral bone loss before and after liver transplantation in women with primary biliary cirrhosis. Hepatology 1991;14(2):296–300.
44. Charatcharoenwitthaya P, Pimentel S, Talwalkar JA, et al. Long-term survival and impact of ursodeoxycholic acid treatment for recurrent primary biliary cirrhosis after liver transplantation. Liver Transpl 2007;13(9):1236–45.
45. Sylvestre PB, Batts KP, Burgart LJ, et al. Recurrence of primary biliary cirrhosis after liver transplantation: histologic estimate of incidence and natural history. Liver Transpl 2003;9(10):1086–93.
46. Neuberger J, Gunson B, Hubscher S, et al. Immunosuppression affects the rate of recurrent primary biliary cirrhosis after liver transplantation. Liver Transpl 2004; 10(4):488–91.
47. Sanchez EQ, Levy MF, Goldstein RM, et al. The changing clinical presentation of recurrent primary biliary cirrhosis after liver transplantation. Transplantation 2003; 76(11):1583–8.
48. Corpechot C, Carrat F, Bahr A, et al. The effect of ursodeoxycholic acid therapy on the natural course of primary biliary cirrhosis. Gastroenterology 2005;128(2): 297–303.
49. Egawa H, Nakanuma Y, Maehara Y, et al. Disease recurrence plays a minor role as a cause for retransplantation after living-donor liver transplantation for primary biliary cirrhosis: a multicenter study in Japan. Hepatol Res 2012. [Epub ahead of print].
50. Kelly DA. Intestinal failure-associated liver disease: what do we know today? Gastroenterology 2006;130(2 Suppl 1):S70–7.
51. Nathan JD, Rudolph JA, Kocoshis SA, et al. Isolated liver and multivisceral transplantation for total parenteral nutrition-related end-stage liver disease. J Pediatr Surg 2007;42(1):143–7.
52. Horslen SP, Sudan DL, Iyer KR, et al. Isolated liver transplantation in infants with end-stage liver disease associated with short bowel syndrome. Ann Surg 2002; 235(3):435–9.
53. Muiesan P, Dhawan A, Novelli M, et al. Isolated liver transplant and sequential small bowel transplantation for intestinal failure and related liver disease in children. Transplantation 2000;69(11):2323–6.
54. Diamond IR, Wales PW, Grant DR, et al. Isolated liver transplantation in pediatric short bowel syndrome: is there a role? J Pediatr Surg 2006;41(5):955–9.
55. McKiernan PJ, Baker AJ, Kelly DA. The frequency and outcome of biliary atresia in the UK and Ireland. Lancet 2000;355(9197):25–9.
56. Yoon PW, Bresee JS, Olney RS, et al. Epidemiology of biliary atresia: a population-based study. Pediatrics 1997;99(3):376–82.
57. Karrer FM, Lilly JR, Stewart BA, et al. Biliary atresia registry, 1976 to 1989. J Pediatr Surg 1990;25(10):1076–80 [discussion: 1081].

58. Nio M, Ohi R, Miyano T, et al. Five- and 10-year survival rates after surgery for biliary atresia: a report from the Japanese Biliary Atresia Registry. J Pediatr Surg 2003;38(7):997–1000.
59. Serinet MO, Broue P, Jacquemin E, et al. Management of patients with biliary atresia in France: results of a decentralized policy 1986-2002. Hepatology 2006;44(1):75–84.
60. Schreiber RA, Barker CC, Roberts EA, et al. Biliary atresia: the Canadian experience. J Pediatr 2007;151(6):659–65, 665.e1.
61. Oh M, Hobeldin M, Chen T, et al. The Kasai procedure in the treatment of biliary atresia. J Pediatr Surg 1995;30(7):1077–80 [discussion: 1080-1].
62. Ryckman F, Fisher R, Pedersen S, et al. Improved survival in biliary atresia patients in the present era of liver transplantation. J Pediatr Surg 1993;28(3): 382–5 [discussion: 386].
63. Barshes NR, Lee TC, Balkrishnan R, et al. Orthotopic liver transplantation for biliary atresia: the U.S. experience. Liver Transpl 2005;11(10):1193–200.
64. Roberts JP, Hulbert-Shearon TE, Merion RM, et al. Influence of graft type on outcomes after pediatric liver transplantation. Am J Transplant 2004;4(3):373–7.
65. Kiuchi T, Kasahara M, Uryuhara K, et al. Impact of graft size mismatching on graft prognosis in liver transplantation from living donors. Transplantation 1999;67(2):321–7.
66. Kasahara M, Kiuchi T, Inomata Y, et al. Living-related liver transplantation for Alagille syndrome. Transplantation 2003;75(12):2147–50.
67. Ovaert C, Germeau C, Barrea C, et al. Elevated right ventricular pressures are not a contraindication to liver transplantation in Alagille syndrome. Transplantation 2001;72(2):345–7.
68. Kamath BM, Schwarz KB, Hadzic N. Alagille syndrome and liver transplantation. J Pediatr Gastroenterol Nutr 2010;50(1):11–5.
69. Shneider BL. Genetic cholestasis syndromes. J Pediatr Gastroenterol Nutr 1999; 28(2):124–31.
70. Davit-Spraul A, Gonzales E, Baussan C, et al. Progressive familial intrahepatic cholestasis. Orphanet J Rare Dis 2009;4:1.
71. Milkiewicz P, Wunsch E, Elias E. Liver transplantation in chronic cholestatic conditions. Front Biosci 2012;17:959–69.
72. Beuers U, Rust C. Overlap syndromes. Semin Liver Dis 2005;25(3):311–20.
73. Lalwani N, Bhargava P, Chintapalli KN, et al. Current update on primary and secondary sclerosing cholangitis. Curr Probl Diagn Radiol 2011;40(6):248–61.
74. Vanatta JM, Modanlou KA, Dean AG, et al. Outcomes of orthotopic liver transplantation for hepatic sarcoidosis: an analysis of the United Network for Organ Sharing/Organ Procurement and Transplantation Network data files for a comparative study with cholestatic liver diseases. Liver Transpl 2011;17(9):1027–34.
75. Casavilla FA, Gordon R, Wright HI, et al. Clinical course after liver transplantation in patients with sarcoidosis. Ann Intern Med 1993;118(11):865–6.
76. Lipson EJ, Fiel MI, Florman SS, et al. Patient and graft outcomes following liver transplantation for sarcoidosis. Clin Transplant 2005;19(4):487–91.
77. Bartlett JR, Friedman KJ, Ling SC, et al. Genetic modifiers of liver disease in cystic fibrosis. JAMA 2009;302(10):1076–83.
78. Molmenti EP, Squires RH, Nagata D, et al. Liver transplantation for cholestasis associated with cystic fibrosis in the pediatric population. Pediatr Transplant 2003;7(2):93–7.
79. Debray D, Kelly D, Houwen R, et al. Best practice guidance for the diagnosis and management of cystic fibrosis-associated liver disease. J Cyst Fibros 2011; 10(Suppl 2):S29–36.

80. Fridell JA, Bond GJ, Mazariegos GV, et al. Liver transplantation in children with cystic fibrosis: a long-term longitudinal review of a single center's experience. J Pediatr Surg 2003;38(8):1152–6.

81. Couetil JP, Houssin DP, Soubrane O, et al. Combined lung and liver transplantation in patients with cystic fibrosis. A 4 1/2-year experience. J Thorac Cardiovasc Surg 1995;110(5):1415–22 [discussion: 1422–3].

82. Couetil JP, Soubrane O, Houssin DP, et al. Combined heart-lung-liver, double lung-liver, and isolated liver transplantation for cystic fibrosis in children. Transpl Int 1997;10(1):33–9.

83. Castro O, Rana SR, Bang KM, et al. Age and prevalence of sickle-cell trait in a large ambulatory population. Genet Epidemiol 1987;4(4):307–11.

84. Ebert EC, Nagar M, Hagspiel KD. Gastrointestinal and hepatic complications of sickle cell disease. Clin Gastroenterol Hepatol 2010;8(6):483–9 [quiz: e70].

85. Banerjee S, Owen C, Chopra S. Sickle cell hepatopathy. Hepatology 2001;33(5):1021–8.

86. Schubert TT. Hepatobiliary system in sickle cell disease. Gastroenterology 1986;90(6):2013–21.

87. Shao SH, Orringer EP. Sickle cell intrahepatic cholestasis: approach to a difficult problem. Am J Gastroenterol 1995;90(11):2048–50.

88. Mekeel KL, Langham MR Jr, Gonzalez-Peralta R, et al. Liver transplantation in children with sickle-cell disease. Liver Transpl 2007;13(4):505–8.

89. Summerfield JA, Nagafuchi Y, Sherlock S, et al. Hepatobiliary fibropolycystic diseases. A clinical and histological review of 51 patients. J Hepatol 1986;2(2):141–56.

90. Desmet VJ. What is congenital hepatic fibrosis? Histopathology 1992;20(6):465–77.

91. Millwala F, Segev DL, Thuluvath PJ. Caroli's disease and outcomes after liver transplantation. Liver Transpl 2008;14(1):11–7.

92. Kassahun WT, Kahn T, Wittekind C, et al. Caroli's disease: liver resection and liver transplantation. Experience in 33 patients. Surgery 2005;138(5):888–98.

93. Habib S, Shakil O, Couto OF, et al. Caroli's disease and orthotopic liver transplantation. Liver Transpl 2006;12(3):416–21.

94. De Kerckhove L, De Meyer M, Verbaandert C, et al. The place of liver transplantation in Caroli's disease and syndrome. Transpl Int 2006;19(5):381–8.

Index

Note: Page numbers of article titles are in **boldface** type.

A

Aagenaes syndrome
  cholestasis related to, 290
Age
  as factor in DILI, 194
AGS. *See* Alagille syndrome (AGS)
AIH. *See* Autoimmune hepatitis (AIH)
AIP. *See* Autoimmune pancreatitis (AIP)
Alagille syndrome (AGS), 152
  cholestasis related to, 279–283
  clinical features of, 280–281
  diagnosis of, 281–282
  incidence of, 279–280
  management of, 282–283
    liver transplantation in, 351–352
  prognosis of, 283
Alpha-1 antitrypsin deficiency (A1ATD)
  cholestasis related to, 291–292
Amoxicillin/clavulanate
  cholestatic liver injury due to, 199
Amyloidosis
  hepatic
    cholestasis related to, 306–307
Antibiotics
  cholestatic liver injury due to, 199–200
Antifungals
  cholestatic liver injury due to, 199–200
Antiinflammatory drugs
  cholestatic liver injury due to, 201
Antiretrovirals
  in PBC management, 237
ARC syndrome. *See* Arthrogryposis-renal dysfunction-cholestasis (ARC) syndrome
Arthrogryposis-renal dysfunction-cholestasis (ARC) syndrome
  cholestasis related to, 289–290
Atresia(s)
  biliary
    liver transplantation for, 350–351
Autoimmune disease(s)
  systemic
    cholestasis related to, 311
Autoimmune hepatitis (AIH)
  clinical spectrum of, 246

Clin Liver Dis 17 (2013) 361–373
http://dx.doi.org/10.1016/S1089-3261(13)00010-X
1089-3261/13/$ – see front matter © 2013 Elsevier Inc. All rights reserved.

Autoimmune hepatitis (AIH) + PBC, 248
    treatment of, 249–250
Autoimmune hepatitis (AIH) + PSC, 248
    treatment of, 250
Autoimmune pancreatitis (AIP), 256
    treatment of, 263–265
Azathioprine
    in PBC management, 234

B

Bacterial infections
    cholestasis related to, 301–304
Bile
    functions of, 147
Bile acid synthesis defects
    cholestasis related to, 285–286
Bile salts
    in pathogenesis of pruritus, 321–322
Biliary atresia
    liver transplantation for, 350–351
Biliary strictures
    dominant
        in PSC
            management of, 219
Budesonide
    in PBC management, 234

C

Cancer(s). *See also specific types*
    PSC and
        management of, 221
CAR
    biology of, 168–169
    in cholestatic liver diseases, 169
    function of, 168–169
    as therapeutic target, 169–171
Cardiac disease
    cholestasis related to, 310
CD. *See* Citrin deficiency (CD)
CFALD. *See* Cystic fibrosis–associated liver disease (CFALD)
Cholangiocarcinoma
    PSC and
        management of, 220–221
            liver transplantation in
                evaluation prior to, 346
Cholangiography
    in PSC, 214–215
Cholangitis
    IgG4-associated, **255–268**. *See also* IgG4-associated cholangitis (IAC)
    secondary sclerosing, **269–277**. *See also* Secondary sclerosing cholangitis (SSC)

Cholestasis, **331–344**
  acute
    in DILI, 196–197
  care of patient with, **331–344**
  causes of
    hereditary, **279–300**. *See also* Niemann-Pick type C (NPC) disease; *specific causes,*
      e.g., Alagille syndrome
    systemic, **301–317**. *See also specific causes, e.g.,* Fungal hepatitis
  chronic
    in DILI, 197–198
    in PSC
      complications of, 219–220
  clinical presentation of, 331–332
  defined, 161–162, 331
  described, 147
  diagnosis of, 331–334
  differential diagnosis of, 334–336
  drug-induced, **191–209**. *See also* Drug-induced liver injury (DILI)
  evaluation of, 332–334
  fatigue in
    management of, 337–338
  genetic determinants of, **147–159**. *See also specific syndromes*
  itch in, 320–321
  management of, 336–340
  osteoporosis and
    management of, 338
  progressive familial intrahepatic, 283–285. *See also* Progressive familial intrahepatic
    cholestasis (PFIC)
  TPN-related
    liver transplantation for, 349–350
Cholestatic liver disease(s)
  CAR in, 169
  FXR in, 165–166
  nuclear receptors as drug targets in, **161–189**. *See also specific types and* Nuclear
    receptors, as drug targets in cholestatic liver diseases
  PPARα in, 170
  PXR in, 169
  UDCA in, 175–176
  VDR in, 171–172
Cholestatic liver disease overlap syndromes, **243–253**. *See also* Overlap syndromes
Cholestatic liver diseases
  liver transplantation for, **345–359**. *See also specific diseases and* Liver transplantation,
    for cholestatic liver diseases
Cholestatic syndromes
  acquired, 153–156
    DILI, 156
    PBC, 153–155
    PSC, 155
  inherited, 149–153
    Alagille syndrome, 152
    cystic fibrosis, 152–153

Cholestatic (*continued*)
 ICP, 151–152
 PFIC, 149–151
Ciliopathy(ies)
 cholestasis related to, 293–294
Circulation
 pruritogen accumulation in
  in pathogenesis of pruritus, 323
Cirrhosis
 primary biliary, **229–242**. *See also* Primary biliary cirrhosis (PBC)
Citrin deficiency (CD)
 cholestasis related to, 288–289
Citrullinemia type II
 cholestasis related to, 288–289
Colchicine
 in PBC management, 233–234
Colorectal cancer
 PSC and
  management of, 221
Computed tomography (CT)
 in PSC, 214
CT. *See* Computed tomography (CT)
Cystic fibrosis, 152–153
Cystic fibrosis–associated liver disease (CFALD)
 liver transplantation for, 353

D

Dietary factors
 in pathogenesis of pruritus, 323
DILI. *See* Drug-induced liver injury (DILI)
Drug-induced cholestasis, **191–209**. *See also* Drug-induced liver injury (DILI)
Drug-induced liver injury (DILI), 156, **191–209**. *See also specific drugs*
 acute cholestasis in, 196–197
 antibiotics and, 199–200
 antifungals and, 199–200
 antiinflammatory drugs and, 201
 chronic cholestasis in, 197–198
 differential diagnosis of, 249
 drugs against HIV, 201
 incidence of, 193
 introduction to, 191–192
 mechanisms of, 191–192
 pathology of, 195–198
 pathophysiology of, 198–199
 prognosis of, 202–203
 psychotropics and, 200
 risk factors for, 193–195
  age, 194
  chemical properties of drugs, 193–194
  disease states, 194

genetic determinants, 194–195
suspected
approach to patient with, 192–193
vanishing bile duct syndrome, 195
Dyslipidemia
cholestasis and
management of, 339

E

EHBA. *See* Extrahepatic biliary atresia (EHBA)
Endocrine dysfunction
cholestasis related to, 310
Environment
in pathogenesis of pruritus, 323
6α-Ethyl-chenodeoxycholic acid
in PBC management, 237
Extrahepatic biliary atresia (EHBA)
in childhood liver disease, 279

F

Fat-soluble vitamin deficiencies
chronic cholestasis and, 220
Fatigue
in cholestasis
management of, 337–338
Female steroid hormones
in pathogenesis of pruritus, 324–325
Fibrates
in PBC management, 236
Fibropolycystic disease of liver
liver transplantation for, 354
Fungal hepatitis
cholestasis related to, 304
FXR
biology of, 162–164
in cholestasis
therapeutic potential of, 166–168
in cholestatic liver diseases, 165–166

G

Gallbladder cancer
PSC and
management of, 221
Gender
as factor in PSC, 229
Genetic(s)
in cholestasis, **147–159**
in DILI, 194–195
in pruritus, 323

GR
  biology of, 174
  as therapeutic target, 175
Graft-versus-host disease
  hepatic
    cholestasis related to, 309–310

H

Hemophagocytic syndrome
  cholestasis related to, 307–308
Hepatic amyloidosis
  cholestasis related to, 306–307
Hepatic graft-versus-host disease
  cholestasis related to, 309–310
Hepatic sarcoidosis
  cholestasis related to, 305–306
Hepatitis
  autoimmune. *See* Autoimmune hepatitis (AIH)
  fungal
    cholestasis related to, 304
Hepatocellular carcinoma
  PSC and
    management of, 221
Histamine
  in pathogenesis of pruritus, 321
HIV. *See* Human immunodeficiency virus (HIV)
Hormone(s)
  female steroid
    in pathogenesis of pruritus, 324–325
Human immunodeficiency virus (HIV)
  drugs against
    cholestatic liver injury due to, 201
3β-Hydroxy-Δ5-C27-steroid dehydrogenase deficiency (MIM607765), 286
Hypertension
  portal
    cholestasis and
      management of, 339–340
    PSC and
      management of, 220

I

IAC. *See* IgG4-associated cholangitis (IAC)
IBD. *See* Inflammatory bowel disease (IBD)
ICP. *See* Intrahepatic cholestasis of pregnancy (ICP)
IgG4-associated cholangitis (IAC), **255–268**. *See also* IgG4-associated systemic disease (ISD)
  described, 255–256
  diagnosis of, 260–262
  differential diagnosis of, 248–249

    introduction to, 255–256
    natural history of, 262–263
    treatment of, 263–265
IgG4-associated systemic disease (ISD). *See also* IgG4-associated cholangitis (IAC)
    clinical features of, 256–260
    clinical manifestations of, 257
    demographics of, 256–257
    described, 255
    diagnosis of, 260–262
    histologic features of, 259–260
    laboratory features of, 257
    natural history of, 262–263
    pathophysiology of, 256
    radiographic features of, 257–258
    treatment of, 263–265
Inflammatory bowel disease (IBD)
    in PSC patients
        features of, 222
Intrahepatic cholestasis of pregnancy (ICP), 151–152
Ischemia
    SSC due to, 272
ISD. *See* IgG4-associated systemic disease (ISD)
Itch
    in cholestasis, 320–321
    pain as inhibitor of
        in pathogenesis of pruritus, 324

    L

Liver biopsy
    in PSC, 215–216
Liver diseases
    cholestatic. *See* Cholestatic liver disease(s)
Liver injury
    drug-induced. *See* Drug-induced liver injury (DILI)
Liver transplantation
    for cholestatic liver diseases, **345–359**. *See also specific diseases*
        AGS, 351–352
        biliary atresia, 350–351
        CFALD, 353
        cholestasis associated with TPN, 349–350
        fibropolycystic disease of liver, 354
        overlap syndromes, 352–353
        PBC, 348–349
        PFIC, 352
        PSC, 221–222, 345–348
        sickle cell disease, 354
        SSC, 274, 353
    orthotopic
        in PBC management, 235–236

Lymphoma(s)
    cholestasis related to, 300–309
Lysophosphatidate
    in pathogenesis of pruritus, 322

M

Macrolides
    cholestatic liver injury due to, 200
Malignancy(ies)
    cholestasis and
        management of, 340
Metabolic bone disease
    chronic cholestasis and, 220
Methotrexate
    in PBC management, 233
MMF. *See* Mycophenolate mofetil (MMF)
Mycobacterial infections
    cholestasis related to, 305
Mycophenolate mofetil (MMF)
    in PBC management, 234–235

N

NAIC. *See* North American Indian childhood cirrhosis (NAIC)
Neonatal ichthyosis-sclerosing cholangitis (NISCH) syndrome
    cholestasis related to, 290–291
Niemann-Pick type C (NPC) disease
    cholestasis related to, 286–288
    clinical features of, 287
    described, 286–287
    diagnosis of, 287–288
    management of, 288
    prognosis of, 288
NISCH syndrome. *See* Neonatal ichthyosis-sclerosing cholangitis (NISCH) syndrome
North American Indian childhood cirrhosis (NAIC)
    cholestasis related to, 292
Nuclear receptors
    as drug targets in cholestatic liver diseases, **161–189**
        CAR, 168–171
        future perspectives on, 176
        FXR, 162–168
        GR, 174–175
        introduction to, 161–162
        PPARs, 172–174
        PXR, 168–171
        UDCA, 175–176
        VDR, 171–172
Nutrition
    total parenteral. *See* Total parenteral nutrition (TPN)

O

Obstruction
    SSC due to, 271
Opioidergic tone
    in pathogenesis of pruritus, 324
Orthotopic liver transplantation
    in PBC management, 235–236
Osteoporosis
    cholestasis and
        management of, 338
Overlap syndromes, **243–253**
    AIH, 246
    defined, 247–248
    described, 243–244
    differential diagnosis of, 248–249
    management of
        liver transplantation in, 352–353
    PBC, 244–246
    prevalence of, 247–248
    treatment of, 249–250
Δ4-3-Oxosteroid 5b-reductase deficiency (MIM235555), 286

P

Pain
    as inhibitor of itch
        in pathogenesis of pruritus, 324
PBC. See Primary biliary cirrhosis (PBC)
Penicillin-resistant penicillins
    cholestatic liver injury due to, 199–200
PFIC. See Progressive familial intrahepatic cholestasis (PFIC)
PFIC1/FIC1 deficiency, 150
PFIC2/BSEP deficiency, 150–151
PFIC3/MDR3 deficiency, 151
Portal hypertension
    cholestasis and
        management of, 339–340
    PSC and
        management of, 220
PPARs
    biology of, 172–173
    in cholestatic liver diseases, 173
    described, 172–173
    as therapeutic targets, 173–174
Pregnancy
    intrahepatic cholestasis of, 151–152
Pregnane X receptor (PXR)
    biology of, 168–169
    in cholestatic liver diseases, 169
    function of, 168–169
    in pathogenesis of pruritus, 322

Pregnane (*continued*)
  as therapeutic target, 169–171
Primary biliary cirrhosis (PBC), 153–155, **229–242**
  cholestasis in
      management of, 336
  clinical spectrum of, 244–246
  defined, 229
  diagnosis of, 230
      histology in, 245–246
      laboratory studies in, 244–245
  epidemiology of, 229–230, 244
  gender predilection for, 229
  introduction to, 229–231
  management of, 231–238
      antiretrovirals in, 237
      azathioprine in, 234
      budesonide in, 234
      colchicine in, 233–234
      6α-ethyl-chenodeoxycholic acid in, 237
      fibrates in, 236
      liver transplantation in, 348–349
      methotrexate in, 233
      MMF in, 234–235
      new approaches to, 236–238
      orthotopic liver transplantation in, 235–236
      pharmacologic, 231–235
      rituximab in, 237–238
      tetrathiomolybdate in, 235
      UDCA in, 231–233
      vitamin D in, 238
Primary biliary cirrhosis (PBC) + AIH, 248
  treatment of, 249–250
Primary sclerosing cholangitis (PSC), 155, **211–227**
  with cholangiocarcinoma
      liver transplantation for
          evaluation prior to, 346
  clinical presentation of, 213
  clinical spectrum of, 246–247
  diagnosis of, 213–216
      cholangiography in, 214–215
      considerations in, 216
      CT in, 214
      histology in, 246–247
      laboratory findings in, 213
      laboratory studies in, 246
      liver biopsy in, 215–216
      US in, 214
  epidemiology of, 212–213, 246
  etiopathogenesis of, 211–212
  IBD in patients with
      features of, 222

management of, 216–222, 336–337
    for cholangiocarcinoma, 220–221
    for colorectal cancer, 221
    for dominant biliary strictures, 219
    for gallbladder cancer, 221
    for hepatocellular carcinoma, 221
    liver transplantation in, 221–222, 345–348
        disease recurrence after, 347–348
        evaluation for, 346
        outcomes following, 346–347
    pharmacologic, 217–219
    for portal hypertension, 220
natural history of, 212–213
Primary sclerosing cholangitis (PSC) + AIH, 248
    treatment of, 250
Progressive familial intrahepatic cholestasis (PFIC), 149–151
    cholestasis related to, 283–285
    clinical features of, 284
    diagnosis of, 284–285
    management of, 285
        liver transplantation in, 352
    nomenclature associated with, 284
Progressive familial intrahepatic cholestatic (PFIC) syndromes, 149–151
    PFIC1/FIC1 deficiency, 150
    PFIC2/BSEP deficiency, 150–151
    PFIC3/MDR3 deficiency, 151
Pruritogen
    in pathogenesis of pruritus
        accumulation in circulation, 323
        accumulation in skin, 323
Pruritus
    chronic cholestasis and, 219–220
    described, 319–320
    management of, 337
        advances in, **319–329**
    pathogenesis of
        advances in, **319–329**
        bile salts in, 321–322
        dietary factors in, 323
        environmental factors in, 323
        female steroid hormones in, 324–325
        genetic factors in, 323
        histamine in, 321
        lysophosphatidate in, 322
        opioidergic tone in, 324
        pain as inhibitor of itch in, 324
        pruritogen accumulation in
            in circulation, 323
            in skin, 323
        PXR in, 322
        serotonergic tone in, 324

PSC. *See* Primary sclerosing cholangitis (PSC)
Psychotropic drugs
    cholestatic liver injury due to, 200
PXR. *See* Pregnane X receptor (PXR)

R

Rituximab
    in PBC management, 237–238

S

Sarcoidosis
    hepatic
        cholestasis related to, 305–306
    liver transplantation for, 353
Secondary sclerosing cholangitis (SSC), **269–277**
    causes of, 269–273
        immunologic, 273
        infectious, 271–272
        inflammatory, 271–272
        ischemia, 272
        obstruction, 271
    clinical symptoms of, 273
    complications of, 274
    in critically ill patients, 272–273
    described, 269
    diagnosis of, 273
    epidemiology of, 270
    introduction to, 269–270
    management of, 274
        liver transplantation in, 353
    pathogenesis of, 270
    radiologic differentiation in, 273–274
Serotonerglc tone
    in pathogenesis of pruritus, 324
Sickle cell disease
    cholestasis related to, 308
    liver transplantation for, 354
Skin
    pruritogen accumulation in
        in pathogenesis of pruritus, 323
Smith-Lemli-Opitz syndrome
    cholestasis related to, 294
Solid organ malignancies
    cholestasis related to, 309
SSC. *See* Secondary sclerosing cholangitis (SSC)
Systemic autoimmune diseases
    cholestasis related to, 311
Systemic viral infections
    cholestasis related to, 305

T

Tetracyclines
  cholestatic liver injury due to, 200
Tetrathiomolybdate
  in PBC management, 235
Total parenteral nutrition (TPN)
  cholestasis associated with
      liver transplantation for, 349–350
  cholestasis related to, 311–313
TPN. *See* Total parenteral nutrition (TPN)
Transplantation
  liver. *See* Liver transplantation
Trimethoprim/sulfamethoxazole
  cholestatic liver injury due to, 200

U

UDCA. *See* Ursodeoxycholic acid (UDCA)
Ultrasound (US)
  in PSC, 214
Ursodeoxycholic acid (UDCA)
  in cholestatic liver diseases, 175–176
  in PBC management, 231–233
US. *See* Ultrasound (US)

V

Vanishing bile duct syndrome, 195
Variant syndromes. *See* Overlap syndromes
VDR
  biology of, 171
  in cholestatic liver diseases, 171–172
  function of, 171
  as therapeutic target, 172
Viral infections
  systemic
      cholestasis related to, 305
Vitamin D
  in PBC management, 238
Vitamin deficiencies
  cholestasis and
      management of, 338–339
  fat-soluble
      chronic cholestasis and, 220

Z

Zellweger syndrome
  cholestasis related to, 293

Moving?

Make sure your subscription moves with you!

To notify us of your new address, find your **Clinics Account Number** (located on your mailing label above your name), and contact customer service at:

Email: journalscustomerservice-usa@elsevier.com

800-654-2452 (subscribers in the U.S. & Canada)
314-447-8871 (subscribers outside of the U.S. & Canada)

Fax number: 314-447-8029

Elsevier Health Sciences Division
Subscription Customer Service
3251 Riverport Lane
Maryland Heights, MO 63043

*To ensure uninterrupted delivery of your subscription, please notify us at least 4 weeks in advance of move.

Printed and bound by CPI Group (UK) Ltd, Croydon, CR0 4YY

03/10/2024

01040442-0004